*Student Study Guide
to Accompany*

NURSING CARE
OF ADULTS

by Monahan, Drake, and Neighbors

Karen L. Burger, M.S., R.N.,C.
Professor
Department of Nursing
Columbus State Community College
Columbus, Ohio

W.B. Saunders Company
A Division of Harcourt Brace and Company
Philadelphia London Toronto Montreal Sydney Tokyo

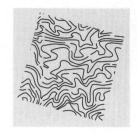

*Student Study Guide
to Accompany*

NURSING CARE
OF ADULTS

by Monahan, Drake, and Neighbors

W.B. SAUNDERS COMPANY
A Division of Harcourt Brace & Company

The Curtis Center
Independence Square West
Philadelphia, Pennsylvania 19106

Student Study Guide to Accompany Nursing Care of Adults
ISBN 0-7216-2725-0

Printed in the United States of America.

Last digit is the print number: 9   8   7   6   5   4   3   2   1

Preface

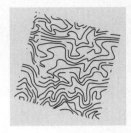

This study guide was developed to accompany *Nursing Care of Adults* by Monahan, Drake, and Neighbors. Its goal is to assist you in comprehending basic information, concepts, disease processes, and nursing interventions as presented in the textbook. It will also help you develop problem-solving and decision-making skills.

This guide is primarily intended for self-directed learning. Its main purpose is to teach you to identify key points and other relevant material from the text. It may also prove to be a valuable tool in reviewing class materials and preparing for examinations, including state board examinations.

Each study guide chapter corresponds to its respective chapter in the text. Study guide chapters are organized using a consistent format with the following features:

Learning Objectives
Definitions
Short Answer
Identification
Fill-in
Matching
True or False
Multiple Choice

After reviewing the learning objectives in the study guide, studying the specific textbook chapters, and drawing from related clinical experience, you will be ready for the learning activity exercises that follow.

For chapters concerned with basic knowledge, the exercises will help you review anatomy and physiology, define terminology, identify diagnostic procedures, and answer questions relevant to specific disorders.

For chapters concerned with the nursing care of adults with specific disorders, the application of theory to practice is tested. In addition to understanding and recalling basic content and disorders, you will be asked to apply that knowledge in making appropriate decisions and choosing appropriate nursing interventions.

You will also have the opportunity to apply problem-solving and decision-making skills as you answer the questions on the clinical situations that are included at the end of the chapters. Most chapters include an opportunity for the student to write nursing care plans relevant to the concepts. The answers for all questions are found at the end of the book.

Karen L. Burger

Contents

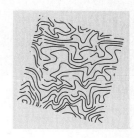

Chapter Thirteen

Nursing Care of Adults with Upper Respiratory Disorders 99

Chapter Fourteen

Nursing Care of Adults with Lower Respiratory Disorders 105

Unit Five

Adults with Dysfunction of the Blood and Blood-Forming Organs

Chapter Fifteen

Knowledge Basic to the Nursing Care of Adults with Dysfunction of the Blood and Blood-Forming Organs 119

Chapter Sixteen

Nursing Care of Adults with Disorders of the Blood and Blood-Forming Organs 125

Unit Six

Adults with Circulatory Dysfunction

Chapter Seventeen

Knowledge Basic to the Nursing Care of Adults with Cardiac Dysfunction 133

Chapter Eighteen

Nursing Care of Adults with Cardiac Disorders 139

Chapter Nineteen

Knowledge Basic to the Nursing Care of Adults with Vascular Dysfunction 145

Chapter Twenty

Nursing Care of Adults with Vascular Disorders 151

Unit Seven

Adults with Gastrointestinal Dysfunction

Chapter Twenty-one

Knowledge Basic to the Nursing Care of Adults with Gastrointestinal Dysfunction 161

Chapter Twenty-two

Nursing Care of Adults with Disorders of the Upper Gastrointestinal System 173

Chapter Twenty-three

Nursing Care of Adults with Disorders of the Lower Gastrointestinal System 181

Chapter Twenty-four

Nursing Care of Adults with Disorders of the Accessory Organs of Digestion 193

Unit Eight

Adults with Urinary Tract Dysfunction

Chapter Twenty-five

Knowledge Basic to the Nursing Care of Adults with Urinary Tract Dysfunction 203

Chapter Twenty-six

Nursing Care of Adults with Urinary Tract Disorders 211

Unit Nine

Adults with Hepatic Dysfunction

Chapter Twenty-seven

Knowledge Basic to the Nursing Care of Adults with Hepatic Dysfunction 223

Unit Ten
Adults with Endocrine Dysfunction

Unit Eleven
Adults with Musculoskeletal Dysfunction

Unit Twelve
Adults with Neurologic Dysfunction

Unit Thirteen
Adults with Sensory Dysfunction

Unit Fourteen

Adults with Reproductive System Dysfunction

Unit One

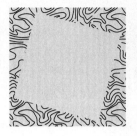

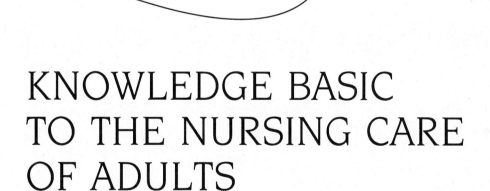

KNOWLEDGE BASIC TO THE NURSING CARE OF ADULTS

Chapter One

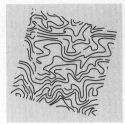

INTRODUCTION TO THE PRACTICE OF MEDICAL-SURGICAL NURSING

Learning Objectives

1.0 Demonstrate an Understanding of the Professional Aspects of Nursing.

1.1 List Five Areas of Practice for Nurses.
1.2 List Two Specialized Roles for Nurses.
1.3 Define the Practice of Nursing.
1.4 Define the Standards of Practice.

2.0 Examine Current and Future Trends in Nursing.

2.1 Describe Changes in Society that Will Impact Nursing.
2.2 Describe Ways that Nurses Can Influence the Changes in Health Care.

3.0 Demonstrate an Understanding of the Nursing Process.

3.1 List the Five Phases of the Nursing Process.
3.2 Describe the Nursing Diagnosis Statement.
3.3 Explain the Planning Process.
3.4 Identify the Reasons for Using the Nursing Process.

Learning Activities

Questions

1. List five areas of employment for nurses today.
   1.
   2.
   3.
   4.
   5.

2. List two of the specialized roles available in nursing.
   1.
   2.

3. Describe what you believe to be the nature of the nursing practice today.

4. Define the term *standards of practice* and explain why it is important.

5. What organization was responsible for the development of the Standards of Medical/Surgical Nursing Practice?

6. List several changes in society that you believe will influence the future practice of nursing.

7. Based on the societal changes you have identified, describe how nurses can influence these changes.

8. What group was responsible for developing a system for nursing diagnoses?

9. List the five phases of the nursing process.
   1.
   2.
   3.
   4.
   5.

10. Define the term *nursing diagnosis*.

11. List and define the three components of the nursing diagnosis.
    1.

    2.

    3.

12. List the four steps of the planning phase of the nursing process.
    1.
    2.
    3.
    4.

13. How can the nurse determine whether the expected patient outcome has been achieved?

14. How would you determine which of the patient's health problems has the highest priority?

15. If after the nursing care plan has been implemented, the expected patient outcome has not been achieved, what questions should be asked?

True or False

16. _____ The nursing process can be described as the essence of nursing.

17. _____ The nursing process allows the nursing care to be individualized.

18. _____ The nursing process only includes the patient in the nurse's care.

19. _____ The nursing diagnosis promotes continuity of care.

20. _____ Each nursing diagnosis can have only one patient outcome.

Chapter Two

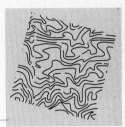

KNOWLEDGE BASIC TO THE NURSING CARE
of the Elderly: The Normal Aging Process

Learning Objectives

1.0 Demonstrate an Understanding of the Changes Associated with the Normal Aging Process.

1.1 Identify Normal Assessment Findings in Elderly Patients.
1.2 Identify Changes in the Body's Systems Related to Aging.
1.3 Identify Nutritional Needs of Elderly Patients.
1.4 Identify Important Considerations Related to Drug Metabolism in Elderly Patients.

2.0 Plan Appropriate Interventions for Elderly Patients with Changes Related to the Normal Aging Process.

2.1 Identify Some Teaching Needs of Elderly Patients.
2.2 Write Nursing Interventions to Help Elderly Patients Cope with Changes Related to Aging.
2.2 List Appropriate Interventions Related to the Self-Administration of Medication.

Learning Activities

Questions

1. Why is it important to understand the physical changes associated with the aging process?

2. Alterations in appetite in the elderly are often due to:

   A. Diminished taste and smell

   B. Loss of teeth

   C. Poor sight

   D. Chronic illnesses

3. The current recommended dietary allowance (RDA) standards for the elderly recommend a diet that contains:

   A. 70% carbohydrates, 15% protein, 15% fat

   B. 60% carbohydrates, 25% protein, 15% fat

   C. 55% carbohydrates, 20% protein, 25% fat

   D. 40% carbohydrates, 40% protein, 20% fat

4. Vitamin deficiencies may occur in the elderly because of poor dietary habits. Symptoms of night blindness would suggest a lack of:

   A. Vitamin C

   B. Vitamin A

   C. Vitamin B_{12}

   D. Vitamin E

5. Changes in the skin have been related to environmental factors, of which the most significant is:

   A. Smoking

   B. Exposure to cold

   C. Exposure to sun

   D. Changes in diet

6. Loose, wrinkled skin in the elderly is due to:

   A. Increase in collagen fibers

   B. Changes in pigmentation

   C. Loss of subcutaneous adipose tissue

   D. Increase in fat cells

7. List three factors that cause an increased sensitivity to cold in the elderly.

   1.

   2.

   3.

8. Because of the visual changes associated with aging, the nurse might suggest which of the following?

   A. Turning the head to compensate for the loss of peripheral vision

   B. Holding reading materials closer to improve vision

   C. Avoiding driving in bright sunlight

   D. Using low-level lighting

True or False

9. _____ Malnutrition is a common problem in the elderly.

10. _____ Dryness of the skin is caused by decreased activity of sebaceous glands.

11. _____ Lotions that contain lanolin are useful for treating dry skin.

12. _____ Appearance of gray hair has nothing to do with genetics.

13. _____ Presbyopia is common in individuals over 50 years of age.

Questions

14. Forgetfulness and short-term memory loss in the elderly may be due to:

    A. Changes in physiologic status.

    B. Decrease in blood flow to the brain.

    C. Decrease in the number of neurons.

    D. All of the above.

15. All of the following are considered part of the normal aging process EXCEPT:

    A. Inappropriate behavior

B. Forgetting names

C. Occasional confusion

D. Slowing of reaction time

16. Mr. Brown, age 82, states that he goes to bed at 11 P.M. and still wakes up at 5:30 A.M. He asks for some advice. As the nurse, you reply:

A. A sleeping pill would probably be helpful.

B. This is a normal sleep pattern for your age.

C. You should drink wine before you go to bed.

D. You should exercise more just before sleep.

17. Because the elderly have a slowed response to the autonomic nervous system, they are at risk for:

A. Heart attacks

B. Transient ischemic attacks

C. Orthostatic hypotension

D. Respiratory insufficiency

18. Constipation is a common problem in the elderly. A recommended treatment might be:

A. Eat large meals that are high in fiber.

B. Increase fluids and fibers, and exercise more.

C. Take laxative daily.

D. Increase milk intake and eat bland foods.

19. A patient in the hospital is having problems with stress incontinence. The nurse is aware that:

A. Loss of urinary control is a normal part of aging.

B. Loss of renal function is progressive and irreversible.

C. Restricting fluids helps this problem.

D. Pelvic exercises can help in treating this problem.

20. Changes in skeletal structure occur with aging. Kyphosis produces:

A. Increase in anteroposterior chest diameter

B. Decrease in anteroposterior chest diameter

C. Thinning of joint cartilage

D. Increase in elasticity and loss of function of the spine

21. Because of the increased incidence of osteoporosis in elderly women, the following daily dietary intake is recommended:

A. 4 g of calcium, 400 units of vitamin D

B. 2 g of calcium, 800 units of vitamin D

C. 1 g of calcium, 400 units of vitamin D

D. 1 g of calcium, 100 units of vitamin D

22. All of the following statements related to the aging process are true EXCEPT:

A. Sexual activity gradually decreases and usually ceases after age 85.

B. Painful intercourse can result from decreased vaginal lubrication.

C. Sperm production will decrease with aging.

D. Men have a slower arousal time as they age.

23. The way that the elderly absorb and metabolize medications will alter the action of some drugs.

List three reasons why drugs may be more potent and have more toxic effects in the elderly.

1.

2.

3.

24. One of the earliest manifestations of drug toxicity in the elderly may be:

A. Nausea and vomiting

B. Diarrhea

C. Mental confusion

D. Dizziness and weakness

25. Correct administration of medications is very important for the elderly individual. List five factors related to the administration of medication that the nurse would teach.

1.

2.

3.

4.

5.

CLINICAL SITUATIONS

Situation ■ 1

Mrs. Barker, age 78, is a recent widow. She has symptoms of depression, loneliness, and lack of motivation following the death of her spouse.

1. An important developmental task of late adulthood for Mrs. Barker would be:

    A. Reestablish a relationship with a male partner.

    B. Begin the process of life review.

    C. Develop dependence on her children.

    D. Understand that social isolation needs to be accepted.

2. A nurse at the local clinic notices that Mrs. Barker is pale and listless and has lost weight. A possible reason for this may be:

    A. She has a chronic illness.

    B. She lacks the motivation to prepare well-balanced meals.

    C. She lacks transportation to the store.

    D. She is exhibiting normal aging traits.

3. The nurse visits Mrs. Barker several weeks later. She notices that her appearance is unkempt, that she is unable to follow directions, and that she keeps asking for her husband. This may be a result of:

    A. The normal process of aging

    B. The grieving process

    C. Malnutrition

    D. Alteration in physiologic status

4. An appropriate nursing intervention would be to:

    A. Have her evaluated by a physician.

    B. Have her admitted to a nursing home.

    C. Call her son.

    D. Take her to the emergency room.

Situation ■ 2

Mr. Mendelson is 85 years old. He has heart disease, high blood pressure, and peripheral vascular disease. He is admitted to the hospital with shortness of breath and chest pain.

1. During the initial assessment, the following findings are made. Place a * next to those findings that are considered to be part of the normal aging process.

    a. _____ color is pale

    b. _____ feet are cool to the touch

    c. _____ pulses in feet are weak

    d. _____ breathing is labored

    e. _____ neck veins are distended

    f. _____ heart rate is irregular

    g. _____ breath sounds are slightly diminished

    h. _____ decreased sensation in toes

2. Mr. Mendelson is diagnosed as having congestive heart failure. He is treated successfully and will be discharged with two new medications, Lasix (a diuretic) and Lanoxin (to increase the strength of heart contractions). Write a nursing care plan that deals with his need to understand how and why to take these medications.

Nursing Diagnosis:

Patient Outcome:

Nursing Interventions:

Situation ■ 3

Mrs. Brown is seen by the nurse from a home health agency to evaluate her ability to care for herself at home. She states that she often gets dizzy when she gets up to go to the bathroom at night. She also has a history of irregular bowel movements with frequent laxative use. Physical examination reveals a frail, thin 82-year-old female with changes consistent with aging. Abnormal findings include reddened areas on the scapula and coccyx.

1. The dizzy spells are most likely due to:

    A. Orthostatic hypotension

    B. Congestive heart failure

    C. Poor food intake

    D. Decreased vision

2. Write three nursing interventions to help solve this problem.

   1.

   2.

   3.

3. The irregular bowel movements may be due to:

   A. Low fiber in the diet

   B. Inadequate fluid intake

   C. Lack of exercise

   D. All of the above

4. Write three nursing interventions to help solve this problem.

   1.

   2.

   3.

5. The reddened areas on the bony prominence may be due to:

   A. Prolonged bed rest and the inability to turn

   B. Limited mobility and pressure, which impairs circulation

   C. Poor vision and potential for a falling injury

   D. Poor nutrition and inability to cook

6. Write three nursing interventions to help solve this problem.

   1.

   2.

   3.

Chapter Three

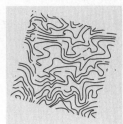

KNOWLEDGE BASIC TO THE NURSING CARE
of Adults with
Fluid, Electrolyte, and Acid-Base Imbalances

Learning Objectives

1.0 Demonstrate an Understanding of Extracellular Fluid Volume Deficits (ECFVDs).

1.1 Identify Conditions that Lead to an ECFVD.
1.2 Identify Symptoms of an ECFVD.
1.3 Identify Appropriate Interventions for a Patient with an ECFVD.
1.4 Plan the Nursing Care for the Patient with an ECFVD.

2.0 Demonstrate an Understanding of Extracellular Fluid Volume Excesses (ECFVEs).

2.1 Identify Conditions that Lead to an ECFVE.
2.2 Identify Symptoms of an ECFVE.
2.3 Identify Appropriate Interventions for a Patient with an ECFVE.
2.4 Identify Characteristics of the Appropriate Diet for a Patient with an ECFVE.
2.5 Plan the Nursing Care for the Patient with an ECFVE.

3.0 Demonstrate an Understanding of Third Space Volume Shift.

3.1 Identify Conditions that Can Lead to a Shift in Fluid to the Third Space.
3.2 Identify Appropriate Nursing Interventions for the Treatment of Third Space Volume Shift.
3.3 Plan the Nursing Care for the Patient with a Third-Spacing of Fluid.

4.0 Demonstrate an Understanding of Intracellular Fluid Volume Excess (ICFVE).

4.1 Identify Conditions that Lead to ICFVE.
4.2 Identify Symptoms of ICFVE.
4.3 Identify Appropriate Nursing Interventions for the Treatment of ICFVE.
4.4 Plan the Nursing Care for the Patient with an ICFVE.

5.0 Demonstrate an Understanding of Electrolyte Imbalances, Which Can Occur as a Result of Fluid Shifts.

5.1 Identify Values for Normal Electrolytes.
5.2 Identify Symptoms of Imbalances.
5.3 Identify Treatments for Electrolyte Imbalances.
5.4 Identify Appropriate Food Choices for Individuals with Electrolyte Imbalances.
5.5 Plan the Nursing Care for the Patient with an Electrolyte Imbalance.

6.0 Demonstrate an Understanding of the Acid-Base System.

6.1 Identify Normal and Abnormal Laboratory Findings.
6.2 Identify Conditions that Can Lead to Abnormalities in the Acid-Base System.

Learning Activities

Questions

1. Extracellular fluid volume deficit is defined as a loss of fluid from the

   A. Interstitial and intravascular spaces

   B. Intracellular and vascular space

   C. Extracellular and extravascular space

   D. Intracellular and interstitial space

2. When extracellular fluid volume loss is present, the patient will probably exhibit signs of:

   A. Hyponatremia

   B. Hypernatremia

   C. Hyperkalemia

   D. Hypomagnesia

3. Signs that would alert the nurse to a severe fluid volume deficit are

   A. Thirst, apprehension

   B. Hot dry skin, hypotension

   C. Marked thirst, lethargy, cold skin, tachycardia

   D. Dyspnea, tachycardia, hypertension

4. If a patient is vomiting, has diarrhea, and is very diaphoretic, the nurse would be aware of the potential for:

   A. Fluid volume deficit

   B. Fluid volume excess

   C. Metabolic alkalosis

   D. Dehydration

5. A patient has exhibited signs of mild fluid volume deficit. The nurse notices a loss of weight of 2 kg. This corresponds to a change in fluid balance of:

   A. 1 L

   B. 2 L

   C. 3 L

   D. 4 L

6. If a patient has a moderate or severe ECFVD, the nurse would expect the physician's orders to include:

   A. Force 4–6 glasses of water

   B. Maintain IV with D_5W at 50 ml/hour

   C. Maintain D5/.9 normal saline at 100 ml/hour

   D. Administer one unit of whole blood

7. During admission, the nurse notices that a patient is dyspneic and has a rapid pulse, elevated blood pressure, and peripheral edema. These are symptoms of:

   A. Fluid volume excess

   B. Fluid volume deficit

   C. Dehydration

   D. Acidosis

8. The nurse is aware that management of a fluid volume excess will probably include:

   A. Diazepam, digoxin, morphine

   B. Diuretics, digitalis, low-sodium diet

   C. IV fluids, potassium

   D. Morphine, high-sodium diet

9. The nurse is caring for a group of patients. She is aware that the _____ is most at risk for third-spacing of fluid.

   A. Patient who had a heart catheterization

   B. Patient with cirrhosis and low serum albumin

   C. Patient with a urinary infection

   D. Patient with a respiratory infection

10. The nurse is assessing a burn patient for signs of fluid shift 3 to 5 days after the injury. Which of the signs, if present, would alert the nurse of a potential problem?

   A. Bradycardia, hypertension

   B. Tachycardia, hypotension

   C. Dyspnea, crackles in chest, positive jugular vein distention (+JVD)

D. Peripheral edema, diminished pulses, hypotension

11. Which of the following laboratory results, if abnormal, can be used to diagnose an extracellular fluid shift?

A. Low serum albumin

B. Low serum potassium

C. Low serum magnesium

D. High serum blood sugar

12. A diet _____ would be most appropriate for a patient with severe fluid overload.

A. Low in protein and low in sodium

B. High in protein and high in sodium

C. High in protein and low in sodium

D. Low in protein and high in sodium

13. The management of a patient with increased secretion of antidiuretic hormone would be aimed at identifying signs of:

A. Extracellular fluid volume excess.

B. Third-spacing of fluid.

C. Intracellular fluid volume excess.

D. Extracellular fluid volume deficit.

14. Signs of cerebral edema in a patient diagnosed with water intoxication would include:

A. Anorexia, projectile vomiting, blurred vision

B. Nausea, hypotension, tachycardia

C. Weight loss, hypertension, tachycardia

D. Weight gain, lethargy, fever

15. An appropriate nursing intervention for the patient with an ICFVE would be:

A. Provide stimulation

B. Maintain seizure precautions

C. Decrease stimulation

D. Force fluids

16. A patient is admitted to the hospital with severe vomiting and diarrhea. The nurse will monitor for loss of serum

A. Sodium

B. Potassium

C. Albumin

D. Protein

17. Hypokalemia is a frequent problem with patients receiving:

A. Aldactone

B. Digoxin

C. Furosemide

D. Verapamil

18. A patient is admitted to the ICU with a potassium level of 2.6. On the cardiac monitor, the nurse might see:

A. Prolonged PR interval

B. Premature atrial contractions

C. Prolonged ST segment and inverted T wave

D. Atrial fibrillation

19. The nurse would observe for physical signs of low potassium, which would include:

A. Lethargy, confusion, diminished sense of touch

B. Anxiety, hallucinations, convulsions

C. Hyperactive bowel sounds, diarrhea

D. Dyspnea, edema, positive JVD

20. The nurse would anticipate that the physician would order which of the following therapies?

A. 100 mEq of KCl in 100 ml to run in 1 hour

B. IV of 5% dextrose in water at 150 ml/hour

C. 25 mEq of KLyte orally

D. 50 mEq of KCl in 250 ml of D_5W to run over 4 hours

21. An ominous sign for a patient with low potassium would be:

A. Heart rate of 52

B. Blood pressure of 90/60

C. Respirations 12, shallow and irregular

D. Lethargy, cool skin

22. A patient with hypokalemia is receiving digoxin. Before administering the medication, the nurse should check:

A. Serum potassium level

B. Serum sodium level

C. Serum digoxin level

D. Serum chloride level

23. In caring for a patient with hyperkalemia, the nurse would be carefully assessing for any effects on which system?

A. Cardiovascular

B. Renal

C. Respiratory

D. Cerebral

24. In caring for a patient with a serum potassium of 6.0, the nurse would expect to see which treatment ordered?

A. Low-potassium diet

B. Blood transfusions

C. Sodium polystyrene

D. Dialysis

25. Which of these conditions would NOT cause hyponatremia?

A. Cardiac failure

B. Renal failure

C. Hepatic failure

D. Respiratory failure

26. The nurse would check for hyponatremia if a patient exhibited which of the following symptoms?

A. Headache, drowsiness, confusion

B. Hyperreflexia, muscle spasms

C. Hypoactive bowel sounds, nausea

D. Lethargy, hypertension, bradycardia

27. A primary goal for the patient with a low sodium level would be to:

A. Maintain airway patency

B. Prevent injury

C. Maintain fluid restriction

D. Prevent skin breakdown

28. Part of the nursing care for the patient with a low sodium level might involve:

A. Administering narcotics

B. Maintaining fluid restrictions

C. Administering laxatives

D. Maintaining IV fluid with 5% dextrose in water

29. When caring for a renal patient, the nurse would expect laboratory values to show:

A. Hypokalemia

B. Hypocalcemia

C. Hypernatremia

D. Hypercalcemia

30. Which nursing action should be included in the plan of care for a patient with a low calcium level?

A. Monitor for signs of tetany

B. Monitor for hypoglycemia

C. Monitor for bradycardia

D. Monitor for constipation

31. A patient with a high serum calcium might develop:

A. Vomiting, diarrhea

B. Excessive blood clotting

C. Muscle twitching

D. Renal failure

32. When the magnesium level is elevated this results in a _____ of acetylcholine and a _____ in excitability of the nerve fibers.

A. Decrease, decrease

B. Increase, increase

C. Decrease, increase

D. Increase, decrease

33. When a patient has a low pH (acidosis) and a rise in CO_2, the nurse would expect:

A. Decrease in respiratory rate and depth

B. Increase in respiratory rate and depth

34. When the patient has a high pH, the nurse would expect:

A. Increase in respiratory rate

B. Decrease in respiratory rate

35. Nursing care for a patient who has a nasogastric tube that is putting out 800 ml of fluid each shift would include:

A. Monitor for signs of fluid overload

B. Monitor for signs of respiratory acidosis

C. Monitor for signs of metabolic alkalosis

D. Monitor for signs of metabolic acidosis

36. Nursing care for a patient who has chronic obstructive pulmonary disease would include:

A. Monitoring for signs of respiratory acidosis

B. Monitoring for signs of respiratory alkalosis

C. Monitoring for signs of metabolic acidosis

D. Monitoring for signs of metabolic alkalosis

37. A patient is admitted for surgery. He is very nervous and begins to pace in the room and hyperventilate. The nurse would monitor for signs of:

A. Respiratory acidosis

B. Respiratory alkalosis

C. Metabolic acidosis

D. Metabolic alkalosis

38. Determine what type of imbalance is present:

A. Metabolic acidosis

B. Respiratory acidosis

C. Metabolic alkalosis

D. Respiratory alkalosis

	CO_2	pH	HCO_3^-
1. _____	40	7.30	18
2. _____	30	7.56	23
3. _____	43	7.48	32
4. _____	65	7.18	26

39. Write the normal laboratory values for the following:

Potassium:

Sodium:

Serum calcium:

Ionized calcium:

Magnesium:

True or False

40. _____ Hypotonic fluid has low osmolality.

41. _____ Dehydration occurs when loss of water exceeds the loss of sodium.

42. _____ The blood urea nitrogen will be low with a fluid volume deficit.

43. _____ With a fluid volume excess, serum osmolality is low.

44. _____ Fluid is constantly shifting between the intravascular and interstitial spaces.

45. _____ 5% dextrose in water is an isotonic solution.

46. _____ Excess potassium is stored in the body.

47. _____ Excess potassium in the body can be life threatening.

48. _____ Potassium supplements may be given subcutaneously.

49. _____ Hyperkalemia is seen more frequently than hypokalemia.

50. _____ Most Americans consume 2–4 g of sodium daily.

51. _____ Digoxin is more effective when potassium levels are increased.

52. _____ Twitching of the facial muscle indicates a positive Trousseau's sign.

53. _____ Renal control of H^+ can occur in a matter of minutes.

CLINICAL SITUATIONS

Situation ■ 1

A patient is admitted to the ICU with extreme shortness of breath, rales in the lungs, blood pressure 190/102, pulse 104, respiratory rate 32, pitting edema in the legs, and positive JVD. A diagnosis of pulmonary edema is made. The following questions relate to this situation.

1. This patient is exhibiting signs of fluid volume excess, probably as a result of:

A. Left-sided heart failure

B. Emphysema

C. Renal insufficiency

D. Sepsis

2. Treatment would involve administration of a diuretic and cardiac glycosides. Which would be the drug of choice to remove fluid rapidly?

   A. HydroDIURIL

   B. Micronase

   C. Furosemide

   D. Digoxin

3. The purpose of administering digoxin is:

   A. Decrease force of myocardial contraction

   B. Lower heart rate and increase force of contraction

   C. Raise heart rate and help excrete potassium

   D. Prevent cardiac arrhythmias

4. Write a care plan for this patient.

   Nursing Diagnosis:

   Patient Outcome:

   Nursing Interventions:

Situation ■ 2

A patient is admitted to the hospital with renal failure. On admission he has periorbital and ankle edema. Blood pressure is 160/104, pulse is 96, respiration is 24, BUN is 40, and creatinine is 3.2.

1. The nurse would expect which electrolyte to be elevated in this patient?

   A. Potassium

   B. Sodium

   C. Calcium

   D. Albumin

2. Physical assessment findings indicate that this patient is showing signs of:

   A. Fluid volume excess (extracellular)

   B. Fluid volume deficit (extracellular)

   C. Third spacing of fluid

   D. Intracellular excess

3. Which condition, if present, would cause a worsening of his condition?

   A. Metabolic acidosis

   B. Metabolic alkalosis

   C. Respiratory acidosis

   D. Respiratory alkalosis

4. If the serum potassium level for this patient was 7.2, the nurse would be aware that the patient is at risk for:

   A. Respiratory failure

   B. Total renal shutdown

   C. Cardiac arrest

   D. Cerebrovascular accident

Situation ■ 3

A patient is admitted to the hospital with an extracellular fluid overload because of heart failure. He receives digoxin to strengthen his heart rate and large doses of Lasix to remove fluid. Because of this, he develops hypokalemia. He will be discharged on these medications.

1. The patient should be instructed to eat a variety of foods that are rich in potassium. From the list below, put a * next to those foods that would be recommended.

   Oranges   Yellow squash   Broccoli
   Spinach   Turkey   Tomatoes
   Potatoes   Fish

2. Because of its effect on the gastrointestinal system, the patient with a low potassium level would be instructed to:

   A. Eat a low-fiber diet

   B. Avoid use of laxatives

   C. Eat a high-fiber diet

   D. Restrict fluids

3. Signs of low potassium, which should be reported at once, would include:

   A. Muscle cramps

   B. Diarrhea

   C. Anxiety

   D. Tachycardia

4. The physician orders a potassium supplement to be taken orally three times a day. The nurse would explain that side effects might include:

   A. Headache, dizziness, hypotension

   B. Nausea, vomiting, GI bleeding

   C. Muscle cramping, spasticity

   D. Diaphoresis

Situation ■ 4

Ms. Parker is admitted to the hospital with a sodium level of 150. She appears lethargic and confused. Her breathing is rapid. She is diaphoretic. Her medical history reveals that she has been vomiting for several days. She is admitted and treatment is started.

1. During the initial assessment, other symptoms the nurse finds that are caused by the high sodium level are:

   A. Muscle twitching, hyporeflexia

   B. Moist, clammy skin

   C. Increased urine output

   D. All of the above

2. The nurse would expect this patient to be treated with:

   A. Digoxin

   B. Furosemide

   C. Diuril

   D. Potassium

3. Which information from the patient's medical history would be a contributing factor to this problem?

   A. Patient has a history of seizures

   B. Patient takes prednisone for arthritis

   C. Patient takes Theo-Dur for emphysema

   D. Patient takes an estrogen replacement

4. Ms. Parker recovers and is ready to be discharged. She will need to monitor her sodium intake carefully until she is seen 3 weeks later by the physician. Foods she should avoid would include:

   A. Milk, green and yellow vegetables

   B. Whole grains, cheese

   C. Lunch meats, snack foods

   D. All of the above

5. Ms. Parker is readmitted 2 months later with a hip fracture. The nurse would monitor for an increase in which laboratory value?

   A. Potassium

   B. Sodium

   C. Calcium

   D. Magnesium

Situation ■ 5

A patient is admitted to the hospital with acute renal failure. The patient appears acutely ill with a pale color, sacral and peripheral edema, high blood pressure, and a distended abdomen. He is somewhat confused and irritable. The following questions relate to this situation.

1. This patient appears to be showing signs of:

   A. Extracellular fluid deficit

   B. Intracellular fluid deficit

   C. Extracellular fluid overload

   D. Dehydration

2. Which laboratory value if elevated is most significant?

   A. Sodium

   B. Calcium

   C. Potassium

   D. Magnesium

3. The nurse reviews the chart and finds this patient has a high phosphorus level. She would also expect to find a low level of:

   A. Calcium

   B. Chloride

   C. Magnesium

   D. Potassium

4. The patient has not had a bowel movement for 1 week. All of the following could be ordered except:

   A. Colace

   B. Dulcolax

C. Milk of magnesia

D. Metamucil

5. Arterial blood gases for this patient are: pH 7.28, CO_2 45, HCO_3 20, O_2 90 %. This would be interpreted as

A. Respiratory acidosis

B. Respiratory alkalosis

C. Metabolic acidosis

D. Metabolic alkalosis

6. The anticipated treatment for this patient would be:

A. Place on ventilator

B. Begin dialysis

C. Give oxygen

D. Increase IV fluid

Chapter Four

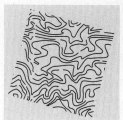

KNOWLEDGE BASIC TO THE NURSING CARE
of Adults Undergoing Surgery

Learning Objectives

1.0 Demonstrate an Understanding of the Legal Parameters Associated with Surgical Procedures.

1.1 Define Types of Consent Required for Surgery.
1.2 Demonstrate an Understanding of the Role of the Nurse in Caring for the Surgical Patient.

2.0 Identify the Needs of the Patient during the Preoperative Period.

2.1 List Diagnostic Tests Done Prior to Surgery.
2.2 Identify Teaching Needs of the Patient Having Surgery.
2.3 Identify Patients Who Have Increased Risk for Complications following Surgery.

3.0 Demonstrate an Understanding of the Needs of the Patient in the Perioperative Period.

3.1 List Preoperative Medications.
3.2 Demonstrate an Understanding of the Types of Anesthetic Agents.
3.3 List Complications Associated with Anesthetic Agents.

4.0 Demonstrate an Understanding of the Needs of the Patient during the Postoperative Period.

4.1 List the Criteria Used to Move a Patient Out of the Postanesthesia Care Unit (PACU).
4.2 Identity Complications that Can Occur during the Postoperative Period.
4.3 Choose Appropriate Nursing Interventions for Patients Who Have Had Surgery.
4.4 Demonstrate an Understanding of the Needs of the Elderly Patients Having Surgery.
4.5 Demonstrate Use of the Nursing Process when Caring for Patients Who Have Had Surgery.

Learning Activities

Define

1. Informed consent

2. Implied consent

3. Regional anesthesia

4. General anesthesia

5. Malignant hyperthermia

Questions

6. Explain the role of the nurse when witnessing consent forms.

7. The _____ is responsible for explaining the benefits and risks of the intended procedure before consent is given.

8. The _____ requires that all health care provider agencies receiving Medicare payments must inform patients over 18 of their right to plan in advance for their own care.

9. List three ways that surgeries have been classified.
   1.
   2.
   3.

10. List four diagnostic tests that would be done prior to surgery.
    1.
    2.
    3.
    4.

11. List three types of medications that may be given prior to surgery and explain their use.
    1.
    2.
    3.

12. List the members of the surgical team.
    1.
    2.
    3.
    4.
    5.

13. List three different types of regional anesthesia. Explain how each might be used.
    1.
    2.
    3.

14. List three of the most common complications of general anesthesia.
    1.
    2.
    3.

15. List five criteria that would be used in determining when a patient is ready to be discharged from PACU.
    1.
    2.
    3.
    4.
    5.

16. When a patient is in PACU, the nurse is aware of the need to monitor for adequate tissue perfusion. List four patient outcomes that would indicate adequate tissue perfusion.
    1.
    2.
    3.
    4.

17. A patient with a poor nutritional status would have an increased risk of:

    A. Poor wound healing, infection

B. Fluid volume overload

C. Decreased peristalsis

D. Cardiovascular collapse

18. A patient who is obese has a higher incidence of postoperative complications such as:

    A. Urinary retention

    B. Neurologic impairment

    C. Poor wound healing, pulmonary complications

    D. Fluid volume deficit, dehydration

19. A cardiovascular exam and clearance for surgery is necessary because:

    A. Poor status compromises the patient's ability to adjust to changes in fluid balance

    B. Poor status makes it harder to recover from blood loss and shock

    C. The patient may be at increased risk of emboli formation

    D. All of the above

20. The nurse knows that a patient who is a heavy smoker is at increased risk after surgery because:

    A. They are less likely to be able to cough effectively

    B. They often have a poor state of nutrition

    C. They are usually overweight

    D. They have a low tolerance for pain

21. The patient with liver disease has an increased surgical risk since adequate liver function is needed for:

    A. Metabolism of carbohydrates

    B. Detoxifying drugs and anesthetic agents

    C. Eliminating electrolytes

    D. Maintaining blood pressure

22. The nurse who is caring for a patient with renal insufficiency who is having surgery would pick the following nursing diagnosis as a priority:

    A. Potential for alteration in skin integrity

    B. Potential for fluid and electrolyte imbalance

C. Potential for alteration mobility

D. Potential for injury

23. If the nurse observes nervousness, tremors, insomnia, and agitation in a patient after surgery, he or she may want to consider the possibility of:

    A. Respiratory insufficiency

    B. Nutritional deficit

    C. Substance abuse

    D. All of the above

24. The nurse is aware that intravenous fluids may be initiated before or during surgery to:

    A. Provide calories since the patient is on NPO status

    B. Prevent urinary retention

    C. Prevent dehydration because of fluid restrictions

    D. All of the above

25. The purpose of skin preparation prior to surgery is:

    A. To make it easier to do dressing changes

    B. To prevent wound contamination

    C. To sterilize the skin

    D. To reduce the number of microorganisms on the skin

26. Surgery is performed during which stage of anesthesia?

    A. Stage 1

    B. Stage 2

    C. Stage 3

    D. Stage 4

27. In the immediate postoperative period, the nurse would promptly report a rapid, thready pulse and drop in blood pressure since these changes may indicate:

    A. Hypertensive crises

    B. Shock

    C. Infection

    D. Respiratory distress

28. If during the postoperative period, the patient exhibits signs of fever, tachypnea, tachycardia, decreased breath sounds, and rales, the nurse would suspect:

    A. Atelectasis

    B. Aspiration

    C. Pneumonia

    D. Pulmonary embolism

29. The reason that antiembolic stockings are applied in the immediate postoperative period is:

    A. To prevent pulmonary emboli

    B. To maintain adequate blood pressure

    C. To prevent venous stasis

    D. To support surgical incisions

30. The nurse is aware of the high risk for ineffective breathing patterns following surgery. This risk is due to:

    A. Effects of general anesthesia

    B. Postoperative pain

    C. Immobility

    D. All of the above

31. If a patient is having respiratory difficulty, the nurse would see signs of:

    A. Tachypnea, tachycardia, rapid, shallow breathing

    B. Bradycardia, seizures

    C. Fever, diaphoresis, hypotension

    D. Respiratory alkalosis, hypertension

32. A patient had a thoracotomy 3 days ago. He still has an IV and patient-controlled analgesia for pain. He has been slow to progress. Today he is exhibiting signs of respiratory depression, oversedation, nausea, and urinary retention. The nurse suspects:

    A. Pneumonia

    B. Narcotic side effects

    C. Problems resulting from immobility

    D. Fluid volume deficit

33. Following surgery, the nurse would monitor for signs of wound infections, which include:

    A. Edema, serosanguineous drainage

    B. Redness, edema

    C. Persistent pain, purulent drainage, delayed healing

    D. Partial separation of the wound edges

34. The nurse will carefully monitor an elderly patient who has had surgery because elderly patients are at greater risk for complications. This is due to _____ cardiac output, _____ peripheral circulation, and _____ vasculomotor response.

True or False

35. _____ Anticoagulants are continued when surgery is planned.

36. _____ Only emergency operations are performed during pregnancy.

37. _____ Corticosteroids will increase the patient's ability to deal with the stress of surgery.

38. _____ Alcohol can interact with medications given perioperatively.

39. _____ All patients having surgery will routinely have an enema to clean out the bowel.

40. _____ Preoperative medication will usually put the patient to sleep.

41. _____ The nurse should change the initial surgical dressing when it becomes saturated.

42. _____ The first responses that the patient will make after surgery are reflex motor responses.

43. _____ The elderly patient over 75 years old has three times as many postoperative complications.

44. _____ Operative time usually is increased with elderly patients.

45. _____ Postoperative confusion is more common in the elderly.

CLINICAL SITUATIONS

Situation ■ 1

A patient is scheduled for exploratory abdominal surgery in the morning. She is anxious and scared about what may be found. The following questions relate to this situation.

The nurse uses the following nursing diagnosis: Anxiety related to hospitalization, surgery, and outcome of surgery.

1. Write two patient outcomes.

    1.

    2.

2. Write several nursing interventions.

    1.

    2.

    3.

    4.

3. Prior to surgery the nurse would anticipate the following orders. Check all that apply.

    A. NPO after midnight

    B. Laxatives and possible enema

    C. Antibiotics

    D. Orders to draw blood for CBC, electrolytes

    E. Pain medication every 4 hours

4. Knowing the potential complications with this type of surgery, the nurse would be sure to include information about _____ in the preoperative period.

    A. Coughing and deep breathing exercises

    B. Chest tubes and heart monitor

    C. Intensive care unit

    D. All of the above

5. The patient has a history of diabetes and hepatitis. Knowing this, the nurse is aware that use of _____ would be contraindicated.

    A. Nitrous oxide

    B. Halothane

    C. Isoflurane

    D. Methoxyflurane

6. During the surgery a partial colectomy is performed and the patient is sent to PACU. With this type of surgery, the nurse monitors for _____ complications.

    A. Cardiovascular

    B. Neurologic

    C. Respiratory

    D. Urinary

Situation ■ 2

Mr. Morrison has just returned to the unit from the PACU. He had an appendectomy for a ruptured appendix. He has a history of chronic obstructive pulmonary disease and hypertension. This condition is stable.

1. Write four nursing diagnoses that would be important during the immediate postoperative period.

    1.

    2.

    3.

    4.

2. While assessing Mr. Morrison on the second postoperative day, the nurse notices abdominal distention and an absence of bowel sounds. The patient is not passing any flatus. The nurse would suspect:

    A. Wound infection

    B. Bowel obstruction

    C. Paralytic ileus

    D. Stress ulcer

3. Mr. Morrison is kept on NPO status, and a nasogastric tube is inserted and attached to low wall suction. Later that evening, the nurse notices hypotension, tachycardia, decrease in level of consciousness, decreased urine output, and poor skin turgor. She suspects:

    A. Ineffective breathing pattern

    B. Alteration in nutrition

    C. Fluid volume deficit

    D. Pain related to surgical incision

4. Mr. Morrison makes steady progress and is ready for discharge after 5 days. He will be monitoring the incision and taking antibiotics on discharge. The nurse would:

   A. Talk with Mr. Morrison the day before he leaves

   B. Provide all discharge information in writing

   C. Schedule an appointment with the surgeon in 1 week

   D. Encourage a full return to normal activity.

Chapter Five

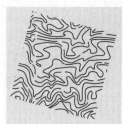

DEATH, DYING, BEREAVEMENT, AND SPIRITUAL DISTRESS

Learning Objectives

1.0 Demonstrate an Understanding of Death as a Developmental Stage of Life.

1.1 List the Five Stages of Grief and Dying.
1.2 List Several of the Final Tasks to Be Achieved if One is to Achieve Acceptance of Death.
1.3 Develop a Nursing Care Plan that Reflects the Psychosocial Care of the Dying Patient.
1.4 Demonstrate an Understanding of the Nurse's Role in Working with Individuals Who Are Dying.

2.0 Demonstrate an Understanding of the Bereavement Process.

2.1 Apply the Nursing Process to the Person Suffering Bereavement.
2.2 Demonstrate an Application of the Nursing Process to the Care of the Person with Dysfunctional Grieving.

3.0 Demonstrate an Understanding of How Religious Beliefs and Practices Relate to Death and Bereavement.

3.1 Identify Characteristics of Several Religious Beliefs.
3.2 Demonstrate Application of the Nursing Process to the Care of the Dying Patient in Spiritual Distress.

4.0 Review Other Aspects of Death and Dying.

4.1 List the Characteristics Found in an Ideal Hospice.
4.2 List Several of the Core Experiences of a Near-Death Experience.
4.3 List the Legal Criteria for Death.
4.4 Examine Your Own Personal Beliefs about Death and Dying.

Learning Activities

Questions

1. List the five stages of grief and dying as identified by Elisabeth Kubler-Ross.

   1.

   2.

   3.

   4.

   5.

2. List four of the final tasks that the dying person must accomplish to reach the final stage of acceptance of death.

   1.

   2.

   3.

   4.

3. Write a nursing care plan that addresses the needs of the dying patient.

   Nursing Diagnosis: Anticipatory grieving related to impending death

   Patient Outcome:

   Nursing Interventions:

4. Write a nursing care plan that addresses the needs of the person suffering bereavement.

   Nursing Diagnosis: Grieving related to the recent death of a loved one.

   Patient Outcome:

   Nursing Interventions:

5. It is essential that nurses provide hope because this is the antidote to:

   A. Depression

   B. Grief

   C. Fear

   D. Anger

6. The stage of death and dying in which the individual promises to do a particular thing in exchange for a longer life is:

   A. Anger

   B. Depression

   C. Decision making

   D. Bargaining

7. The first emotion that is felt by the bereaved individual after the death of a loved one is usually:

   A. Anger

   B. Shock

   C. Depression

   D. Disbelief

8. During a conversation with the nurse, a patient says, "Why bother getting dressed or eating? It won't make any difference." This indicates a stage of:

   A. Depression

   B. Grief

   C. Indifference

   D. Melancholy

9. As a health care professional, the nurse is aware that the grieving process can last as long as:

   A. 3–6 months

   B. 6–12 months

   C. 1–2 years

   D. 2–4 years

10. Which of the individuals listed would be most at risk for developing dysfunctional grieving?

    A. Parent who has lost a young child in an accident

    B. Daughter who has emotional problems and fought frequently with mother who has died

C. Wife who lost her husband after having cancer for 2 years.

D. Son who loses his father from a stroke at age 64.

11. After an unexpected death, survivors often show signs of emotional stress. This is often due to the fact that:

A. The survivor feels guilty

B. Opportunities for closure are denied

C. The survivor wishes he or she had died instead

D. Death is always stressful

12. Write a nursing care plan for a young adult with symptoms of dysfunctional grieving following the death of his father.

Nursing Diagnosis: Dysfunctional grieving related to an ambivalent feeling resulting from unresolved conflict with the deceased

Patient Outcome:

Nursing Interventions:

True or False

13. _____ All dying patients will experience all the stages of grief and dying.

14. _____ The stages of death and dying follow the same sequence for all.

15. _____ Acceptance of death is not fully experienced by many persons.

16. _____ Nurses should examine their own philosophy about death to be better equipped to care for dying patients.

17. _____ Spiritual needs do not significantly impact during a time of illness.

18. _____ To meet the spiritual needs of patients, nurses must be very religious themselves.

19. _____ Dying is the final developmental stage of life.

20. _____ To live fully and freely, individuals must understand that death is a reality.

21. _____ After the death of a child, parents are often overwhelmed by feelings of guilt.

22. _____ The Living Will is a legally binding document.

Matching

A. Buddhism
B. Hinduism
C. Judaism
D. Christianity
E. Islam
F. Jehovah's Witnesses
G. Mennonites
H. Mormons

23. _____ Believe Jesus Christ is a perfect expression of God.

24. _____ Their life goal is to reach Nirvana.

25. _____ Express opposition to organ transplantation and blood transfusion.

26. _____ Believe in reincarnation and believe that death is the nonfunctioning of the body and mind.

27. _____ Worship in Tabernacles, believe that faith keeps one well, and value health prevention.

28. _____ Life goal is the mystical union with the Brahma.

29. _____ Strong belief in Karma and the beauty of the soul.

30. _____ Express belief in an omnipotent, caring, and ethical God.

31. _____ Pacifist, don't believe in insurance; practice passive euthanasia.

32. _____ Believe in reincarnation, and that the ways to reach God are via worship, yoga, meditation.

33. _____ Worship Allah as the Divine Being and believe in eternal life.

34. _____ Prohibited from eating pork, consuming alcohol, and gambling.

35. _____ Value education and family; worship Jehovah as a just, merciful and omnipotent God; believe humans are immortal.

Questions

36. Write a nursing care plan for the person who is exhibiting signs of spiritual distress.

    Nursing Diagnosis: Spiritual distress related to the inability to engage in usual religious practices

    Patient Outcome:

    Nursing Interventions:

37. List several of the characteristics that would be found in an ideal hospice.

38. List some of the common characteristics of the phenomena that have been called near-death experiences.

39. List four of the six criteria for the definition of brain death that are commonly used today.

    1.

    2.

    3.

    4.

Food for Thought

Examine your own personal beliefs about death and dying. Have any of your beliefs changed since studying nursing? Can you successfully interact with a dying patient?

CLINICAL SITUATIONS

Situation ■ 1

Mrs. Fletcher is 78 years old and has terminal cancer. She is expected to live less than 2 weeks. She is very weak and in constant pain. She lives alone and has no family.

1. If Mrs. Fletcher should suddenly stop breathing, what would be an appropriate intervention by the nurse?

    A. Start CPR

    B. Call the physician

    C. Do nothing

    D. Get the chart

2. Mrs. Fletcher has made out a living will. Which of the following statements applies?

    A. If sudden death occurs, the nurse would do nothing.

    B. It is an expression of her wishes only and is not legally binding in all states.

    C. The nurse must follow her wishes or risk prosecution.

    D. It is meaningless; the nurse would still resuscitate her.

3. Mrs. Fletcher says, "I was very angry when I first found out I had cancer, but now I just don't care about anything at all." What stage of dying is she in?

    A. Bargaining

    B. Denial

    C. Depression

    D. Acceptance

4. In order for this patient to reach the final stage of acceptance, what should the patient do?

    A. Develop awareness of impending death

    B. Balance hope and fear

    C. Detach herself from former experiences

    D. All of the above

5. The nurse notices a Bible and a crucifix at the patient's bedside. What would be an appropriate question to determine whether the patient is in need of spiritual comfort?

    A. Would you like to tell me about your spiritual beliefs?

    B. What can I do to help you spiritually?

    C. Would you like to see a spiritual advisor?

    D. Any of the above

6. Mrs. Fletcher says that she wants a peaceful death without pain. A do not resuscitate (DNR) order is written. Which of the following statements is NOT TRUE about a DNR order?

   A. It should not be written unless the patient is consulted and approves of the order.

   B. The responsible attending physician writes the order in the chart.

   C. Once a DNR order is written, no further medical treatment is begun.

   D. The DNR order can be rescinded at any time.

Unit Two

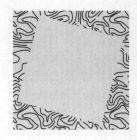

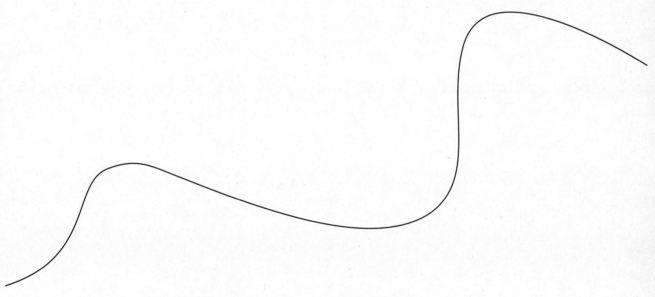

ADULTS WITH INTEGUMENTARY DYSFUNCTION

Chapter Six

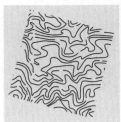

KNOWLEDGE BASIC
TO THE NURSING CARE
of Adults with Skin Dysfunction

Learning Objectives

1.0 Review the Anatomy and Physiology of the Skin.

1.1 Identify the Layers of the Skin.
1.2 Match the Skin Structures with Their Functions.

2.0 Demonstrate an Understanding of the Assessment Data Related to Skin Dysfunction.

2.1 Identify the Clinical Manifestations of Various Skin Diseases.
2.2 Identify Specific Types of Skin Lesions.
2.3 Identify Diagnostic Procedures Used to Identify a Variety of Skin Alterations.
2.4 Apply the Nursing Process in Caring for a Patient Who Is Having a Skin Biopsy.

3.0 Demonstrate an Understanding of Interventions Used to Treat Alterations in Skin Function.

3.1 Identify the Pharmacologic Treatments Used.
3.2 Identify the Surgical Management for Patients with Skin Dysfunction.
3.3 Identify Complications of Surgical Procedures Used to Treat Skin Dysfunctions.
3.4 Utilize the Nursing Process in Planning the Care for the Patient Who Has Had Treatment for a Skin Dysfunction.
3.5 Demonstrate an Understanding of the Needs of Patients Having Surgical Management of Skin Dysfunction.

Learning Activities

Identify

1. On the following drawing, identify the following:

   Epidermis   Subcutaneous layer

   Dermis   Sweat gland

   Hair shaft

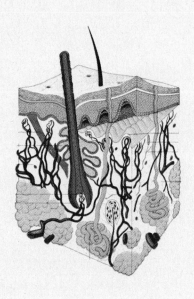

Matching

Match the skin structure with the appropriate function.

A. Epidermis   E. Melanocyte
B. Dermis   F. Blood vessels
C. Subcutaneous fat tissue G. Sebaceous glands
D. Sweat glands

2. _____ Provide skin pigment and color

3. _____ Outer layer of skin, protective barrier

4. _____ Provide nourishment

5. _____ Provides support and elasticity

6. _____ Provides insulation from cold and trauma

7. _____ Help with temperature regulation

8. _____ Gives bulk to the skin

9. _____ Oil-producing glands

Questions

10. List four areas that could be affected when an individual has a skin dysfunction.

    1.

    2.

    3.

    4.

Define

11. Macule:

12. Papule:

13. Cyst:

14. Ulcer:

15. Wheal:

16. Vesicle:

Identify

Write the name of the skin lesion shown in each of the following illustrations.

17.

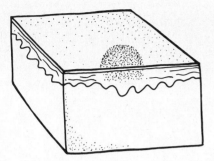

18.

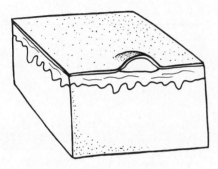

19.

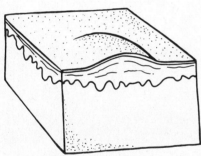

20.

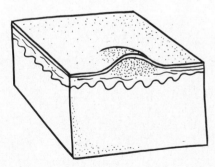

21.

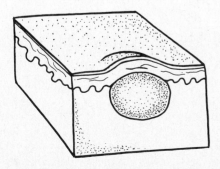

22.

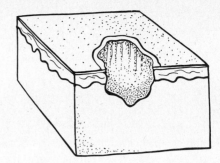

Fill In

23. A wart or mole is an example of a _____.

24. A skin abscess is often caused by a _____ infection.

25. Pustules are common in _____.

26. A wheal is also known as a _____.

27. Crusts are often seen with conditions such as _____.

28. Loss of subcutaneous tissue can result in _____.

Questions

29. The potassium hydroxide mount is an office procedure used to diagnose:

    A. Viral infections

    B. Fungal infections

    C. Bacterial infections

    D. Scabies

30. A Tzanck smear is done to diagnose:

    A. Herpes viral infections

    B. Fungal infections

    C. Staphylococcal infections

    D. Syphilis infection

31. A darkfield microscope examination is done to diagnose:

    A. Fungal infections

    B. Viral herpes

    C. Active syphilis infection

    D. Scabies

32. The type of skin biopsy that would be done when malignant melanoma is suspected is:

    A. Shave biopsy

    B. Punch biopsy

    C. Needle biopsy

    D. Excision biopsy

33. The nurse is aware that coal tar agents are usually used to treat a patient with:

    A. Psoriasis

    B. Scabies

    C. Poison ivy

    D. Fungal infection

34. A topical skin preparation that is used for its antiproliferative and anti-inflammatory effect is:

    A. Anthralin

    B. Corticosteroid

    C. Hibiclens

    D. Betadine

35. A topical agent that is known to be effective against fungal infections is:

    A. Nystatin

    B. Acyclovir

    C. Retinoid

    D. Hydrocortisone

36. The antiviral drug that is the treatment of choice for herpes simplex is:

    A. Hydrocortisone

    B. Tetracycline

    C. Retin-A

    D. Acyclovir

37. An antimetabolite medication that has been found to be useful in the treatment of psoriasis is:

    A. Fluorouracil

    B. Leukeran

    C. Methotrexate

    D. Cytotoxin

True or False

38. _____ A cream is an oil-in-water emulsion.

39. _____ An ointment is a water-in-oil emulsion.

40. _____ A lotion is a liquid suspension.

41. _____ Systemic effects can result from the use of topical steroids.

42. _____ Hydrocortisone cream 0.5% has no side effects.

43. _____ Hexachlorophene can be used on any open skin lesion.

44. _____ Occlusive dressings are used to enhance penetration of medications.

45. _____ Occlusive dressing increases the risk of skin irritation and toxic side effects.

Questions

46. The most common procedure used for the removal of early basal cell cancer is:

    A. Curettage and desiccation

    B. Punch biopsy

    C. Scraping

    D. Radiation treatment

47. The type of procedure that uses liquid nitrogen application to destroy lesions such as warts is known as:

    A. Radiation treatment

    B. Cryosurgery

    C. Nitrogen scraping

    D. Dermabrasion

48. The nurse is aware that the CO_2 laser works by:

    A. Chemical irritation to the tissue

B. Freezing of tissue and subsequent destruction

C. Vaporizing of tissue by causing cells to swell and burst

D. Causes death to tissue by direct penetration of beam

49. The type of graft in which skin is transplanted from one person to another is called:

A. Autograft

B. Homograft

C. Heterograft

D. Dermograft

50. The most common donor site for a split-thickness skin graft is the:

A. Upper arm

B. Scapula

C. Anterior thigh

D. Abdomen

51. The nurse caring for a patient with a skin graft is aware that the first dressing change is done in approximately:

A. 24 hours

B. 48 hours

C. 72 hours

D. 1 week

52. The nurse would teach the patient how to care for the donor site. Instructions would include all the following EXCEPT:

A. Maintaining immobility of the site

B. Preventing pressure on the site

C. Changing the dressing every 4 hours

D. Keeping the site free of contamination

53. For the patient with a skin graft: Using the following diagnosis, write a patient outcome and several nursing interventions:

Nursing Diagnosis: High risk for infection related to multiple routes of possible invasion by microorganisms caused by breaks in the skin

Patient Outcome:

Nursing Interventions:

54. A surgical procedure that involves sanding the epidermis is known as:

A. Skin sanding

B. Skin grafting

C. Dermabrasion

D. Chemical peeling

55. A procedure that consists of the application of an irritant chemical solution to soften and dissolve the horny layer of the epidermis is called:

A. Skin sanding

B. Dermal abrasion

C. Face peel

D. Dermabrasion

56. The nurse would observe for complications of dermabrasion, which include:

A. Infection

B. Pigment changes

C. Scarring

D. All of the above

57. Which of the following individuals would be a candidate for a dermabrasion?

A. Teenager with severe acne

B. Young adult with squamous cell carcinoma

C. Middle-aged adult with basal cell carcinoma

D. Older adult with wrinkles

58. Which of the following individuals would be a candidate for a chemical skin peeling?

A. Young adult with acne scars

B. Older adult with basal cell carcinoma

C. Child with burns on the legs

D. Teenage girl with wrinkles

59. The nurse is aware that because phenol is used as the chemical during a facial peel, the patient would be at risk for which of the following complications?

A. Cardiac arrhythmias

B. Infection

C. Pigment changes

D. Keloid formation

60. The nurse would tell the patient that the erythema after a skin peeling usually disappears in

A. 7–10 days

B. 2–3 weeks

C. 4–6 weeks

D. 10–12 weeks

61. A surgical procedure that is done to remove areas of alopecia is called:

A. Dermabrasion

B. Blepharoplasty

C. Scalp reduction

D. Hair transplant

62. A surgical procedure that is done to correct sagging or baggy eyelids is called:

A. Skin reduction

B. Skin grafting

C. Blepharoplasty

D. Rhytidoplasty

63. A procedure that is done to remove facial wrinkles that are the result of aging skin is called:

A. Blepharoplasty

B. Rhytidoplasty

C. Dermal abrasion

D. Skin reduction

64. Which of the following is a true statement about a face lift done to remove wrinkled skin?

A. Effect will be permanent.

B. Younger patients have better results than older patients.

C. Complications are minimal.

D. Surgery is always successful.

65. A complication that the nurse would observe for after liposuction would be:

A. Fat embolism

B. Hypotension

C. Cardiac arrhythmia

D. Infection

CLINICAL SITUATIONS

Situation ■ 1

A patient is admitted with psoriasis. It has been a problem for several months, and she is seeking relief.

1. The nurse examines the skin. It is irregular and thick with flaky exfoliation. A word that may be used to describe this condition is

A. Crusty

B. Ulceration

C. Atrophy

D. Scaly

2. One type of medication that has been found to be useful in the management of this condition is:

A. Hydrocortisone

B. Anthralin

C. Tetracycline

D. Penicillin

3. The physician orders a hydrating therapeutic bath for this patient. The proper procedure would be to

A. Have the patient soak in hot water for 1 hour, then rinse and pat dry.

B. Place the patient in a whirlpool to which oils have been added.

C. Place the patient in warm water for 30 minutes, then wash her with a soft cloth to gently debride the scales.

D. Place the patient in cool water, then brush away rough skin vigorously with a brush.

4. The patient also has signs of psoriasis on her scalp. What type of agent would the nurse expect the physician to order to aid in debriding the lesions?

A. Keratolytic agents

B. Steroidal agents

C. Antibiotic agents

D. Coal tar products

5. A example of this type of agent would be:

A. Hydrocortisone

B. Tetracycline ointment

C. Salicylic acid in oil base

D. Acyclovir

6. The physician also sets up a series of treatments with ultraviolet radiation. The nurse would instruct the patient on all of the following EXCEPT:

A. She must wear blocking goggles.

B. She will be asked to stand nude in the cabinet.

C. The time of treatment is gradually increased.

D. Receiving a sunburn is not a problem.

Situation ■ 2

The nurse working in a clinic setting is caring for a patient who is having a basal cell cancer on the upper back removed by curettage and desiccation.

1. Following the treating, information that the nurse would tell the patient would be:

A. Healing takes place in 1–3 weeks; the crust forms and sloughs in 7–10 days.

B. Healing takes 3–5 days; the crust drops off in 2–3 days.

C. Healing may take as long as 6 months; infection is a big problem.

D. Scabs drop off in 3 days; healing is complete in 1 week.

2. The patient asks if this type of cancer is going to be fatal. The nurse would reply:

A. "You need to discuss that with your physician."

B. "The cure rate of early basal cell cancer with this procedure is excellent."

C. "The outcome with any type of cancer is very uncertain."

D. "Don't worry about that now."

Unfortunately the cancer recurs. Micrographic surgery is recommended.

3. The patient is worried and asks how the physician will know if all the cancer is removed. The nurse replies:

A. The physician takes out all the abnormal tissue that he can see.

B. The lesion is removed and the tissue is examined. If malignant cells are present, more tissue is removed until it is free of abnormal cells.

C. An area twice the size of the cancer is removed so that the physician is sure that all the abnormal cells have been removed.

4. The area that is removed is large enough to require the use of a skin flap. The best explanation of what a skin flap involves is:

A. Tissue is raised from one area of the body and transferred to an adjacent area.

B. Tissue is cut out from an area that is highly vascular.

C. A flap of skin is taken from the leg and placed on the back.

D. A piece of skin is cut from the leg with a razor and then laid on the area where the cancer was.

5. The patient asks how the donor site will heal. The nurse would reply:

A. By scar formation

B. By revascularization

C. By reepithelialization

D. By forming a crust

Situation ■ 3

Mr. Potter had a skin graft to his upper arm after a burn. The nurse is instructing him on home management. Write four discharge instructions for Mr. Potter to help protect the graft.

1.

2.

3.

4.

Chapter Seven

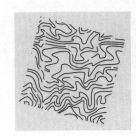

NURSING CARE
of Adults
with Skin Disorders

Learning Objectives

1.0 Demonstrate an Understanding of Infectious Processes of the Skin.

1.1 Match Several Types of Skin Disorders with the Correct Definition.
1.2 Identify the Clinical Manifestations of Several Infections of the Skin.

2.0 Demonstrate an Understanding of the Types of Treatment Options Available for Adults with Skin Disorders.

2.1 Identify Medical Treatment Options for an Adult with a Skin Disorder.
2.2 Identify the Surgical Treatment Options for an Adult with a Skin Disorder.
2.3 Demonstrate an Understanding of the Information Needs of the Patient with a Skin Disorder.

3.0 Apply the Nursing Process in Caring for Adults with Skin Disorders.

3.1 Plan the Nursing Care for the Patient with Eczema.
3.2 Plan the Nursing Care for the Patient with a Viral Infection.
3.3 Plan the Nursing Care for the Patient with a Bacterial Infection.

4.0 Demonstrate an Understanding of the Needs of the Patient with Skin Cancer.

4.1 Identify Characteristics of Benign Neoplasms of the Skin.
4.2 Identify Characteristics of Malignant Neoplasms of the Skin.
4.3 Identify Ways to Prevent Development of Skin Cancer.
4.4 Plan the Nursing Care for a Patient with a Benign Skin Lesion.
4.5 Plan the Nursing Care for a Patient with a Malignant Skin Lesion.

Learning Activities

Matching

A. Pyoderma
B. Folliculitis
C. Furuncle
D. Abscess
E. Impetigo

F. Cellulitis
G. Dermatophyte infections
H. Eczematous dermatitis
I. Acne
J. Pemphigus vulgaris

1. _____ Skin disorder that affects the sebaceous gland

2. _____ Superficial fungal infection of the skin (ringworm)

3. _____ Bacterial skin infections

4. _____ Similar to furuncle except caused by direct invasion of bacteria

5. _____ Autoimmune disease characterized by flaccid, easily ruptured bullae

6. _____ Deep folliculitis, also known as a boil

7. _____ Deep infection of the skin and subcutaneous tissue

8. _____ Superficial inflammation of the skin characterized by itching, erythema, and edema

9. _____ Superficial infection of the hair follicle

10. _____ Superficial skin infection

Fill In

11. A furuncle is caused by infection of the _____.

12. Bacterial skin infections are most commonly caused by _____.

13. Fungal infections are classified as _____ infections.

14. Warts are caused by the _____.

True or False

15. _____ Cellulitis is caused when a pathogen enters the dermis via an external route.

16. _____ The lymphatic system is rarely involved in cellulitis.

17. _____ Dermatophyte infections are spread through indirect contact.

18. _____ *Candida albicans* is normally present on the skin.

19. _____ Warts cannot be transmitted by touch.

20. _____ Herpes simplex virus is not contagious.

21. _____ Eczema is caused by a bacterial infection.

22. _____ Drug eruptions are the most common cause of generalized erythematous eruptions.

23. _____ Acne is the most common skin disease seen by dermatologists.

24. _____ Neoplasms of the skin are very common.

Questions

25. A patient seen in a clinic has been diagnosed with a furuncle. The treatment might include all of the following EXCEPT:

A. Application of hot compresses four times daily

B. Squeezing gently

C. Local antibiotics

D. Surgical excision

E. Systemic antibiotics

26. The nurse is aware that the medical treatment for impetigo would involve:

A. Oral antibiotics for 7–10 days

B. Topical antibiotics

C. Gentle cleansing of the skin with antiseptic ointment

D. All of the above

27. When caring for a patient with cellulitis, the nurse would expect to implement which of the following orders?

    A. Oral and topical antibiotics

    B. Warm compresses, oatmeal bath

    C. Bed rest, parenteral antibiotics

    D. Surgical debridement, antibiotics

28. Medical management for the patient who has a severe tinea infection of the scalp would include:

    A. Topical antifungal agents, daily cleansing with soap and water

    B. Cleansing, wet soaks, systemic antifungal agents

    C. Oral antifungal agents, daily scrubbing with coal tar agents

    D. Surgical debridement followed by wet to dry compresses

29. Presence of _____ in a skin culture would confirm the presence of a fungal infection in a patient.

    A. Streptococcus

    B. Staphylococcus

    C. Candidiasis

    D. *Escherichia coli*

30. Which of these factors, if present, would predispose a patient to the development of candidiasis?

    A. Pregnancy

    B. Diabetes

    C. Antibiotic therapy

    D. Steroid therapy

    E. Any of the above

31. The nurse is aware that certain patients are more at risk for developing candidiasis, such as:

    A. Child with ringworm

    B. Elderly male with leukemia

    C. Young adult pregnant with her first child

    D. Middle-aged male with prostate cancer

32. The most common method of treating warts is:

    A. Laser surgery

    B. Cytotoxic agents

    C. Cryosurgery

    D. Surgical incision

33. A patient is admitted to the hospital with pneumonia and shingles. The nurse is aware that shingles is caused by:

    A. Reactivation of herpes simplex

    B. Activation of varicella-zoster in individuals who have had varicella

    C. Exposure to individuals with genital herpes

    D. Compromised immune system

34. A patient with shingles is complaining of severe pain and itching. Treatment might involve administration of:

    A. Antibiotics and analgesics

    B. Antifungals and steroids

    C. Analgesics and antipruritics

    D. Antibiotics and steroids

35. The nurse would expect a patient being treated for an acute flare-up of eczema to receive:

    A. Prednisone

    B. Acyclovir

    C. Penicillin

    D. Tetracycline

36. While working on the oncology unit, the nurse accidentally spills some of the chemotherapeutic medication on her hands. A possible result might be:

    A. Contact dermatitis

    B. Seborrheic dermatitis

    C. Dermatophyte infection

    D. Stasis dermatitis

37. If the nurse did develop a reaction, which of the following clinical manifestations would occur?

    A. Pustules, macule

    B. Skin erosion followed by abscess

    C. Vesicles, fluid-filled papules

    D. Erythema following linear tracts

38. When checking a patient with peripheral vascular disease, the nurse notices edema, brown pigmentation, and thickened skin on the extremities. This would suggest:

    A. Allergic dermatitis

    B. Seborrheic dermatitis

    C. Stasis dermatitis

    D. Contact impetigo

39. A nurse is about to administer the second dose of gentamicin to a patient. The patient complains of pruritus and the nurse notices a generalized macular/papular rash on the body. An appropriate nursing action is:

    A. Administer the medication and then call the physician

    B. Hold the medication and call the physician

    C. Administer an antipyretic, then administer the medication

    D. Administer the medication and then recheck patient in 1 hour

40. A type of antibacterial and keratolytic agent that is used in the treatment of acne vulgaris is:

    A. Tretinoin

    B. Isoretinoin

    C. Benzoyl peroxide

    D. Prednisone

41. The nurse would instruct a patient with psoriasis to take which precaution to avoid an exacerbation?

    A. Avoid overexposure to sun

    B. Avoid over-the-counter medications

    C. Wash hands frequently

    D. Avoid exposure to cold

42. Which nursing action would be a priority in treating a patient who has a known allergy to hymenoptera?

    A. Monitor skin integrity

    B. Monitor for infection

    C. Monitor breathing patterns

    D. Monitor fluid status

Define

43. Seborrheic keratosis:

44. Epidermal cyst:

45. Xanthelasma:

46. Keloid:

47. Lipoma:

Questions

48. List six ways to avoid overexposure to ultraviolet radiation.

    1.

    2.

    3.

    4.

    5.

    6.

49. List the warning signs of malignant melanoma.

50. Write a nursing care plan for the patient with a bacterial skin infection.

    Nursing Diagnosis: Impaired skin integrity

    Patient Outcome:

    Nursing Interventions:

51. Write a nursing care plan for the patient with eczema:

    Nursing diagnosis: Body image disturbance related to the presence of skin lesions

    Patient Outcome:

    Nursing Interventions:

52. Write a nursing care plan for the patient with a benign skin lesion.

    Nursing Diagnosis: Anxiety related to procedures to be done and possibility of skin cancer

    Patient Outcome:

    Nursing Interventions:

53. Write a nursing care plan for the patient with a malignant melanoma.

    Nursing Diagnosis: Impaired skin integrity

    Patient Outcome:

    Nursing Interventions:

CLINICAL SITUATIONS

Situation ■ 1

Mrs. Perry is being treated for Crohn's disease. She is receiving systemic antibiotics and steroids. Because of this, the nurse realizes that the patient is at risk for developing candidiasis.

1. Factors that decrease host resistance and are present in this patient include:
   A. Immunosuppressive therapy
   B. Nutritional problems
   C. Diabetes
   D. Cancer

2. If candidiasis is present, the nurse would notice what type of lesions?
   A. Skin is brownish white with vesicles
   B. Skin is pink and surrounded by white scales and pustules
   C. Skin is red with purple patches and pustules
   D. Skin is whitish with pustules and cysts

3. Treatment would involve:
   A. Parenteral antibiotic agents
   B. Oral antibiotic agents
   C. Topical antifungal agents
   D. Parenteral antiviral agents

4. The patient shows she has an understanding of the cause and treatment of this disorder when she states,
   A. I understand that this is contagious.
   B. I will leave the shampoo on for 10 minutes before I rinse.
   C. I will take my antibiotics for 10 days.
   D. I will avoid sunlight in the future.

Situation ■ 2

Greg, age 18, is seen by a dermatologist for treatment of severe acne vulgaris.

1. As the nurse assesses Greg, she or he would expect to see which type of characteristic lesions?
   A. Papules, pustules, cysts, erythema
   B. Macule, suppurative cysts, scaling
   C. Vesicles, erythema
   D. Cysts, abscess formation

2. Greg has been treated with topical keratolytic agents and systemic antibiotics. The physician now recommends using low-dose glucocorticoids. The reason is to:
   A. Suppress estrogen formation
   B. Decrease the inflammatory reaction
   C. Suppress androgen secretion
   D. Speed the turnover of epithelial cells

3. Which of the following nursing diagnoses would have priority?

   A. High risk for infection

   B. Altered skin integrity

   C. Body image disturbance

   D. Altered health maintenance

4. The nurse would instruct Greg on the principles of skin care. These would include:

   A. Cleaning the skin with abrasive soap four times daily

   B. Washing the face with mild soap twice a day

   C. Eating a healthy diet with no restrictions

   D. Shampooing the hair only twice a week

5. The physician is also using isoretinoin (a vitamin A derivative) to treat Greg. The nurse is aware that side effects of this medication often include:

   A. Nausea, vomiting, diarrhea

   B. Visual changes, dizziness

   C. Cheilitis, dry skin, nosebleeds

   D. Postural hypotension

Situation ■ 3

Mary, age 35, has had psoriasis for many years. She has another flare-up. She is being evaluated in a clinic to determine other possible therapies. Mary is upset and wonders why this had to happen to her.

1. The nurse asks Mary if she knows what factors aggravate this problem. Mary answers correctly:

   A. Using alcohol; trauma to the skin

   B. Exposure to people with the disease

   C. Reaction to insect bites

   D. Allergic reaction to chemical irritants

2. The nurse reviews the current treatment protocol, which involves:

   A. Use of occlusive dressing over infected areas

   B. Therapeutic baths once a week

   C. Use of coal tar or corticosteroids three times a day

   D. All of the above

3. A nursing diagnosis which is a priority for Mary at this time would be:

   A. Individual ineffective coping

   B. High risk for infection

   C. High risk for impaired skin integrity

   D. Impaired skin integrity

4. Using the priority diagnosis, an appropriate nursing intervention would be:

   A. Provide Mary with information about support groups

   B. Refer Mary to another dermatologist

   C. Give Mary some written material on this disorder

   D. Suggest that Mary see a psychiatrist

Situation ■ 4

Mr. Oldman, age 88, is admitted to the surgical unit for treatment of squamous cell carcinoma.

1. The nurse is aware that the most common and effective method of treatment for this disorder is:

   A. Cryotherapy

   B. Laser therapy

   C. Curettage and desiccation

   D. Radiation therapy

2. Which information in Mr. Oldman's history would give the nurse information about the etiology of this disorder?

   A. Patient had actinic keratosis for several years

   B. Patient has a history of sebaceous cysts

   C. Patient has a history of psoriasis

   D. Patient has peripheral vascular disease

3. Because of his age and other medical problems, surgical resection is too risky. Another treatment option would be:

   A. Radiation therapy

   B. Chemotherapeutic agents

   C. Steroidal agents

   D. Immunosuppressive agents

Chapter Eight

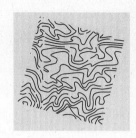

NURSING CARE
of Adults
with Burn Injuries

Learning Objectives

1.0 Demonstrate the Ability to Assess the Patient with a Burn Injury.

1.1 Identify Factors that Determine the Severity of a Burn.
1.2 Define Types of Burn Injury.
1.3 Match Types of Burns with Their Identifying Characteristics.

2.0 Demonstrate Application of the Nursing Process When Caring for the Patient with a Burn Injury.

2.1 Demonstrate an Understanding of Patient Needs during the Immediate Phase of the Burn Injury.
2.2 Demonstrate an Understanding of Patient Needs during the Emergent Phase of the Burn Injury.
2.3 Apply the Nursing Process to the Care of the Patient with a Burn Injury.
2.4 Identify Problems that Can Occur as a Result of a Burn Injury.
2.5 Demonstrate an Understanding of the Patient Needs during the Acute Phase of the Burn Injury.
2.6 Demonstrate an Understanding of the Patient Needs during the Rehabilitation Phase.

3.0 Demonstrate an Understanding of the Interventions Used to Treat Burn Injuries.

3.1 Identify Way to Manage Pain in the Burn Patient.
3.2 Write a Nursing Care Plan for the Burn Patient.
3.3 Describe Types of Wound Care Used in Treating the Patient with a Burn Injury.

4.0 Demonstrate an Understanding of the Special Needs of the Patient with a Severe Burn.

4.1 Demonstrate an Understanding of the Increased Metabolic Needs of the Burn Patient.
4.2 Demonstrate an Understanding of the Fluid and Electrolyte Changes in the Burn Patient.
4.3 Demonstrate an Understanding of the Psychosocial Needs of the Burn Patient.

Learning Activities

Questions

1. List five important questions that the nurse should ask to obtain a history of the cause and circumstances of the burn injury.

   1.

   2.

   3.

   4.

   5.

2. If a patient suffered a burn injury in a small enclosed area, the nurse would assess for signs of:

   A. Cardiac complications

   B. Acute airway obstruction

   C. Severe fluid imbalances

   D. Stress reaction

Fill In

3. During the first 48–72 hours after a burn, fluid shifts from _____ into _____.

4. Children under the age of _____ and adults over the age of _____ are considered to be at high risk when burned.

Questions

5. The nurse is aware that it is important to determine the size of the body area burned in order to:

   A. Medicate for pain appropriately

   B. Prevent serious complications

   C. Determine amount of parenteral fluid replacement

   D. Determine chance of survival

6. The reason that the Lund and Browder chart is a more accurate method of determining burn injury is:

   A. It can be used with children.

   B. It takes into account changes in body proportion that occur with age.

   C. It can predict serious complications.

   D. All of the above.

7. If a patient has a severe burn that damages the stratum germinativum, this would be significant because:

   A. This is the site where new cells are produced.

   B. This tissue cannot regenerate.

   C. Respiratory complications are inevitable.

   D. Fluid shifts cannot be controlled.

Matching

Match the characteristics with the type of burn.

A. Superficial partial-thickness burn

B. Deep partial-thickness burn

C. Full-thickness burn

8. _____ Caused by prolonged contact with flame or a hot object

9. _____ Pink to red, with dry surface and minimal edema

10. _____ Involves total destruction of the epidermis and dermis

11. _____ Can result from contact with a hot object

12. _____ May appear black, waxy white, cherry red, or tan. Appears leathery, dry, and hard

13. _____ Appears red, mottled, or waxy white; fluid-filled surface vesicles form

14. _____ Burn is painless because of destruction of the nerves

15. _____ May blister and peel after 24 hours

16. _____ Causes a great deal of pain

17. _____ Heals spontaneously without scarring

18. _____ Spontaneous healing will not occur

True or False

19. _____ A minor burn has a partial thickness injury of less than 25% in adults.

20. _____ A patient with a major burn should be transported to the nearest hospital.

21. _____ A major burn is a partial thickness injury of >25% of the total body surface area (TBSA) in adults.

22. _____ A major burn is one that involves the face and eyes.

23. _____ Burns >20% TBSA will require parenteral fluid resuscitation.

24. _____ Diuretics are usually given during the early burn period.

25. _____ Debridement is painless.

26. _____ Chemical burns have the same appearance as any burn.

Questions

27. The acute phase of the burn injury is defined as:
    A. The first 48–72 hours after injury
    B. The period of time that begins with reabsorption of interstitial fluid
    C. The period of time when the fluid shifts from the vascular to the interstitial space
    D. The period of time when the patient is unstable

28. The priority in treatment during the immediate care period of a burn is to:
    A. Stop the burning process
    B. Assess for other injuries
    C. Assess circulation
    D. Maintain skeletal alignment

29. After the treatment priority has been accomplished, the next essential step is to:
    A. Cover the burned area
    B. Establish a patent airway
    C. Assess for other life-threatening injuries
    D. Transport to a burn center

30. The emergent phase of burn care is also known as the:
    A. Acute phase of the injury
    B. Critical phase of therapy
    C. Fluid resuscitation stage
    D. Life-threatening stage

31. On assessment, the nurse finds that a burn patient has a pink, flushed appearance, is restless, irritable, and confused. This suggests:
    A. Impaired airway
    B. Smoke inhalation
    C. Carbon monoxide poisoning
    D. Massive fluid shifts

32. A patient has a burn of over 40% TBSA. If this patient exhibits anxiety, restlessness, labored breathing, and cyanosis, the nurse would suspect:
    A. Inhalation injury
    B. Carbon monoxide poisoning
    C. Restrictive disease
    D. Decreased cardiac output

33. If carbon monoxide poisoning is suspected, the nurse would anticipate the following treatment ordered:
    A. Low-flow oxygen and intermittent positive pressure breathing (IPPB) treatments
    B. 100% oxygen
    C. Mechanical ventilation
    D. 50% oxygen and frequent suctioning

34. Following a burn injury, the nurse would expect to see which serum laboratory value changes during the emergent phase?
    A. High sodium, low potassium

B. High sodium, high potassium

C. Low sodium, high potassium

D. Low sodium, low potassium

35. A patient undergoing burn shock would exhibit which symptoms?

A. Dehydration, increased urine output, hypotension

B. Hypotension, tachycardia, decreased cardiac output

C. Hypertension, increased urine output, tachycardia

D. Decreasing consciousness, bradycardia, hypotension

36. To determine the amount of fluid to be replaced following a burn injury, most authorities advocate administration of _____ of the volume in the first 8 hours and _____ during each of the next 8 hours.

A. 33%, 33%

B. 25%, 37%

C. 50%, 25%

D. 75%, 12%

37. The nurse is aware that the fluid shifts stop after the first 24 hours because:

A. Capillary permeability increases

B. Hydrostatic pressure in interstitial space increases

C. Intravascular volume decreases

D. Leakage of protein has reached a maximum

38. In caring for the patient with a burn injury, the nurse would be aware that fluid mobilization is occurring when:

A. Urine output is greater than 30 ml/hour

B. Urine output is greater than 50 ml/hour

C. Urine output is greater than 75 ml/hour

D. Urine output is greater than 100 ml/hour

39. Because burn patients often have severe pain, the nurse would assist in pain management. This would include administration of _____ to control pain.

A. Aspirin

B. Tylenol

C. Codeine

D. Morphine

40. Nursing care of the burn patient is aimed at preventing _____, which is the leading cause of death in the acute burn period.

A. Sepsis

B. Dehydration

C. Electrolyte imbalance

D. Respiratory failure

41. During the acute phase of the burn injury, the nurse is responsible for assessing metabolic needs of the patient, which can increase by:

A. 50%

B. 100%

C. 200%

D. 300%

42. The main reason that the metabolic rate increases after a burn injury is thought to be:

A. The inability of the skin to conserve heat

B. The loss of protein in wound exudate

C. Excessive nitrogen loss

D. All of the above

43. Which laboratory finding if low would indicate that a burn patient has an alteration in nutrition?

A. Sodium

B. Potassium

C. Albumin

D. Creatinine

44. If the nurse detects an absence of bowel sounds in a burn patient, she or he would suspect

A. Curling's ulcer

B. Paralytic ileus

C. Hypovolemic ileus

D. Bowel obstruction

45. Hypertrophic scar formation is often a problem with burn patients. To help prevent this problem, the nurse would assist in:

    A. Applying pressure garments

    B. Debriding wounds daily

    C. Providing adequate nutrition

    D. Splinting all extremities

46. Chemical burns cause destruction of tissue by:

    A. Burning

    B. Coagulation

    C. Heating

    D. Irritation

47. Initial medical management of a chemical injury would involve:

    A. Stopping the burn by covering with sterile dressings

    B. Flushing the wound with copious amounts of water

    C. Covering with analgesic ointment as soon as possible

    D. Transporting to burn unit immediately

Define

Define the type of wound care and give an advantage of each.

48. Open wound care:

49. Closed wound care:

50. Debridement:

Questions

51. Write a nursing care plan for the patient with altered respiratory function following a burn injury.

    Nursing Diagnoses: (1) Impaired gas exchange (2) High risk for ineffective airway clearance

    Patient Outcome:

    Nursing Interventions:

52. Write a nursing care plan that addresses the needs of the patient with hypovolemia and electrolyte imbalance following a major burn injury.

    Nursing Diagnosis: High risk for fluid volume deficit

    Patient Outcome:

    Nursing Interventions:

53. Write a nursing care plan for the patient with pain following a burn injury.

    Nursing Diagnosis: Pain related to open burn wounds.

    Patient Outcome:

    Nursing Interventions:

CLINICAL SITUATIONS

Situation ■ 1

Jeffrey, age 28, was burned in a garage fire. He has burns on 43% of his body, including his face and upper body. He is admitted to the burn unit.

1. The initial examination classified this as a:

    A. Minor burn injury

    B. Moderate burn injury

    C. Major burn injury

2. The nurse working in the burn unit realizes that Jeffrey is at risk for hypovolemia and electrolyte imbalance during the emergent phase, which occurs:

   A. During the first 12 hours

   B. During the first 24–48 hours

   C. During the first 48–72 hours

   D. During the first week

3. When assessing the severity of Jeffrey's burns, the nurse notices soot around his mouth. The nurse would take special precautions because of the risk for:

   A. Respiratory complications

   B. Cardiovascular complications

   C. Gastrointestinal complications

   D. Electrolyte imbalances

4. The nurse realizes that fluid shifts from the intravascular space to the interstitial space because of:

   A. Decrease in the amount of histamine

   B. Loss of red blood cells and hemoglobin

   C. Increase in capillary permeability

   D. Loss of healthy tissue

5. The nurse realizes the patient is in the _____ phase of the burn injury when _____ fluid is reabsorbed.

   A. Critical, vascular

   B. Emergent, extracellular

   C. Acute, interstitial

   D. Rehabilitation, vascular

6. Signs that indicate that Jeffrey is in the emergent phase of the burn injury would be:

   A. Edema, hypotension

   B. Bradycardia, hypertension

   C. Increased urine output

   D. Increased cardiac output, tachycardia

7. The nurse reviews the laboratory results and notes that Jeffrey's serum potassium is 6.0. The nurse would observe carefully for:

   A. Renal failure

   B. Cardiac arrhythmias

   C. Hypovolemic shock

   D. Loss of consciousness

Situation ■ 2

Sally has a severe burn over 50% of her body from a car accident. She is in the burn unit. It has been 8 hours since her injury.

1. The nurse is aware of the importance of fluid replacement during the emergent phase of the injury. If Sally has lost 2000 ml of fluid, how much parenteral fluid would the nurse be replacing?

   A. 500 ml

   B. 1000 ml

   C. 2000 ml

   D. 3000 ml

2. The type of fluid that will most likely be ordered is

   A. 5% dextrose

   B. 0.9% sodium chloride

   C. Lactated Ringer's

   D. Albumin

3. Sally has a full-thickness burn on her upper thighs with eschar formation. Nursing care would include assessing Sally for:

   A. Signs of hypovolemia

   B. Signs of impaired peripheral circulation

   C. Signs of respiratory insufficiency

   D. Signs of infection

4. It is the third postburn day and Sally is in the acute phase of the burn injury. Nursing responsibilities during this period include observing for:

   A. Increase in urine output, vital signs returning to normal

   B. Decrease in urine output, hypertension

   C. Increase in cardiac output, hypotension

   D. Changing level of consciousness, hypertension

5. Sally has the eschar debrided from her legs. The nurse is to apply closed-wound dressings, which might include:

   A. Applying silver sulfadiazine and sterile gauze

   B. Applying bacitracin ointment and leaving the wound open

   C. Applying betadine wet-to-dry dressings

   D. Applying saline wet-to-dry dressings

6. Because of the full-thickness burn injury on Sally's thigh, the nurse anticipates that a _____ will be used.

   A. Homograft

   B. Heterograft

   C. Autograft

Situation ■ 3

Mr. Ferrine, age 70, was burned when he fell asleep while smoking. His wife died of smoke inhalation in the fire. He has burns on his chest and lower body of 38% TBSA.

1. During the acute phase of his recovery, Mr. Ferrine has a serum albumin of 2.0 and has lost 4 lb in 2 days. The priority nursing diagnosis would be:

   A. Alteration in fluid and electrolytes

   B. Alteration in urinary elimination

   C. Alteration in nutrition

   D. Alteration in comfort

2. Mr. Ferrine is unable to tolerate his diet; he is pale; he has absent bowel sounds; and he has severe pain. An appropriate diet would be:

   A. High protein, high fat

   B. Tube feeding with osmolyte at 100 ml/hr

   C. Intravenous hyperalimentation

   D. High-protein, high-carbohydrate diet with supplements

3. Mr. Ferrine is depressed and withdrawn, and he refuses to talk about what has happened. An appropriate nursing diagnosis would be:

   A. Post-trauma response

   B. Body image disturbance

   C. Ineffective individual coping

   D. Impaired home maintenance management

4. To prevent the formation of scars during the rehabilitation period, the nurse would:

   A. Do range-of-motion exercises four times daily

   B. Take patient to hydrotherapy

   C. Do dressing changes as ordered

   D. Give pain medication as ordered

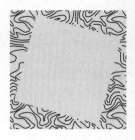

Unit Three

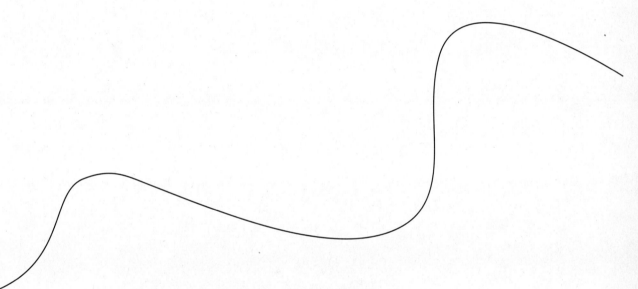

ADULTS WITH IMMUNE DYSFUNCTION

Chapter Nine

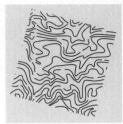

KNOWLEDGE BASIC TO THE NURSING CARE
of Adults with Immune Dysfunction

Learning Objectives

1.0 Review the Anatomy and Physiology of the Immune System.

1.1 Identify the Parts of the Immune System.
1.2 Match Each Type of White Cell with Its Function.
1.3 Identify the Functions of T Cells and B Cells.

2.0 Demonstrate an Understanding of the Specific Immune Responses That Occur in the Body.

2.1 List the Three Stages of the Immune Response.
2.2 Identify Types of Specific and Nonspecific Immune Responses.
2.3 Demonstrate an Understanding of the Types of Immunity.

3.0 Demonstrate an Understanding of Assessment Data Related to Adults with Immune Dysfunction.

3.1 Identify Clinical Manifestations of Immune Dysfunction.
3.2 Review Diagnostic Procedures Used to Identify Immune Dysfunctions.
3.3 Match Each Specific Allergy Test with Its Characteristics.
3.4 Plan the Nursing Care of the Patient Having a Bone Marrow Aspiration.
3.5 Plan the Nursing Care for an Individual With a Bone Marrow Transplant.

4.0 Demonstrate an Understanding of the Interventions Used to Manage Adults with Immune Dysfunction.

4.1 Identify the Types of Medical Treatment Currently Used.
4.2 Demonstrate an Understanding of the Reasons Certain Treatments Are Used.
4.3 Plan the Nursing Care for an Adult with an Immune Dysfunction.
4.4 Identify Ways to Prevent Infection in the Elderly.

Learning Activities

Questions

1. List the three primary functions of the immune system.

   1.

   2.

   3.

2. List four of the peripheral lymphoid organs.

   1.

   2.

   3.

   4.

3. Where are T cells produced?

4. Where are B cells produced?

5. What plays an important role in homeostasis by removing worn out or damaged erythrocytes?

6. The cells of the immune system have special roles in the body's defense. Some cells help defend the body against infection; others mediate allergic reactions. What is the specific function of the T cell?

7. What type of response is evoked as a protective mechanism in the body after exposure to a virus?

8. What are responsible for the production of antibodies?

9. What are responsible for the destruction of other cells and the regulation of the type and intensity of the specific immune response?

Fill In

10. The major serum antibody is _____ , which constitutes about 70% of the total circulating antibodies.

11. The first antibody produced in response to an antigen is _____ .

Matching

Match the leukocyte type with its specific function.

A. Neutrophils   C. Monocytes
B. Eosinophils   D. Lymphocytes

12. _____ Have great phagocytic ability to ingest large numbers of microorganisms.

13. _____ Responsible for the specific immune response.

14. _____ Able to quickly phagocytize bacteria; one of the first lines of defense during infection.

15. _____ Respond primarily to allergic reactions.

Questions

The body can evoke either a specific or a nonspecific response to an invader. Put an S (specific) or an N (nonspecific) next to each of the following defense mechanisms.

16. _____ Physical barrier

17. _____ Interferon

18. _____ Inflammation

19. _____ Antigen

20. _____ Phagocytosis

21. List and describe the three stages of the inflammatory response.

   1.

2.

3.

Define

22. Phagocytosis:

23. Antigen:

24. Antibodies:

25. Complement:

26. Immunosuppression:

Matching

Match each type of allergy test with its description.

A. Scratch test   C. Intradermal test
B. Prick test   D. Radioallergosorbent
                       (RAST) test

27. _____ A drop of antigen is placed on the skin; then the skin is pricked with a small-gauge needle.

28. _____ Done on the back or forearms, antigens can be tested one at a time.

29. _____ Determines the presence of allergen-specific IgE antibodies in the blood.

30. _____ A small amount of antigen is injected under the skin.

Questions

31. An example of a chemical barrier within the body would be:
    A. Lysozyme
    B. Sweat
    C. Urine
    D. Interferon

32. Neoplastic diseases can lead an individual to become more susceptible to infections. This is usually a result of:
    A. Anemia
    B. Neutropenia
    C. Thrombocytopenia
    D. All of the above

33. Choose the statement which best describes the inflammatory response.
    A. It is an attempt to maintain homeostasis and repair injured tissue.
    B. It is an abnormal response to a threat of invasion.
    C. It is a specific response by the body to protect against any threat of invasion.

34. If an individual has abnormal phagocytosis, the nurse would see the following in the patient's history:
    A. Presence of neoplastic disease
    B. Recurrent bacterial infections
    C. Recurrent viral infections
    D. Recurrent colds and fevers

35. What type of immune process is found in the newborn infant?
    A. Maternal immunity
    B. Natural immunity
    C. Active immunity
    D. Acquired immunity

36. Immunity to a disease can develop as the result of exposure to an antigen. This is called:
    A. Natural immunity
    B. Acquired immunity

C. Systemic immunity

D. Lifelong immunity

37. What does the term *artificial exposure* refer to?

A. Immunity received from the mother

B. Immunity received from exposure to a virus

C. Immunity received after receiving a vaccine

D. Immunity received after exposure to bacteria

38. Which lasts longer, active or acquired immunity? Why?

39. When the nurse does the health history on a patient, what information should be gathered that is related to the immune system?

A. History of infections

B. History of cancer

C. History of childhood disease

D. History of immunizations

E. All of the above

True or False

40. _____ Live vaccines can be given safely to pregnant women.

41. _____ Multiple antigens can be administered simultaneously.

42. _____ The preferred injection site for vaccines for adults is the arm.

43. _____ Vaccines should not be given to adults who are allergic to eggs.

44. _____ It is easier to suppress the secondary immune response.

45. _____ Corticosteroids are a type of immunosuppressant agent.

46. _____ Cytotoxic drugs kill immunologically competent cells.

Questions

47. The main reason that immunosuppressive therapy is used is:

A. To treat viral infections that don't otherwise respond

B. To treat adults with allergies

C. To help with the success of organ transplants

D. To treat chronic diseases

48. A specific type of induced immunosuppression would be:

A. Allergy desensitization

B. Administration of antibody from one individual to another

C. Use of RhoGAM

D. All of the above

49. Which of the following statements is NOT true about cytotoxic drugs?

A. They can kill any cell that is replicating.

B. They may affect both the T cells and the B cells.

C. They have few side effects.

D. They have been used to treat rheumatoid arthritis.

50. A patient is having a bone marrow aspiration. She wants to know what site will be used. What is the nurse's reply?

A. The hip

B. The iliac crest

C. The scapula

51. A critical factor in the success of any bone marrow transplant is a compatible _____.

52. Following a bone marrow transplant, new marrow begins to mature and function in:

A. 2–6 days

B. 10–20 days

C. 1–4 weeks

D. 1–2 months

53. After a bone marrow transplant, how long does it take for the body to regain the normal immune function?

    A. 1–3 months

    B. 3–6 months

    C. 6–12 months

    D. 12–18 months

54. For the individual who has had a bone marrow transplant, which of the following gifts would not be allowed?

    A. Flowers

    B. Candy

    C. Cards

    D. Puzzle

55. What is the rationale for this restriction?

56. What is the biggest threat to the individual who has had a bone marrow transplant?

    A. Nutritional deficiency

    B. Interstitial bleeding

    C. Graft-versus-host disease

    D. Infection

57. Write a nursing care plan for the individual who is having a bone marrow transplant.

    Nursing Diagnosis: Knowledge deficit: procedure.

    Patient Outcome:

    Nursing Interventions:

58. There is a gradual decrease in the immunologic competency with aging.

    A. True

    B. False

59. Which of the following statements are most accurate in terms of the clinical manifestation of an infection in an 80-year-old female?

    A. Fever is always present

    B. White blood cell count is always elevated

    C. Behavior changes are often present

    D. Pain and inflammation are often present

60. Why is there an increased incidence of infection among the elderly?

CLINICAL SITUATIONS

Situation ■ 1

The nurse is assigned to care for Kathy, a 19-year-old with leukemia. She is scheduled for a bone marrow transplant. The following questions refer to this situation.

1. Kathy's mother wants to know why the physician wants to insert a Hickman catheter. Your response would be:

    A. It will prevent Kathy from getting infections.

    B. It is always inserted for this procedure.

    C. It makes it easier to administer drugs and draw blood.

    D. It prevents any complications from occurring.

2. Kathy's mother can't understand why Kathy is going to receive chemotherapy before the transplant. "Isn't one procedure enough?" she asks. As the nurse, you explain to her that chemotherapy is done to:

    A. Prevent transplant rejection.

    B. Suppress the patient's immune system.

    C. Prevent side effects of the procedure.

    D. Prevent graft-versus-host disease.

3. Following the procedure, the patient is in the recovery period. What is an appropriate nursing role at this time?

    A. Review behaviors that might indicate a knowledge deficit.

    B. Place the patient in a room with another teenager to allow her to verbalize her concerns.

    C. Encourage family and friends to visit.

Situation ■ 2

Mrs. Potter is admitted to your unit. She is 80 years old and was brought to the hospital by her husband because of fatigue, apathy, and confusion. She has a history of diabetes and angina.

1. As a nurse, you often work with geriatric patients and recognize that these symptoms may indicate:

   A. The patient may have organic brain syndrome.

   B. The patient may have a nutritional deficit.

   C. The patient may have low blood sugar.

   D. The patient may have an infection.

2. Part of your nursing care of this patient will include:

   A. Monitoring for signs of decreased metabolic rate.

   B. Monitoring for signs of hypoglycemia.

   C. Monitoring for signs of adequate oxygenation.

   D. All of the above.

3. Discharge instructions for Mrs. Potter would include which of the following information?

   A. Stay in bed as much as possible

   B. Avoid excessive contact with children

   C. Limit fluids during the day

Chapter Ten

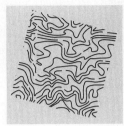

NURSING CARE
of Adults with
Immunodeficiency and
Hypersensitivity Disorders

Learning Objectives

1.0 Demonstrate an Understanding of the Etiology and Pathology of the Disorders of the Immune System.

1.1 Identify Clinical Manifestations of an Immunodeficiency.
1.2 Review the Etiology and Pathophysiology of Several Immunodeficiencies.

2.0 Demonstrate Application of the Nursing Process When Caring for the Patient with Acquired Immunodeficiency Syndrome (AIDS).

2.1 Describe the Etiology and Transmission of AIDS.
2.2 List the Clinical Manifestations of AIDS.
2.3 Identify Several of the Syndromes Associated with AIDS.
2.4 Describe Treatment Options Available for the Patient with AIDS.
2.5 Describe the Psychological Needs of the Patient with AIDS.
2.6 Plan the Nursing Care for the Patient Being Treated for AIDS.

3.0 Demonstrate an Understanding of the Nursing Process When Caring for the Adult with a Hypersensitivity Reaction.

3.1 Identify Several of the Hypersensitivity Disorders.
3.2 Recognize the Medical Management for the Adult with a Hypersensitivity Reaction.
3.3 Plan the Nursing Care for the Patient Who Has a Hypersensitivity Reaction.

4.0 Demonstrate Application of the Nursing Process When Caring for the Adult with a Dysfunction of the Immune System.

4.1 Demonstrate an Understanding of the Needs of the Adult with Asthma.
4.2 Identify the Clinical Manifestations of the Patient with Autoimmune Disorders.
4.3 Plan the Nursing Care for the Patient with Several Autoimmune Disorders.
4.4 Identify the Special Needs of the Geriatric Patient with an Immune Disorder.

Learning Activities

Fill In

1. An immunodeficiency occurs when the immune system fails to _____ .

2. If an adult has acquired a secondary immunodeficiency, reasons for this might be found in the patient's past history. List several precipitating factors:

3. Stem cell deficiency is an example of a _____ deficiency.

4. AIDS is the result of infection with _____ .

5. A vascular neoplasm which causes dermatologic manifestations and occurs in about 25% of the patients with AIDS is known as _____ .

6. The most frequent pulmonary manifestation of AIDS is pneumonia caused by the protozoa _____ .

Questions

7. List four syndromes that have been associated with AIDS.

   1.

   2.

   3.

   4.

8. List the clinical manifestations of human immunodeficiency virus (HIV) infections. Include the four stages.

   1.

   2.

   3.

   4.

9. Identify the primary symptom(s) of an immunodeficient disease.

   A. Failure to thrive

   B. Chronic infection

   C. Weakness and malaise

   D. Chronic pain

10. Stem cell deficiency is characterized by:

    A. Absence of T-cell function

    B. Absence of B-cell function

    C. Absence of both T-cell and B-cell function

    D. Absence of thymic development

11. An individual who has had _____ may be at risk for developing a secondary immunodeficiency.

    A. Tuberculosis

    B. Cytomegalovirus

    C. Acquired immunodeficiency disease

    D. Malignancies

    E. All of the above

12. Education of the patient with an immunodeficiency would include teaching all of the following EXCEPT:

    A. Need to avoid crowds

    B. Ways to avoid infection

    C. Importance of good hygiene

    D. Need to take prophylactic medication

    E. Signs and symptoms of infections

13. What happens within the body when the HIV infects the helper T cells?

    A. RNA is transformed into viral DNA, which destroys the helper T cells if activated by exposure to antigens.

B. DNA is transformed into RNA, which destroys the B cells and T cells and destroys the immune system.

C. RNA is transformed into DNA, which, when transformed, enters the leukocytes, which subsequently multiply rapidly and immaturely.

D. HIV virus infects the entire immune system and renders the individual helpless when exposed to any bacteria or virus.

14. The nurse is aware that HIV is transmitted by:

A. Saliva and droplet infection

B. Sexual contact that involves exchange of body fluids

C. Contaminated food products

D. Prolonged exposure to an AIDS victim

True or False

15. _____ The more sexual partners a person has, the greater the risk of contracting AIDS.

16. _____ Anal intercourse carries a greater risk of HIV transmission than vaginal intercourse.

17. _____ Transmission of HIV often occurs through contaminated blood.

18. _____ Women can pass HIV to their infants.

19. _____ Health care workers are at an increased risk of being infected by HIV.

20. _____ AIDS can be easily diagnosed by laboratory testing for HIV antibodies.

21. _____ Certain sexual practices increase the risk of exposure to body fluids.

22. _____ Use of latex barriers by health care workers will lessen the chance of exposure.

23. _____ There is an increase in infection among the elderly.

24. _____ The elderly patient frequently exhibits classical symptoms of infection.

Questions

25. If an individual infected with HIV develops an acute infection, the nurse might expect to see symptoms such as:

A. Fever, sweats, malaise, anorexia, vomiting

B. Maculopapular rash on the chest

C. Lymphadenopathy, enlarged spleen

D. Any of the above

26. Current medical management for AIDS consists primarily of:

A. Removal of the causative agent

B. Early treatment of infections

C. Antiviral drug therapy

D. Bone marrow transplants

27. The nurse admits a patient who has a diagnosis of AIDS. During the physical assessment, she notices white patches in the buccal cavity. This finding suggests:

A. Kaposi's sarcoma

B. *Candida albicans*

C. *Pneumocystis carinii*

D. *Shigella*

28. Mr. Maters, a 25-year-old patient with AIDS, is admitted with a serious fluid and electrolyte imbalance. When gathering information, it would be important to ask about:

A. History of excessive exercise patterns

B. History of adherence to prescribed medications

C. History of changes in bowel patterns

D. History of changes in fluid intake

29. The nurse is assisting Mr. Maters with his hygienic needs. One important reason for offering a back rub is to:

A. Help him combat the sense of isolation

B. Help him prevent formation of skin lesions

C. Help him bathe since he can't reach his back

D. Help him acknowledge his feelings

30. A patient with AIDS develops fever, dyspnea, tachypnea, and dry cough. These symptoms suggest the patient has:

    A. *Entamoeba histolytica*

    B. *Shigella*

    C. *P. carinii* pneumonia

    D. tuberculosis

31. Write a nursing care plan for an adult with AIDS. Use the following diagnosis.

    Nursing Diagnosis: Knowledge deficit related to the etiology, transmission, clinical course, and treatment protocols

    Patient Outcome:

    Nursing Interventions:

Matching

Match the following hypersensitivity disorders with the appropriate reactions.

A. Type I   C. Type III
B. Type II   D. Type IV

32. _____ Occurs within minutes of the antigen-antibody reaction.

33. _____ Delayed reaction caused by the release of lymphokines by T cells.

34. _____ Cytotoxic reaction that causes cell damage.

35. _____ Occurs when soluble antigens react with antibodies.

Fill In

36. Hayfever is an example of a Type _____ reaction.

37. A transplant reaction is an example of a Type _____ reaction.

38. The patient who has a transfusion reaction is exhibiting a Type _____ hypersensitivity reaction.

39. A patient on erythromycin who develops joint pain, hives, and fever is exhibiting a Type _____ reaction.

40. _____ is a sudden, life-threatening reaction to an antigen.

41. The most useful drugs in the treatment of hayfever are _____ .

42. A form of immunotherapy in which the patient is injected with extracts of the pollen he is allergic to is known as _____ .

43. _____ is an impaired hypersensitivity reaction to an antigen that the patient has been exposed to previously.

44. _____ is a condition in which the body is reacting against itself.

Questions

45. Which of the following clinical manifestations, if present, would indicate a hypersensitivity reaction?

    A. Bronchoconstriction, vasoconstriction, shock

    B. Bronchoconstriction, vasodilation, hypotension

    C. Bronchodilation, vasoconstriction, increased capillary permeability

    D. Bronchodilation, respiratory distress, shock

46. Initial medical treatment for an allergic reaction would most likely include the use of:

    A. Steroids

    B. Dopamine

    C. Benadryl

    D. Epinephrine

True or False

47. _____ Asthma is considered to be the most common chronic disease among children.

48. _____ In extrinsic asthma, the relationship of exposure to agents is not evident.

49. _____ An asthma attack can be life threatening.

50. _____ Lack of sleep and stress can contribute to an asthma attack.

51. _____ It is important to limit fluids during an acute asthmatic attack.

Questions

52. When assessing a patient during an acute asthma attack, the nurse would expect to find:

    A. Rhonchi and rales

    B. Wheezes, tachycardia

    C. Moist cough, diminished breath sounds

    D. Hypotension, tachypnea, bradycardia

53. Aggressive medical treatment for status asthmaticus involves using:

    A. Steroids, epinephrine, aminophylline

    B. Steroids, antibiotics, atropine

    C. Epinephrine, theophylline, morphine

    D. Aminophylline, steroids, antibiotics

54. A patient with asthma is usually placed on bronchodilators for relief of symptoms. An example would be:

    A. Albuterol

    B. Cortisone

    C. Codeine

    D. Cool aerosol

55. During an asthma attack, it is important for the nurse to assess for signs of hypoxia such as:

    A. Bradycardia, diaphoresis

    B. Restlessness, confusion, cyanosis

    C. Wheezing, vomiting

    D. All of the above

56. A patient is admitted with a diagnosis of hypersensitivity pneumonitis. The nurse would expect to find symptoms such as:

    A. Shortness of breath

    B. Fever, chills

    C. Malaise

    D. All of the above

57. The nurse is aware that hypersensitivity pneumonitis results from:

    A. Autoimmune response

    B. Arthus reaction

    C. Antigen-antibody response

    D. Any of the above

58. All of the following are common characteristics of autoimmune disease EXCEPT:

    A. They occur more often in men than women

    B. They tend to run in families

    C. They improve with immunosuppressive therapy

    D. They may involve all of the body systems

59. Write a nursing care plan for a patient who enters the emergency room in anaphylactic shock.

    Nursing Diagnosis:

    List two applicable patient outcomes.

    1.

    2.

60. Systemic lupus erythematosus (SLE) is an autoimmune disease. From the list below, which factors might trigger SLE?

    A. Sulfa drugs   E. Viral infections
    B. Antibiotics   F. Ultraviolet light
    C. Analgesics   G. Stress
    D. Oral contraceptives   H. Pollutants

61. Presence of _____ in the serum is an important diagnostic finding with SLE.

62. When the nurse is assessing an individual with SLE, the typical expected findings would be:

    A. Inflammation of almost every organ system

    B. Inflammation limited to the joints

    C. No inflammation, but symptoms of sepsis

    D. No inflammation, but dermatitis and a butterfly rash

63. Providing which of the following information would meet the educational needs of the patient with SLE?

    A. Explain medical treatments that can cure the disease

    B. Teach how to avoid factors that cause exacerbation

    C. Teach which drugs are given prophylactically

    D. Explain that this disease won't interrupt the patient's lifestyle

64. A patient who has been diagnosed with SLE should be taught to avoid:

    A. Pregnancy

    B. Ultraviolet light

    C. Emotional stress

    D. All of the above

65. If a patient with scleroderma were to exhibit malnutrition and weight loss, the probable cause would be:

    A. Renal failure

    B. Crest syndrome

    C. Esophageal stricture

    D. Pericarditis

66. An autoimmune disorder which is characterized by the increased destruction of red blood cells is:

    A. Aplastic anemia

    B. Thrombocytopenia

    C. Hemolytic anemia

    D. Hemophilia

67. The following statements about chronic fatigue syndrome are all true EXCEPT:

    A. It is also known as Epstein-Barr virus

    B. It occurs in whites and blacks

    C. It occurs mainly in young adults

    D. It is characterized by unrelenting fatigue

68. Plan the nursing care for a patient who is diagnosed with SLE.

    Nursing Diagnosis: Pain

    Patient Outcome:

    Nursing Interventions:

69. Plan the nursing care for the patient with chronic fatigue syndrome.

    Nursing Diagnosis: Fatigue related to chronic fatigue syndrome

    Patient Outcome:

    Nursing Interventions:

CLINICAL SITUATIONS

Situation ■ 1

Tom Brown, a 35-year-old patient, has had AIDS for 8 months. He has tried many types of treatments, even illegally obtained medications. He is admitted for treatment of secondary infections and general debilitation.

1. During assessment, the nurse finds he is 5' 10", and weights 125 lb. He is pale and has poor skin turgor. He has white patches in his mouth. What other information is relevant?

    A. Dietary history

    B. List of medications he is taking

    C. Number of past hospitalizations

    D. List of his intimate contacts

2. The nurse realizes that it is important to perform a thorough neurologic assessment. This is because:

    A. The patient may have had a stroke

    B. The patient may have a pulmonary embolus

    C. The patient may have an adverse effect from medication

    D. The patient may have ineffective coping ability

3. A primary nursing diagnosis is knowledge deficit related to treatment and self-care. Which action by the patient indicates the nurse's intervention has been effective?

    A. Patient describes the correct use of prescribed analgesic.

B. Patient states symptoms that require immediate medical attention.

C. Patient can chew soft foods with minimal discomfort.

D. Patient does not get short of breath with activity.

4. Mr. Brown has had severe diarrhea during the last month. The nurse would carefully assess for signs of:

A. Fluid and electrolyte imbalance

B. Malnutrition

C. Skin breakdown

D. All of the above

5. It would be important to provide a nonjudgmental atmosphere to help Mr. Brown cope with his feelings. An appropriate intervention would be:

A. Help the patient deal with death and dying

B. Help the patient manage home care

C. Help the patient understand his medical care

Situation ■ 2

Kathy Simmons is brought into the emergency room. She is dyspneic and diaphoretic. Her husband states that she was stung by a bee. The physician administers epinephrine.

1. The nurse should consider which action of primary importance when performing the nursing assessment?

A. Calm the patient and reassure her that she will be fine

B. Document her reaction and response to treatment

C. Assess for signs of allergic reaction to epinephrine

D. Insist that her husband wait outside

2. Kathy is breathing much easier now. She asks you if this will ever happen again. What would be an appropriate response?

A. I don't know, ask your doctor.

B. No, these types of reactions generally don't recur.

C. Yes, another sting could cause a similar reaction.

3. The nurse should explain to Kathy that she should:

A. Avoid areas where bees are prevalent.

B. Carry a bee sting kit and know how to use it.

C. Wear a MedicAlert band.

D. All of the above

Situation ■ 3

Ms. Lancing is a 28-year-old computer programmer with a 20-year history of asthma. She is recovering from a severe attack. Her current medications are Theo-Dur, prednisone, and Valium.

1. The nurse enters the room to find the patient crying. Ms. Lancing says, "Why can't I be normal? Everything was fine; I just got a promotion at work, a new apartment, and a new car. Why, just before this happened, my new boyfriend asked me to go away with him." What area would you explore in your communication?

A. Ways to avoid allergens

B. Ways to prevent stressors from being disruptive

C. The importance of a good diet

D. The types of medications she is on

2. How can the physician determine which antigens may be precipitating Ms. Lancing's asthma attacks?

A. Through a series of skin tests

B. Can't be done since asthma is caused by stress

C. Try different medications and see the response

D. A and C

3. Nursing interventions that may be helpful in promoting effective breathing patterns would include:

A. Elevating the head of the bed

B. Changing linens frequently

C. Encouraging a fluid intake of 2 L a day

D. All of the above

4. The nurse prepares to administer Ms. Lancing's morning medication. The patient states she is very nervous and nauseated. Her heart rate is 128, BP 130/88, RR 28. What would be an appropriate action?

   A. Hold her medication and call the doctor.

   B. Give her the medication, then call for an antiemetic.

   C. Stay and talk with her, as she is very stressed.

   D. Give medication, but recheck her in 30 minutes.

Situation ■ 4

A 23-year-old college student is admitted to the hospital with a diagnosis of scleroderma. She has been treated by her family physician until this episode.

1. Which of the following statements best describes this disorder?

   A. It occurs mainly in men.

   B. It is an autoimmune collagen disorder.

   C. It is an allergic reaction to antigens.

   D. It is caused by a bacteria.

2. Specific characteristics that the nurse would ask about would include:

   A. Fibrosis in the skin

   B. Edema in joints

   C. Thickening of dermis

   D. Vasospasmodic episodes

   E. Any of the above

3. The patient is having difficulty breathing and difficulty swallowing. This may be a result of:

   A. Pulmonary fibrosis, esophageal stricture

   B. Pericarditis, heart failure

   C. Formation of plaque

   D. Raynaud's syndrome

4. Because of the systemic nature of this disease, important laboratory findings for the nurse to review would be:

   A. CBC,WBC

   B. BUN, creatinine

   C. CPK, SGOT

   D. ABGs

5. The nurse would expect medical treatment to involve:

   A. Antibiotics

   B. Prednisone

   C. Vasodilators

   D. Vasoconstrictors

Chapter Eleven

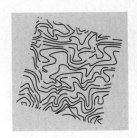

NURSING CARE
of Adults with
Oncologic Disorders

Learning Objectives

1.0 Review the Etiology of Oncologic Disorders.

1.1 Define Current Terminology.
1.2 Describe Current Theories on the Causes of Oncologic Disorders.

2.0 Demonstrate an Understanding of the Diagnostic Testing Used to Identify an Oncologic Disorder.

2.1 Define Staging.
2.2 Identify the Patient Who Is in the High Risk Category.
2.3 Identify Diagnostic Procedures Used When an Oncologic Disorder is Suspected.

3.0 Demonstrate Application of the Nursing Process When Caring for the Patient Receiving Radiation Therapy.

3.1 Compare Internal and External Radiation Therapy.
3.2 Describe Indications for Radiation Therapy.
3.3 Identify the Side Effects Related to Radiation Therapy.
3.4 Plan the Nursing Care for the Adult Receiving Radiation Therapy.

4.0 Demonstrate Application of the Nursing Process When Caring for the Adult Receiving Chemotherapy.

4.1 Describe the Types and Actions of Various Chemotherapeutic Agents.
4.2 Identify Types of Delivery Systems for Chemotherapeutic Agents.
4.3 Identify the Side Effects Related to Chemotherapy.
4.4 Demonstrate an Understanding of the Needs of the Patient Who Has Pain Secondary to Cancer.
4.5 Plan the Nursing Care for the Adult Receiving Chemotherapy.

5.0 Demonstrate an Understanding of the Psychosocial Needs of the Adult Being Treated for an Oncologic Disorder.

5.1 Describe Methods to Meet the Nutritional Needs of the Adult with an Oncologic Disorder.

5.2 Plan the Nursing Care for the Patient Being Treated for Cancer.

Learning Activities

Define

1. Neoplasm:

2. Oncogenesis:

3. Carcinogenesis:

4. "Cancer-prone" personality:

5. Staging:

6. Tumor markers:

Questions

Explain how each of the following factors is thought to contribute to carcinogenesis.

7. Genetic factors:

8. Environmental factors:

9. Smoking:

10. Diet:

11. Immunologic defects:

12. Psychosocial factors:

Matching

Match the following terms with their correct definitions.

A. Benign   D. Sarcoma
B. Carcinoma   E. Leukemia
C. Malignant

13. _____ Malignant cells of connective tissue

14. _____ Cells resembling the tissue of origin

15. _____ Malignant cells of the blood

16. _____ Undifferentiated cells unlike the tissue of origin

17. _____ Malignant cells in the epithelial tissue

Questions

18. List the seven warning signals of cancer.

    1.
    2.
    3.
    4.
    5.
    6.
    7.

19. Cancer cells differ from normal cells in that they are anaplastic, which means:

    A. They are primitive, undifferentiated cells

    B. They grow slowly as they replicate

    C. They closely resemble the original cells

    D. All of the above

20. Malignant tumors can spread through a direct or indirect process. This is known as:

    A. Tissue invasion

    B. Metastasis

    C. Replication

    D. Duplication

21. One way that a tumor can be spread by an indirect process is by way of the _____ . (List all that apply.)

    A. Muscle cells

    B. Vascular system

    C. Lymphatic system

    D. Immune system

    E. Neuron fibers

22. Which of the following would be environmental factors that can contribute to the development of certain oncologic disorders? (List all that apply.)

    A. Arsenic

    B. Asbestos

    C. Nitrogen gas

    D. Smoking

    E. Antibiotics

23. Research has shown that there is a relationship between _____ and onset of illness.

    A. Diet

    B. Smoking

    C. Stress

    D. Alcohol use

24. An example of a blood test that is used to diagnose cancer is the test for carcinoembryonic antigen (an oncofetal protein). What type of cancer has it been associated with?

    A. Cervical

    B. Gastrointestinal

    C. Brain

    D. Bone

25. Which of the following statements is NOT true about magnetic resonance imaging?

    A. The patient is seen in a three-dimensional image.

    B. The patient is not exposed to radiation.

    C. The patient is checked first with a metal detector.

    D. The patient is kept on NPO status after midnight the night before the procedure.

26. The type of diagnostic test that uses high frequency sound waves which are directed over a specific body part is called:

    A. Tomography

    B. Ultrasonography

    C. Mammography

    D. Radionuclide scanning

27. The radiographic procedure which produces a detailed three-dimensional image that can be analyzed by a computer is called:

    A. Radionuclide scanning

    B. Magnetic resonance imaging

    C. Computed tomography

    D. Ultrasonography

28. Mrs. James is scheduled for a PAP smear and biopsy to rule out a neoplasm. From the list below, pick the nursing diagnosis that is most appropriate at this time.

    A. Anxiety related to uncertain outcome of tests

    B. Pain related to diagnostic procedure

    C. Alteration in urinary elimination related to diagnostic procedure

29. In assessing Mrs. James, who was diagnosed as having cancer, which of the following is important to ask?

    A. Have you talked with your family about the diagnosis?

    B. What do you usually do when you have a problem?

C. What kind of medical plan do you have?

D. All of the above are appropriate

30. Write a nursing care plan for the individual who is newly diagnosed with cancer.

    Nursing Diagnosis: Knowledge deficit related to cause, prognosis, type of malignancy, and treatment methods

    Patient Outcome:

    Nursing Interventions:

31. Which statement by the patient would indicate that the above goal has been partially met?

    A. Please explain the purpose of radiation therapy.

    B. Leave me alone, I'm not worried.

    C. My husband doesn't need to know about this.

    D. I've read that cancer is always fatal.

32. A biopsy may be done to _____ a suspicious mass.

    A. Diagnose or remove

    B. Radiate or test

    C. Treat or remove

33. The type of biopsy which removes all of the tumor can best be defined as:

    A. Needle biopsy

    B. Incisional biopsy

    C. Excisional biopsy

    D. Irradiation biopsy

34. Which statement by the nurse would best describe the rationale for radiation therapy? The purpose is:

    A. To remove the neoplasm

    B. To damage and kill cancer cells

    C. To prevent metastasis

    D. All of the above

Matching

Match the following radiation therapy terms with their correct definitions.

A. Particle radiation   D. Rad
B. Isotope   E. Half-life
C. Gamma ray

35. _____ Amount of radiation delivered to tissue

36. _____ Length of time radiation is emitted

37. _____ Radioactive substance

38. _____ Uses high energy beams to destabilize ions

39. _____ High energy used to treat malignancies

Questions

40. When radiation is used in the early stages of cancer, the goal is to cure the neoplasm.

    A. True

    B. False

41. The rationale for giving radiation therapy over a period of several weeks is that:

    A. Normal cells can have time for cellular repair

    B. Costs will be decreased

    C. Alopecia will be prevented

    D. Radiation burns will not occur

42. The nurse is caring for a patient who has an internal radiation implant for uterine cancer. Star each of the nursing measures which should be implemented.

    A. Call for a private room.

    B. Have the same nurse care for the patient.

    C. Cover the patient with a lead apron.

    D. Spend only 30 minutes in the room at a time.

43. It is important for the nurse to provide education to the patient undergoing radiation therapy. List five of the side effects associated with radiation therapy that the patient should be aware of.

    1.

    2.

3.

4.

5.

44. Pick two of the side effects and list an intervention that will help the patient cope with the problem.

1.

2.

45. Which of the following is not a necessary part of the assessment of the patient receiving radiation therapy of the esophagus?

A. Assess for changes in skin color

B. Assess for mouth ulcerations

C. Assess for pain in the chest

D. Assess ability to ambulate

46. Plan the nursing care for the patient who is undergoing external radiation therapy.

Nursing Diagnosis: High risk for altered health maintenance related to lack of knowledge of side effects of treatment

Patient Outcome:

Nursing Interventions:

47. Which of the following explanations would the nurse give to a patient to explain how chemotherapeutic drugs work?

A. They destroy only the abnormal cells.

B. They work quickly and have few side effects.

C. They prevent a recurrence of the cancer.

D. They disrupt the development and reproduction of cells.

48. Which of the following is a major advantage of chemotherapy?

A. It has few side effects.

B. It is less expensive.

C. It is systemic.

D. It prevents a return of the neoplasm.

49. Which of the following statements is NOT true about plant alkaloids?

A. They inhibit DNA and protein synthesis.

B. They come from the periwinkle plant.

C. They are active during the mitosis phase.

D. They are most effective against tumors with increased metabolic rates.

50. The type of chemotherapeutic drugs that interfere with normal biochemical processes are:

A. Antimetabolites

B. Plant alkaloids

C. Hormones

D. Steroids

51. The type of chemotherapeutic drugs which would most likely be given to the individual with prostate cancer would be:

A. Plant alkaloid

B. Steroid

C. Hormonal therapy

D. Antimetabolite

52. A patient wants to know why he has to have a chemotherapy treatment every week. He would rather have them daily to finish sooner. What does the nurse reply?

53. In preparing for the delivery of chemotherapy, a variety of routes may be used. Check each of the possible methods from the list below.

A. Central venous catheter

B. Intra-arterial catheter

C. Intrapleural catheter

D. Orally

54. Following surgery for liver cancer, Mr. Moore is having a method of chemotherapy known as adjuvant therapy. This is done:

    A. For the cure, control, or palliation of the tumor

    B. To stop further cell division of metastatic cells

    C. To prevent a recurrence of the tumor

    D. Because the patient is not a candidate for radiation therapy

55. The reasons that patients undergoing chemotherapy are at risk for side effects is because:

    A. Having cancer causes debilitation

    B. Chemotherapy destroys normal cells

    C. The drugs are very potent

    D. Chemotherapy causes toxic reactions

56. Educating patients about the side effects of chemotherapy is an important nursing responsibility. List five of the possible side effects of chemotherapy.

    1.

    2.

    3.

    4.

    5.

57. Pick two of these side effects and list a specific nursing intervention which the nurse would implement that will help alleviate the problem.

    1.

    2.

58. Since one of the side effects of chemotherapy is irritation of the gastrointestinal tract, the nurse might treat this problem with any of the following EXCEPT:

    A. Administer antiemetic drugs as ordered

    B. Use relaxation therapy with the patient

    C. Administer antihistamines as ordered

    D. Administer anxiolytic drugs as ordered

    E. Administer a small feeding prior to chemotherapy

59. During the intravenous administration of a chemotherapeutic drug, the nurse finds that the medication has infiltrated. What is an appropriate nursing action?

    A. Stop the infusion and give the recommended antidote.

    B. Slow the infusion and call the physician.

    C. Change the infusion site and continue the medication.

    D. Wait and see if problems occur before taking action.

60. Ms. Brown has received chemotherapy for the past 6 weeks. Today she states that she feels uncoordinated, is weak, and has ringing in her ears. A reason might be:

    A. Cardiotoxicity

    B. Neurotoxicity

    C. Pulmonary toxicity

    D. Tissue extravasation

61. Since chemotherapy can cause a variety of side effects, which action by the nurse could help to prevent an infection in a patient?

    A. Monitor for leukopenia

    B. Monitor for signs of anemia

    C. Monitor for energy levels

    D. Monitor for stomatitis

62. If the patient who is undergoing chemotherapy has a low platelet count, the nurse would monitor for:

    A. Infection

    B. Fluid and electrolyte imbalance

    C. Bleeding

    D. Hypoxia

63. The type of treatment for cancer with a chemical or biologic agent which is intended to assist the immune system in destroying cancer cells is known as:

    A. Chemotherapy

    B. Hormonal therapy

    C. Immunotherapy

    D. Radiation therapy

64. Which of the following is NOT an example of a chemotherapeutic agent?

    A. Vincristine

    B. Dobutamine

    C. Doxorubicin

    D. Nitrogen mustard

65. Cancer presents a variety of psychosocial problems. From the list below, which occur most frequently?

    A. Anxiety and fear

    B. Threat to self-concept

    C. Alteration in breathing patterns

    D. Potential for injury

    E. Isolation and alienation

    F. Family stress

When providing support to the cancer patient, the nurse needs to know the prognosis to help the patient deal successfully with the problems. Therefore, it is important to know if the treatment is to cure the disease, control symptoms, or only provide comfort. List two interventions that would be appropriate for each of the treatment focuses:

66. Cure: How will the nurse help the patient cope with anxiety and fear?

    1.

    2.

67. Control: How will the nurse help the patient cope with problems related to sexuality?

    1.

    2.

68. Comfort: How will the nurse help the patient deal with loss of life and helplessness?

    1.

    2.

69. Isolation is often a problem with individuals who have cancer. Which of these would be an appropriate nursing intervention?

    A. Call the local minister

    B. Offer the suggestion of a referral to the Cancer Society.

    C. Bring the patient to a group meeting of the Cancer Society.

    D. Provide a book on hospice care.

70. What is one of the reasons that patients with advanced cancer have pain?

    A. Tissue damage and tissue infiltration

    B. Bleeding into the tissue

    C. Severe infection

    D. All of the above

71. Explain the gate control theory.

72. Chemicals that are produced by the body in response to pain are known as:

    A. Narcotics

    B. Neurotransmitters

    C. Stimulants

    D. Depressants

73. Pharmacologic agents which control pain by acting on the central nervous system are:

    A. Psychotropic agents

    B. Narcotic agents

    C. Anti-inflammatory agents

    D. Nonnarcotic agents

74. A type of cutaneous therapy which stimulates the peripheral nervous system in an attempt to override the pain stimuli is called:

    A. Acupuncture

    B. Skin massage

    C. Transcutaneous electrical nerve stimulation (TENS)

    D. Cold application

75. Plan the nursing care for the patient with severe pain secondary to a malignancy.

    Nursing Diagnosis: Pain related to the malignant process

    Patient Outcome:

    Nursing Interventions:

CLINICAL SITUATIONS

Situation ■ 1

Mr. Donner is 75 years old. He has had surgery for esophageal cancer. This is to be followed by radiation therapy upon discharge

1. All of the following are side effects of radiation therapy that he may experience EXCEPT:

   A. Alopecia

   B. Erythema

   C. Esophagitis

   D. Weakness

2. Mr. Donner develops a sore throat and esophagitis. What is a nursing diagnosis that is most relevant at this time?

   A. Alteration in skin integrity

   B. High risk for infection

   C. Alteration in urinary elimination

   D. Alteration in nutrition

3. At this time it would be important for the nurse to teach Mr. Donner:

   A. How to perform good oral hygiene

   B. How to perform coughing and deep breathing

   C. How to control pain and discomfort

   D. How to apply lotions and compresses

Situation ■ 2

The nurse is caring for a 66-year-old female with a lymphoma. Part of the care for Mrs. Angelo involves giving today's dose of vincristine. The following questions refer to this situation.

1. In order to be certified in the administration of chemotherapy, the nurse must have special training. Which of the following is NOT included in the training?

   A. Starting the intravenous solution with vincristine

   B. Awareness of the possibility of tissue extravasation

   C. Appropriate ways to treat nausea

   D. Understanding of emergency procedures

2. After a course of chemotherapy, Mrs. Angelo is to have several radiation therapy treatments. The purpose of radiation therapy in this case would be:

   A. Adjuvant therapy

   B. Palliative therapy

   C. Primary curative therapy

3. The nurse is explaining to Mrs. Angelo what to expect during the first treatment. Which of the following statements is inaccurate?

   A. You will be required to lie still.

   B. You will have a radiologist with you.

   C. You will not be radioactive after the treatment.

   D. You will hear a noise from the machine.

4. As a result of the treatment, Mrs. Angelo develops dermatitis. All of the following are appropriate nursing measures, EXCEPT:

   A. Apply moisturizer

   B. Apply a water-soluble lubricant

   C. Apply warm compresses

   D. Apply soap

Situation ■ 3

A patient is admitted to the hospital for further chemotherapy to treat lung cancer. Her tumor was resected 2 months ago, which was followed by 4 weeks of radiation therapy.

1. Following the first chemotherapy treatment, she complains of severe nausea and begins to vomit. A medication that has had some effect on minimizing nausea is:

   A. Demerol

   B. Valium

   C. Phenergan

   D. Haldol

2. A common complication of chemotherapy is mucositis. The nurse is aware that the reason for this is:

   A. Chemotherapy attacks cells that grow rapidly.

   B. The drug is taken orally.

C. Unknown

D. The drug is very irritating to tissue.

3. To help prevent this problem, the nurse would:

   A. Offer a soft diet.

   B. Provide good oral hygiene.

   C. Provide pain medication.

   D. Provide diversional therapy.

4. The patient also begins to have severe episodes of diarrhea. The most appropriate interventions would include:

   A. Nutritional interventions

   B. Drugs such as Lomotil

   C. Fluid replacement

   D. All of the above

5. When the patient is discharged, she is told that a common side effect of the medication she received is photosensitivity. Because of this she should:

   A. Avoid crowds

   B. Avoid exposure to sunlight

   C. Avoid any over-the-counter medications

   D. Avoid milk in her diet

Unit Four

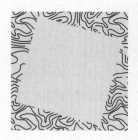

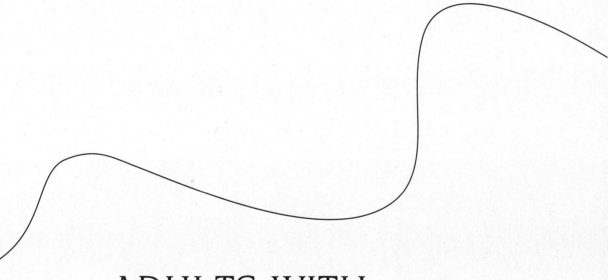

ADULTS WITH RESPIRATORY DYSFUNCTION

Chapter Twelve

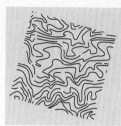

KNOWLEDGE BASIC TO THE NURSING CARE
of Adults with
Respiratory Dysfunction

Learning Objectives

1.0 Review the Anatomy and Physiology of the Respiratory System.

1.1 Identify the Parts of the Respiratory System.
1.2 Explain the Process of Breathing.
1.3 Demonstrate an Understanding of the Process of Ventilation.

2.0 Demonstrate an Understanding of Assessment Data Related to the Respiratory System.

2.1 Identify Clinical Manifestations of Respiratory Dysfunctions.
2.2 Review the Health History of an Adult with a Respiratory Dysfunction.
2.3 Identify Normal and Abnormal Breath Sounds.
2.4 Identify the Tests Which are Used to Diagnose Respiratory Alterations.

3.0 Demonstrate an Understanding of Interventions Used to Treat Adults with Respiratory Dysfunction.

3.1 Identify Nonsurgical Methods of Treating Adult Respiratory Dysfunction.
3.2 State the Purpose of Mechanical Ventilation.
3.2 Identify the Needs of a Patient on a Ventilator.
3.3 Identify the Parts of an Intrapleural Drainage System.
3.4 Utilize the Nursing Process in Planning Care for the Adult Having Thoracic Surgery.

Learning Activities

Questions

1. List the structures of the lower airway.

   1.

   2.

   3.

   4.

   5.

2. List the structures of the upper airway.

   1.

   2.

Identify

3. On the diagram below, label the parts.

Larynx   Diaphragm   Parietal pleura
Visceral pleura   Left bronchus   Trachea

Fill In

4. Inspiration is the _____ phase of ventilation.

5. Expiration is the _____ phase of ventilation.

6. During inspiration, the diaphragm _____. During expiration, the diaphragm returns to its normal position.

7. List one of the mechanisms which controls ventilation and explain how it functions.

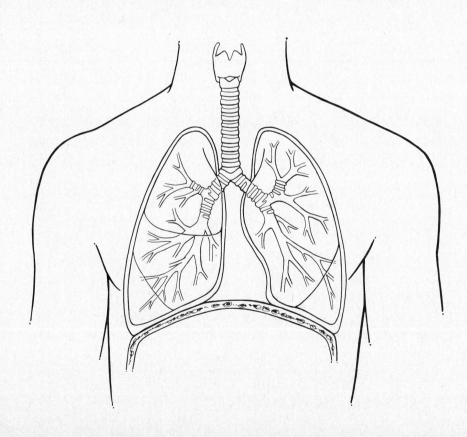

8. Lung tissue is _____.

9. Lung compliance is a measure of how easily the lung can be _____.

10. External respiration takes place at the _____.

11. Internal respiration takes place at the _____.

12. Oxygen is transported by _____ in the blood.

Questions

13. Adequate circulation is essential for tissue oxygenation. List two factors which affect the circulation.

    1.

    2.

14. List four of the signs and symptoms of a respiratory dysfunction that a nurse would look for when assessing a patient.

    1.

    2.

    3.

    4.

15. Surfactant is produced within cells of the alveoli. What purpose does it serve?

    A. It helps stimulate respirations

    B. It minimizes friction during respiration

    C. It prevents collapse of the alveoli

    D. It assists with all of the above

16. How much total body energy is used for normal breathing?

    A. 2–3%

    B. 5–10%

    C. 10–15%

    D. 15–25%

17. Gas exchange depends on the matching of the distribution of air in the lungs and the blood flow in the pulmonary capillaries. When ventilation is present without perfusion, no gas exchange occurs. This is known as:

    A. Dead space

    B. Shunting

    C. Hypoxia

    D. Hypercapnia

18. When capillaries are perfused but no ventilation occurs, this is known as:

    A. Shunting

    B. Dead space

    C. Third spacing

    D. Anoxia

19. The nurse is aware that if a patient has _____, it is an example of a shunt-producing condition.

    A. Atelectasis

    B. Acute respiratory distress syndrome (ARDS)

    C. Pneumonia

    D. All of the above

Matching

Match the following conditions with their descriptions.

A. Hypoxia   C. Hypocapnia
B. Hypercapnia   D. Anoxia

20. _____ Low level of carbon dioxide

21. _____ High level of carbon dioxide

22. _____ Low level of oxygen

23. _____ Absence of oxygen

Questions

24. When reviewing diagnostic tests for an adult with a respiratory dysfunction, the nurse would look at _____ since it is the most reliable indicator of hypoxemia.

    A. Chest x-ray

    B. Ventilation studies

C. Hemoglobin and hematocrit

D. Arterial blood gases

25. The nurse would be alert to a possible hypoxic condition if a patient exhibited which of the following symptoms?

A. Decrease in heart rate and blood pressure

B. Changes in level of orientation

C. Change in urinary output

D. Increase in respiration, cough

26. When assessing the respiratory system, the nurse is aware that the main respiratory stimulant is:

A. Hypocapnia

B. Hypoxemia

C. Hypercapnia

D. Anoxia

27. An adult with chronic hypoxemia might exhibit the following symptoms:

A. Cyanosis, palpitations

B. Fatigue, apathy, muscle twitching

C. Confusion, irritability

D. Low heart rate and respiratory rate

28. A patient exhibits a sudden loss of consciousness. The nurse is aware that this may be due to:

A. Hypercapnia

B. Hypocapnia

29. A patient who shows signs of hyperventilation is at risk for developing:

A. Hypocapnia

B. Hypercapnia

C. Hypoxemia

30. The nurse is obtaining a patient history. The patient is complaining of hemoptysis. This symptom may be related to which of the following diseases?

A. Tuberculosis

B. Emphysema

C. Asthma

D. Pneumonia

31. In obtaining the history for the patient with a respiratory disorder, the nurse would be sure to obtain information in which of the following areas?

A. Smoking history

B. Exposure to occupational pollutants

C. Exposure to carcinogens

D. Presence of cough, pain

E. All of the above

32. Which of the following postures in a patient would indicate a respiratory problem?

A. Lying prone

B. Sitting in a chair with the feet elevated

C. Sitting up in bed with the arms on a table

D. Walking in the hall with a slow gait

Define

Define the following respiratory terminology.

33. Hyperpnea:

34. Hyperventilation:

35. Kussmaul's breathing:

36. Cheyne-Stokes respirations:

37. Biot's breathing:

38. Pigeon breast:

39. Barrel chest:

40. Kyphosis:

41. Lordosis:

42. Scoliosis:

Questions

43. Breath sounds are heard as a result of:

    A. Vibrations produced in the larynx which are transmitted to the chest wall

    B. Transmission of vibration of air from larynx to alveoli

    C. Transmission of the air exchange in the alveoli

    D. None of the above

44. Adventitious breath sounds can be defined as:

    A. Extra sounds heard during inspiration

    B. Harsh sounds heard during expiration

    C. Abnormal sounds superimposed over breath sounds

    D. Abnormal sounds heard instead of normal breath sounds

Assessment of Respiration

Matching—Normal Breath Sounds

A. Bronchial
B. Bronchovesicular
C. Vesicular

45. _____ Quiet, low pitched

46. _____ High pitched, loud, over the trachea

47. _____ Medium pitched, between the trachea and the lung

Matching—Abnormal Breath Sounds

A. Rales
B. Friction rub
C. Wheezing

48. _____ Creaking, grating sound

49. _____ Discrete, non-continuous sound

50. _____ Continuous, musical sound

Questions

51. The purpose of pulmonary function studies is:

    A. To measure the tidal capacity

    B. To measure the functional ability of the lungs

    C. To measure the ventilation capacity of the lungs

    D. To evaluate the diaphragmatic excursion

52. Arterial blood gases are used to measure the blood oxygenation. Abnormal blood gases would indicate:

    A. Respiratory dysfunction

    B. Cardiac dysfunction

    C. Metabolic imbalance

53. A painless, noninvasive procedure that can monitor arterial oxygen saturation is called:

    A. Pulse oximetry

B. Arterial blood gas measurement

C. Venous blood sampling

D. Pulmonary function testing

Identify

Identify the cause of each of these abnormal states.

A. Metabolic acidosis   C. Metabolic alkalosis
B. Respiratory alkalosis   D. Respiratory acidosis

54. _____ Hypoventilation

55. _____ Diabetic ketoacidosis

56. _____ Diarrhea

57. _____ Hyperventilation

58. _____ Nasogastric suctioning

59. _____ Renal failure

60. _____ Chronic obstructive pulmonary disease

Matching—Diagnostic Testing

A. Sputum test   D. Lung scan
B. Angiography   E. Mediastinoscopy
C. Thoracentesis   F. Bronchogram

61. _____ Visualizes pulmonary vessel

62. _____ Determines presence of infection

63. _____ Removes fluid from the lung

64. _____ Evaluates pulmonary perfusion

65. _____ Visualizes lymph nodes

66. _____ Radiopaque material is inserted into the trachea to allow visualization

Questions

67. To determine adequate tissue oxygenation when evaluating arterial blood gases, what should be measured?

    A. Oxygen gas tension

B. Oxyhemoglobin saturation

C. Tissue capillary pressure

D. Carrying capacity of the body

68. Nursing care of a patient receiving a perfusion lung scan would include explaining all of the following EXCEPT:

A. You will be required to lie still and breathe quietly.

B. You will receive less radiation than with a chest x-ray.

C. You will have no discomfort during the procedure.

D. You may be required to use a mouthpiece and a noseclip.

69. The most appropriate diagnostic procedure for the adult who is suspected of having a foreign body in the respiratory tract would be:

A. Lung scan

B. Thoracentesis

C. Bronchoscopy

D. Pulmonary function test

70. A diagnostic test that is used primarily in the diagnosis of bronchiectasis is called a:

A. Bronchoscopy

B. Bronchogram

C. Laryngogram

D. Esophagoscope

71. Following a bronchoscopy, the nurse would observe for possible complications. These would include:

A. Hyperventilation

B. Infection

C. Aspiration

D. Desaturation

72. A patient has just had a thoracentesis. The physician orders a chest x-ray. What is the rationale?

A. To assess for pneumonia

B. To check for a pneumothorax

C. To evaluate lung perfusion

D. To visualize the pulmonary vessels

73. List several potential complications that the nurse would observe for in a patient who has had a thoracentesis.

74. Medical management of the individual with breathing difficulty would include teaching ways to improve the quality of breathing. Two methods used for this are:

1.

2.

75. The type of oxygen therapy in which oxygen is administered through a small catheter inserted directly into the trachea through the lower neck is:

A. Tracheostomy

B. Laryngoscopy

C. Transtracheal

D. Pericardial

76. The advantages of the above method over continuous oxygen therapy include:

A. Decreases work of breathing

B. Doesn't interfere with eating

C. Doesn't lead to sore throat

D. All of the above

Fill In

77. A technique which involves applying manual compression and tremor to the chest wall during exhalation is called _____.

78. A technique that uses the effect of gravity to assist in draining secretions from the lung is _____.

79. In caring for the patient with an endotracheal tube, which part of the assessment is a priority?

    A. Assessing heart rate

    B. Assessing for bilateral breath sounds

    C. Assessing for peripheral pulses

    D. Assessing for ascites

80. List four nursing interventions which would prevent any impaired tissue integrity when the patient has an endotracheal tube.

    1.

    2.

    3.

    4.

81. A rationale for the insertion of a tracheostomy tube would be: (star all that apply)

    A. To allow for long-term ventilation

    B. To decrease the respiratory effort

    C. To facilitate removal of secretion

    D. To prevent aspiration of gastric secretions

    E. All of the above

82. The nurse is aware that the presence of cough, sharp chest pain, and tachycardia after insertion of a tracheostomy tube may be an indication of:

    A. Cardiac tamponade

    B. Cardiac arrhythmias

    C. Pneumothorax

    D. Pneumonia

83. Signs of dizziness after a patient has received an intermittent positive pressure breathing treatment are most likely related to:

    A. Hypoxemia

    B. Hypoventilation

    C. Hyperventilation

    D. Hypercapnia

84. The emergency room calls to give the nurse information about an admission. Mrs. Kelly was admitted in respiratory distress. She was intubated and placed on a ventilator. What is one indication for mechanical ventilation?

Define

85. Mrs. Kelly is placed on an MA1 ventilator with an assist control of 10; a tidal volume of 750; and FIO_2 of 45%.

Assist control:

Tidal volume:

Questions

86. The nurse auscultates breath sounds. There is no air moving on the left side. This may mean:

    A. The endotracheal tube needs to be repositioned.

    B. The patient has a pleural effusion.

    C. The ventilator has malfunctioned.

87. An appropriate nursing intervention would be:

88. Because the patient has scattered coarse rales throughout the lung fields, suctioning is indicated. Pre- and postoxygenation is done to:

    A. Prevent complications of hypoxia

    B. Prevent increase in secretions

    C. Stimulate the cough reflex

89. Tracheal suctioning should not be continued more than _____ seconds.

90. Suction is applied when:

    A. The catheter is introduced

B. The catheter is removed

C. The catheter is inserted and removed

91. An important part of the nursing care of a patient on a ventilator should involve developing a method of communication. What are some ways that communication can be established?

92. The physician changes the ventilator mode to intermittent mandatory ventilation (IMV) of 8. The nurse is aware that the main difference between the IMV and assist-control modes is that with IMV:

A. The patient's respiratory effort triggers the machine

B. The volume is delivered at a constant rate

C. The ventilator responds to every patient effort

D. The patient can breathe spontaneously as desired

93. Which of the ventilator modes is used as a weaning mode?

A. Assist-control

B. Assist

C. Intermittent mandatory ventilation

D. Positive end-expiratory pressure (PEEP)

94. While assessing the patient, the nurse notices that she is restless, tachycardiac, and confused. The nurse is aware that this may indicate:

A. Hypoxia

B. Hypercapnia

C. Hypocapnia

D. Hyperventilation

95. When a patient is on PEEP on a ventilator, the nurse is aware that it is important to observe for signs of decreased cardiac output. Signs of this would be:

A. Hypertension, tachycardia

B. Weak pulses, slow capillary refill, low urine output

C. Cyanosis, chest pain

D. Lethargy, diaphoresis, headache

96. One of the priorities in caring for the patient on a ventilator is to ensure effective breathing patterns. Write an appropriate nursing care plan that addresses this need.

Nursing Diagnosis:

Patient Outcome:

Nursing Interventions:

97. Look at the parts of the thoracic drainage system. Label each part.

Drainage tube
Underwater seal chamber

Tube-to-suction device
Suction control chamber
Drainage collection chamber

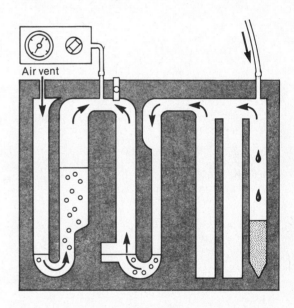

Air vent

Questions

98. The essential parts of an intrapleural drainage system are:

A. Chest tube, collection bottle, suction

B. Chest tube, one-way valve, collection bottle

C. Collection bottles, one-way valve, suction

D. Drainage tube, air vent, collection bottle

99. The main reason that suction is added to an intrapleural drainage system is:

   A. To drain the air faster

   B. To help the patient breathe easier

   C. Because the underwater seal is not effective

   D. Because the patient has had thoracic surgery

100. When checking the patient's intrapleural drainage system with 20 cm of suction, the nurse notices bubbling in the suction control chamber. This most likely indicates:

   A. The system is malfunctioning

   B. The system is set up correctly

   C. There is a large air leak

101. List several measures that would be included as part of the nursing care for a patient with a chest tube.

102. The patient who has had a chest tube inserted following thoracic surgery has a problem with decreased lung expansion. Write a nursing care plan that addresses this problem.

   Nursing Diagnosis:

   Patient Outcome:

   Nursing Interventions:

103. Chest tubes are used to allow for lung re-expansion following thoracic surgery. A chest tube would not be inserted following:

   A. Pneumonectomy

   B. Lobectomy

   C. Open heart surgery

   D. Wedge resection

104. Following thoracic surgery, the nurse is aware that it is important for the patient to cough frequently to bring up secretions. This is done to prevent:

   A. Hemorrhage

   B. Bronchopleural fistula

   C. Empyema

   D. Atelectasis

105. On the second postoperative day, the nurse finds crepitation around the chest tube insertion site. This finding is indicative of:

   A. Hemorrhage into the tissue

   B. Presence of a fistula

   C. Persistent air leak into the tissue

   D. Presence of infection

106. A patient who has a chronic cough and dyspnea on exertion is admitted to the unit. He is scheduled for a mediastinoscopy. What questions that are relevant to his condition should the nurse ask during the health history?

107. Describe this procedure as the nurse would explain it to the patient.

108. Nursing care of the patient having a mediastinoscopy includes prevention of complications. These can include:

   A. Gastrointestinal bleeding

   B. Myocardial infarction

   C. Thrombophlebitis

   D. Cerebral vascular accident

109. Plan the nursing care for the patient who has had a pneumonectomy. Keep in mind the information that the patient needs to ensure recovery.

Nursing Diagnosis:

Patient Outcome:

Nursing Interventions:

CLINICAL SITUATIONS

Situation ■ 1

Mrs. Rosen had a right upper lobectomy to remove a lung mass. She returns to the unit after surgery. She has a chest tube to underwater seal with 20 cm suction; oxygen at 2l/nasal cannula; and an IV to KVO (keep vein open) or 30 ml/hour. During assessment, the nurse notices fluctuation in the tubing with respirations. The surgical dressing is dry and intact. Vital signs are stable. She has no complaints at present.

1. The physician has ordered blood gases to be drawn and wants to be called with the results. The laboratory calls. The values are pH 7.32; P_{CO_2} 48%; P_{O_2} 90%; HCO_3 25; O_2 saturation 92%. The nurse is aware that this patient is in:

   A. Respiratory alkalosis

   B. Respiratory acidosis

   C. Metabolic alkalosis

   D. Metabolic acidosis

2. The physician orders respiratory therapy to start breathing treatments with cool aerosol. Mrs. Rosen asks you why she has to have these treatments. The nurse explains:

   A. You need the treatment to promote ventilation.

   B. You need the treatment because you may have pneumonia.

   C. You need the treatment since you can't ambulate yet.

   D. You need the treatment to remove secretions.

3. Mrs. Rosen wants to know if she will be able to walk to the bathroom while she has the chest tube in place. The nurse replies:

   A. No, it is too dangerous; the bottle could break.

   B. Yes, if we clamp off the chest tube.

   C. Yes, if proper safety measures are taken.

4. It is now 3 days after the operation. There is no longer any fluctuation in the tubing when the patient breathes. What might this indicate?

   A. The system has malfunctioned; you should call the doctor.

   B. The lung has expanded and the tube can be pulled.

   C. The patient is lying on the tubing.

Situation ■ 2

The nurse is assigned to Mr. Bartly, 78 years old, who is in acute respiratory failure. He has had chronic obstructive pulmonary disease for many years. He was admitted, intubated, and placed on a ventilator with settings of IMV, 12; FIO_2, 40%; tidal volume (TV), 700. He is confused and combative. Laboratory results confirm *Pseudomonas* in his sputum. He is placed on antibiotics.

1. Which of the following nursing diagnoses would be the most relevant at this time?

   A. Alteration in nutrition related to lack of food intake.

   B. Ineffective breathing patterns related to inflammatory process.

   C. Self-care deficit related to impaired thought process.

   D. Alteration in tissue perfusion related to disease process.

2. Which of the following statements is NOT true about the type of ventilator support Mr. Bartly is receiving?

   A. The patient can initiate his own respirations.

   B. This setting is often used to wean patients.

   C. The ventilator delivers a TV of 700 each time the patient breathes.

   D. The ventilator has alarms built in to detect malfunction.

3. Which of the following would give you the best indication that you should suction this patient?

   A. It has been 4 hours since you suctioned him.

   B. The alarm on the ventilator goes off.

   C. During auscultation, you hear wheezing.

   D. During auscultation, you hear coarse rales.

4. Mr. Bartly is scheduled to have a bronchoscopy to determine if he is retaining secretions. Nursing responsibilities prior to the procedure would include all of the following EXCEPT:

A. Restricting food or fluid intake for 6 hours

B. Obtaining suction equipment for the room

C. Explaining to the patient that biopsies may be taken

D. Explaining that the procedure is not uncomfortable

5. Mr. Bartly's wife is very concerned that this procedure will be very painful. What does the nurse say to reassure her?

A. This is an easy and painless procedure.

B. This procedure is done under general anesthesia.

C. This is done with a local anesthesia.

6. After the procedure, which assessment finding by the nurse would be indicative of a complication that should be reported immediately to the physician?

A. Hypotension

B. Respiratory stridor

C. Tachycardia

D. Any of the above

Chapter Thirteen

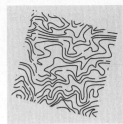

NURSING CARE
of Adults with
Upper Respiratory Disorders

Learning Objectives

1.0 Demonstrate an Understanding of the Infections and Inflammations of the Upper Respiratory Tract.

1.1 Identify the Clinical Manifestations of Several Upper Respiratory Disorders.
1.2 Recognize Types of Medical Treatment Used with Adults Who Have Upper Respiratory Infections.
1.3 Describe the Nursing Care for the Adult Who is Having Sinus Surgery.
1.4 Identify Complications That Can Occur for the Adult with an Upper Respiratory Infection.
1.5 Plan the Nursing Care of the Adult Having a Tonsillectomy.
1.6 Write Nursing Interventions for the Adult with an Upper Respiratory Infection.

2.0 Demonstrate an Understanding of the Obstructive Disorders of the Upper Respiratory Tract.

2.1 Identify Several Obstructive Disorders.
2.2 Identify Treatment Options for the Patient with an Obstructive Disorder.
2.3 Plan Nursing Interventions when Caring for the Adult with an Obstructive Disorder.
2.4 Review the Emergency Treatment of Laryngeal Trauma.

3.0 Demonstrate an Understanding of the Types of Neoplasms That Can Affect the Upper Respiratory Tract.

3.1 Identify the Clinical Manifestations of Laryngeal Cancer.
3.2 Review the Surgical Interventions Used in the Treatment of Laryngeal Cancer.
3.3 Plan the Nursing Care for the Adult with Cancer of the Larynx.

Learning Activities

Matching

A. Laryngitis   E. Tonsillitis
B. Sinusitis   F. Pharyngitis
C. Rhinitis   G. Epistaxis
D. Common cold

1. _____ Infectious process of the upper respiratory tract that can be caused by any of 100 viruses.

2. _____ Caused by an obstruction of the drainage tracts.

3. _____ Caused by a bacterium and often seen secondary to an upper respiratory infection.

4. _____ Inflammation of the throat.

5. _____ An inflammation of the mucous membrane of the nose.

6. _____ Inflammation of the voice box.

7. _____ Bleeding from the nose.

True or False

8. _____ Medical management is required for a cold.

9. _____ Pharyngitis is often caused by a streptococcal organism.

10. _____ Tetracycline is the drug of choice for treating hemolytic streptococcal infections.

11. _____ Warm saline irrigations are used to treat pain associated with a peritonsillar abscess.

12. _____ Another name for allergic rhinitis is hay fever.

13. _____ Abuse of the voice cannot cause laryngitis.

Questions

14. Why would a geriatric patient with a common cold be more likely to have complications than a young adult?

A. Atrophy and weakness of respiratory muscle slows the cough reflex.

B. Hypertrophy of the diaphragm increases susceptibility to infection.

C. Atrophy of the extremities causes immobility and leads to increased risk of infection.

D. Changes in white blood cell production cause elderly patient to acquire infections easily.

15. The nurse would urge the patient with a cold to seek medical advice if he had which of the following symptoms?

A. Low-grade fever for more than 48 hours

B. Cough productive of yellow sputum

C. High fever and greenish sputum production

D. Diaphoresis, weakness, and loss of appetite

16. Symptoms of sinusitis such as fever, chills, and pain over the affected sinuses are a result of:

A. Obstruction of drainage

B. Bacterial infection

C. Surgery

D. Ineffective antibiotic therapy

17. The most appropriate medication to treat the symptoms of sinusitis would be:

A. Tylenol

B. Darvocet

C. Phenylephrine

D. Phenergan

18. Pharyngitis may be caused by beta hemolytic streptococcus. If an adult has this type of infection, the nurse would carefully monitor for complications of which systems?

A. Respiratory and cardiac

B. Cardiac and urinary

C. Gastrointestinal and neurologic

D. Endocrine and respiratory

19. Presence of which of the following symptoms would indicate to the nurse that an adult has

complications secondary to a streptococcal infection?

A. Wheezing with breathing

B. Hyperactive bowel sounds

C. Diminished sensation in the lower extremities

D. Systolic heart murmur

20. Choose the most appropriate nursing diagnosis for the patient with acute pharyngitis.

A. Decreased cardiac output

B. High risk for fluid volume deficit

C. Altered tissue perfusion

D. Impaired gas exchange

21. Why would a vasoconstriction drug such as phenylephrine be used for the individual with sinusitis?

A. To prevent postural hypotension

B. To maintain adequate cardiac output

C. To promote drainage of the sinuses

D. To prevent spread of the infection to the brain

22. Symptoms such as persistent headache, chronic cough, and purulent nasal drainage are indicative of which of the following conditions?

A. Meningitis

B. Bacterial endocarditis

C. Emphysema

D. Chronic sinusitis

23. Presence of persistent postnasal discharge following chronic sinusitis can predispose the patient to:

A. Bronchiectasis

B. Pneumonia

C. Sepsis

D. Meningitis

24. In caring for a patient with tonsillitis, which of the following goals would be primary?

A. Patient sleeps 12 hours per day.

B. Patient has adequate urinary output.

C. Patient has understanding of antibiotic therapy.

D. Patient avoids irritating foods.

25. For the patient with tonsillitis, presence of unilateral pain radiating to the ear with swallowing may indicate:

A. Mastoiditis

B. Peritonsillar abscess

C. Esophagitis

D. Laryngitis

26. A major complication of a tonsillectomy in the immediate postoperative period would be:

A. Hemorrhage

B. Shock

C. Sepsis

D. Infection

27. Based on your knowledge of the importance of careful assessment of the patient who has had a tonsillectomy, which laboratory values would the nurse be certain to assess?

A. CBC, platelets, clotting time

B. CBC, WBC, BUN and creatinine

C. CPK, SGOT, LDH, electrolytes

D. Electrolytes, PT, PTT

28. Write two nursing diagnoses that would be appropriate when caring for an adult who has had a tonsillectomy.

1.

2.

29. Which of the following would be an appropriate nursing intervention to help alleviate pain following tonsillectomy?

A. Analgesics as ordered

B. Warm saline gargles

C. Ice collar as ordered

D. All of the above

30. A common condition caused by the overuse of nose drops is known as:

A. Vasomotor rhinitis

B. Rhinitis medicamentosa

C. Medicatisus allergitis

D. Nasal pharyngitis

31. Which of the following diseases has been associated with episodes of epistaxis?

    A. Laryngitis

    B. Hypertension

    C. Pneumonitis

    D. Hyperglycemia

32. The first intervention for an episode of epistaxis that the nurse would implement would be:

    A. Administer an anticoagulant

    B. Apply iced compresses

    C. Apply pressure to the nares for 10 minutes

    D. Insert nasal packing

Fill In

33. Benign tumors in the nasal mucosa that are freely moveable are known as _____

34. An operative procedure that straightens and reduces the nasal septum is known as a _____ .

35. An operative procedure that involves surgical reconstruction of the nose is known as a _____ .

Questions

36. A patient is admitted to the emergency room after a motorcycle accident. His neck is swollen and bruised. Hoarseness and respiratory stridor are present. What is a probable cause of these symptoms?

    A. Laryngeal trauma

    B. Fracture of the neck

    C. Pneumothorax

    D. Esophageal trauma

37. Because of the possible complications of this condition, what equipment would the nurse have available?

    A. Endotracheal tube

    B. Tracheostomy set

    C. Chest tube

    D. Nasogastric tube

38. List two risk factors that have been associated with laryngeal cancer.

    1.

    2.

39. Which of the following would be a late symptom of laryngeal cancer?

    A. Dyspnea

    B. Dysphagia

    C. Weight loss

    D. All of the above

True or False

40. _____ Speech is possible following a partial laryngectomy.

41. _____ Danger of aspiration is a big risk following a total laryngectomy.

42. _____ All patients will learn esophageal speech after a total neck resection.

43. _____ Morphine is the drug of choice for postoperative pain following a laryngectomy.

Questions

44. As the nurse caring for the patient who has had a total laryngectomy, the diagnosis you choose is: Ineffective airway clearance related to altered airway.
    Write an appropriate patient outcome and three nursing interventions.

    Patient Outcome:

    Nursing Interventions:

CLINICAL SITUATIONS

Situation ■ 1

Mr. Archer has had sinusitis for several years. He often wakes with headaches and suffers from nasal discharge and chronic fatigue. He is admitted for possible surgery.

1. Although sinusitis may be attributed to a specific organism, other factors may be indicated. These would include:

   A. Irritating gases

   B. Tobacco smoke

   C. Irritating dusts

   D. All of the above

2. Which of the following symptoms if exhibited by this patient would indicate to the nurse a possible side effect of his medication (Neo-Synephrine)?

   A. Tachycardia, hypertension, shortness of breath

   B. Anxiety, tremors, chest pain

   C. Lethargy, confusion

   D. Urinary or bowel incontinence

3. Mr. Archer has surgery to remove the diseased mucous membrane. Following surgery, which of the following would be an appropriate intervention in view of the fact that nasal packing is in place?

   A. Potential alteration in the oral mucous membrane

   B. Potential for sensory perceptual deficit

   C. Knowledge deficit related to outcome of surgery

   D. Alteration in body image

4. Nasal packing after this type of surgery would be removed in:

   A. 6–8 hours

   B. 12 hours

   C. 24 hours

   D. 48 hours

5. Which of the following instructions would the nurse give to the patient following the removal of the nasal packing?

   A. Do not blow your nose

   B. Avoid any activity for 2 days

   C. Do not drink hot beverages

   D. Do not engage in sexual activity

Situation ■ 2

Mr. Kelson has been diagnosed with laryngeal cancer and has just returned to the unit following a total laryngectomy.

1. As a nurse, you are aware that the patient will undergo many changes following the surgery. Which of the following would not occur?

   A. Loss of normal speech

   B. Loss of normal respiratory patterns

   C. Loss of normal eating habits

   D. Loss of normal olfactory sensations

2. Which of the following health care professionals should be consulted since they have a critical role in the recovery of Mr. Kelson?

   A. Occupational therapist

   B. Speech therapist

   C. Pharmacist

   D. Dietitian

3. The nurse will need to do health teaching for Mr. Kelson so that he can care for himself after discharge. Which of the following would not be important to teach him?

   A. How to suction the tracheostomy

   B. How to perform tracheostomy care

   C. How to care for his feeding tube

   D. How to contact a support group

Situation ■ 3

Ms. Oldman has had recurrent episodes of tonsillitis and is being evaluated by her physician for the most appropriate treatment.

1. During the physical exam, which of the following symptoms would most likely be present?

   A. Tonsils red and swollen with white patches

   B. Tonsils whitish or gray with reddish lesions

   C. Throat red and the cervical lymph nodes swollen

   D. Tongue and gums red with white patches

2. The office nurse would pick which of the following

nursing diagnoses as having the highest priority with this patient?

A. Pain related to inflammation of the tonsils.

B. High risk for fluid volume deficit related to inability to swallow.

C. Knowledge deficit related to treatment of tonsillitis

D. Ineffective family coping

3. When Ms. Oldman is seen 1 week later for a recheck, she is complaining of sore throat with pain radiating to her ear. On examination, there is swelling of the soft palate. A possible explanation is:

A. The antibiotics were not effective

B. She has pharyngitis

C. She has a peritonsillar abscess

D. She has become reinfected

4. Because of her recurrent infections, the physician decides to perform a tonsillectomy. The nurse is aware that a major complication is:

A. Infection

B. Bleeding

C. Aspiration

D. Septicemia

5. In the immediate postoperative period, which of the following nursing diagnoses would have the highest priority?

A. Pain related to the surgical procedure.

B. High risk for fluid volume deficit.

C. High risk for aspiration

D. Anxiety related to the procedure

Chapter Fourteen

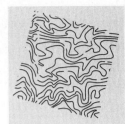

NURSING CARE
of Adults with
Lower Respiratory Disorders

Learning Objectives

1.0 Demonstrate an Understanding of the Infections and Inflammations of the Lower Respiratory Tract.

1.1 Define Several Respiratory Tract Infections.
1.2 Review the Etiology and Clinical Manifestations of Several Infectious Disorders.
1.3 Identify the Nursing Interventions for the Adult with an Infectious Process.
1.4 Identify the Medical Management of Several Types of Infectious Processes.
1.5 Plan the Nursing Care for an Adult with an Inflammatory Disorder.

2.0 Demonstrate an Understanding of Obstructive Disorders of the Lower Respiratory Tract.

2.1 Define Several Obstructive Disorders.
2.2 Review the Etiology of Several Obstructive Disorders.
2.3 Identify the Medical Management of Adults with Obstructive Disorders.
2.4 Plan the Nursing Care for Adults with Obstructive Disorders.

3.0 Demonstrate an Understanding of Disorders of the Pulmonary Circulation.

3.1 Identify the Pathophysiology of Pulmonary Embolism.
3.2 Review the Clinical Manifestation of Disorders of the Pulmonary Circulation.
3.3 Describe the Medical Management for an Adult with a Pulmonary Embolism.
3.4 Plan the Nursing Care for an Adult with Disorders of the Pulmonary Circulation.

4.0 Demonstrate an Understanding of Traumatic Injuries to the Lower Respiratory Tract.

4.1 Identify the Clinical Manifestation of the Adult with a Chest Injury.
4.2 Describe the Medical Management of Chest Injuries.
4.3 Pick Appropriate Nursing Interventions for the Adult With Chest Trauma.

5.0 Demonstrate an Understanding of the Types of Neoplasms Which Can Affect the Lower Respiratory Tract.

5.1 Identify Clinical Manifestations of Lung Cancer.
5.2 Identify the Medical Management of Lung Cancer.
5.3 Assess the Needs of the Adult with Lung Cancer.
5.4 Plan the Nursing Interventions for the Adult with Lung Cancer.

Learning Activities

Define

1. Bronchitis:

2. Pneumonia:

3. Empyema:

4. Pleurisy:

5. Emphysema:

Questions

6. Assessment of the patient with a respiratory infection would include which of the following? Check all that apply.

    A. Monitor vital signs

    B. Check results of arterial blood gases

    C. Check for Homans' sign

    D. Assess for presence of cough

    E. Assess breathing patterns

    F. Check results of chest x-ray

    G. Check for cyanosis

    H. Assess mucous membranes

7. A patient is being discharged after therapy for acute bronchitis and pneumonia. Which patient behavior would alert the nurse to the need for further education?

    A. Patient asks for prescriptions

    B. Patient asks how long before he can smoke again

    C. Patient asks for instruction in diet

    D. Patient asks if there are any activity limits

8. Paroxysmal attacks of coughing and wheezing in acute bronchitis may be precipitated by:

    A. Exposure to irritants

    B. Exposure to heat

    C. Exposure to cold

    D. A & C

    E. A,B,C

9. Assessment data of the individual with pneumonia would most likely produce the following findings:

    A. Fever, chills, productive cough

    B. Purulent sputum, signs of shock

    C. Diminished breath sounds, wheezes

    D. Absent breath sounds over the involved area

10. Common causes of pneumonia are known to include:

    A. Viruses

    B. Bacteria

    C. Aspiration

    D. All of the above

11. Which statement best describes the physiologic changes associated with pneumonia?

    A. They result from specific injury to the cells in the alveoli.

    B. They result in permanent destruction of lung tissue.

    C. They result from reduced functioning of lung volume and alteration of ventilation and blood flow.

    D. They result from aspiration of chemical irritants.

12. Nonbacterial atypical pneumonia is commonly caused by:

    A. *Staphylococcus aureus*

    B. *Haemophilus influenzae*

    C. *Mycoplasma pneumoniae*

    D. *Legionella pneumophila*

13. List four of the most important nursing interventions necessary when caring for the adult with pneumonia.

    1.

    2.

    3.

    4.

14. The choice of the proper antibiotic for the adult with a lower respiratory disorder is best determined by:

    A. Physician's orders

    B. Patient allergies

    C. Results of blood culture

    D. All of the above

15. Which individual would have the highest risk for developing influenza?

    A. Sixteen-year-old teenager

    B. Fifty-year-old male executive

    C. Seventy-year-old female with cardiac disease

    D. Sixty-five-year-old male recently retired

16. A 75-year-old lethargic patient has a fever, chills, and productive cough. The nurse suspects _____ pneumonia.

    A. Viral

    B. Aspiration

    C. Bacterial

    D. Fungal

17. A patient has developed a lung abscess and is admitted for evaluation and treatment. The nurse would expect to see which of the following medical therapies?

    A. Oral analgesics and antibiotics

    B. Surgical intervention

    C. Intravenous antibiotic, postural drainage

    D. All of the above

18. The nurse is caring for a patient with empyema. The laboratory results reveal that the pH of the exudate is 7.16. The nurse would be ready to:

    A. Assist with chest tube insertion

    B. Start oxygen therapy

    C. Discharge the patient

    D. Start IV antibiotics

19. Empyema is often a recurrent condition. Upon the patient's discharge, the nurse instructs the patient and family the signs and symptoms that should be reported. These would include:

    A. Cough, expectorating whitish sputum

    B. Shortness of breath, painful breathing

    C. Weight gain, increased appetite

    D. Lack of energy, increased thirst

20. Plan the nursing care for the adult with pneumonia and list four nursing interventions.

    Nursing Diagnosis: Impaired gas exchange related to inflammation and production of exudate.

    Patient Outcome:

    Nursing Interventions:

21. An elderly debilitated patient is receiving tube feeding through a nasogastric tube. List three nursing measures which the nurse would implement in order to prevent aspiration pneumonia.

    1.

    2.

    3.

22. A patient is admitted with fever, right-sided chest pain, dyspnea, and anorexia. He has a recent history of bacterial pneumonia. His symptoms suggest:

    A. Empyema

    B. Tuberculosis

    C. Septicemia

    D. Emphysema

23. What is the best method for obtaining a culture and sensitivity of the pleural exudate?

    A. Blood culture

    B. Skin culture

    C. Thoracentesis

    D. Bronchoscopy

24. In caring for a patient with influenza, it is important to be aware of the route it is transmitted, which is:

    A. Direct contact

    B. Aerosol

    C. Body secretions

    D. Indirect contact

25. To prevent a complication of influenza, the nurse would carefully assess for symptoms of which of the following? Check all that apply.

    A. Pneumonia

    B. Renal disease

    C. Cardiac disease

    D. Encephalitis

26. Annual influenza vaccination is recommended for which population group? Check all that apply.

    A. Anyone over the age of 50

    B. Anyone over the age of 65

    C. Anyone with a chronic illness

    D. Anyone who has already had influenza

27. The clinic nurse is doing health education at a senior citizen's group. Ways to prevent contracting influenza are explained. The nurse realizes that teaching is effective when a participant says:

    A. I never realized that I needed to stay in all winter.

    B. I shouldn't go to the mall during a flu epidemic.

    C. I never realized everyone harbors this virus.

    D. I guess getting the flu is a risk I'll have to take.

28. Individuals in which environment would be most susceptible to developing tuberculosis?

    A. Crowded, inner city, lower socioeconomic area

    B. Rural areas with septic system and well

    C. Inner city, living in apartments

    D. Suburbs with crowded school system

Fill In

29. The causative agent of tuberculosis is

    _____ .

True or False

30. _____ Tuberculosis (TB) is controllable by chemotherapy.

31. _____ TB requires close prolonged contact for transmission.

32. _____ Symptoms of TB occur within 2 weeks of exposure.

33. _____ TB always results in granulomatous consolidation of lung areas.

34. _____ Presumptive diagnosis for TB is based on a skin test.

Questions

35. The main treatment of tuberculosis is chemotherapy. The most effective drug is considered to be:

    A. Streptomycin

    B. Rifampin

    C. Isoniazid

    D. Penicillin

36. For the patient who is receiving drug therapy for tuberculosis, the nurse would provide the following information:

    A. You will take this medication until the symptoms subside.

    B. You may take as many as four different medications for 2 months.

    C. You may have intermittent drug therapy for a total of 6 months.

    D. You may take a combination of medication for a period of 9 months to as long as 2 years.

37. Knowing the therapeutic regimen required for the treatment of tuberculosis, what is an appropriate nursing diagnosis?

    A. Potential alteration in mobility

    B. Potential noncompliance

    C. Potential fluid volume overload

    D. Potential alteration in elimination

38. Write a nursing care plan for the patient with active pulmonary tuberculosis.

    Nursing Diagnosis: High risk for infection related to lack of understanding of the method of the spread of disease

    Patient Outcome:

    Nursing Interventions:

39. A patient is admitted with a respiratory disorder. During auscultation of breath sounds, the nurse hears an audible friction rub. This is most indicative of:

    A. Pneumonia

    B. Lung abscess

    C. Influenza

    D. Pleurisy

40. When a patient has chronic obstructive pulmonary disease (COPD), the highest nursing priority should be to prevent:

    A. Hypoxia

    B. Infection

    C. Sepsis

    D. Altered nutrition

41. Pick the statement that best explains the immediate effect of COPD in a patient.

    A. Expiration is restricted, causing hypoxia.

    B. Alveoli are insufficiently ventilated and cannot provide the normal oxygen to surrounding blood.

    C. Airway obstruction leads to hypoxia and hypocapnia.

    D. Elastic recoil of the alveoli is hampered by excessive secretions.

42. Why is the expiratory phase longer than the inspiratory phase in the individual with COPD?

    A. There is loss of lung recoil, and it is harder to get trapped air out.

    B. The drive to breathe has been lost.

    C. The muscles of the diaphragm are beginning to hypertrophy.

    D. The passive process of inspiration and expiration is impaired because of loss of elasticity.

43. The nurse is aware that prolonged hypoxemia causes the body to produce more red blood cells. This condition is known as:

    A. Anemia

    B. Leukopenia

    C. Polycythemia

    D. Hypercapnia

44. Which of following factors has been implicated in the development of chronic bronchitis?

    A. Smoking

    B. Air pollution

    C. Dust

    D. Toxic fumes

    E. All of the above

45. The continual inflammation associated with chronic bronchitis makes the patient susceptible to:

    A. Dehydration

    B. Infection

    C. Cyanosis

    D. Hypocapnia

46. Which of the following best describes the pathophysiology involved in pulmonary emphysema?

    A. Alveoli are insufficiently ventilated because of obstruction.

    B. Prolonged exposure to irritants results in excessive mucus production.

    C. Inflammation of large and small airways leads to infection and scarring.

    D. Alveoli lose elasticity, lungs become stiff, and compliance decreases with loss of lung recoil.

47. What mechanism in the individual with emphysema results in the barrel-chest appearance?

    A. Chronic hypoxia

    B. Pulmonary hypertension

    C. Cor pulmonale

    D. Loss of lung recoil

48. During the assessment of the patient with emphysema, typical symptoms that are often present include:

    A. Dyspnea, pursed lip breathing, barrel chest, diminished breath sounds

    B. Cyanosis, labored breathing, hyperresonance

    C. Weight gain, edema, rhonchi and wheezing throughout

    D. Anorexia, weight loss, pallor

49. In emphysema, high levels of carbon dioxide can result in which of the following symptoms?

    A. Anorexia, weakness, lethargy

    B. Headache, lack of ability to concentrate

    C. Dyspnea, cyanosis

    D. Pursed lip breathing, dyspnea

50. Medical management of the individual with emphysema is designed to:

    A. Cause remission of the disease

    B. Control symptoms and prevent further deterioration

    C. Prevent development of pneumothorax

    D. Return the normal respiratory function

51. For the patient with emphysema and chronic bronchitis, there is a risk of developing:

    A. Pulmonary hypertension and cor pulmonale

    B. Pneumonia and renal failure

    C. Pleurisy and peripheral vascular disease

    D. Pulmonary embolus and hypoxia

52. The nurse would check which of the following diagnostic tests to determine the severity of the patient's obstructive disease?

    A. Lung function studies

    B. Arterial blood gases

    C. Ventilation and perfusion scan

    D. Chest x-ray

53. Along with influenza, this is the leading infectious cause of death among the elderly:

    A. Bronchitis

    B. Emphysema

    C. Lung cancer

    D. Pneumonia

54. A patient with COPD who is experiencing dyspnea may be taught which of the following to assist in controlling the dyspnea? Check all that apply.

    A. How to control the inspiratory to expiratory (I:E) ratio to prolong expiration

    B. How to control the I:E ratio to prolong inspiration

    C. How to do diaphragmatic breathing

    D. How to do pursed lip breathing

55. Medical management of the patient with an obstructive lung disorder would be designed to prevent further deterioration of the condition. The nurse would expect the patient to be taking:

    A. Antibiotics

    B. Antihypertensives

    C. Bronchodilators

    D. Beta blockers

True or False

56. _____ A patient with COPD can do aerobic exercise to train skeletal muscles.

57. _____ Patients with COPD should get as much rest as possible.

58. _____ Antibiotics are often given at the first sign of any cold symptoms.

59. _____ To aid in weight gain, patient should drink milk and eat ice cream.

60. _____ Sustained hypoxemia can result in pulmonary hypertension.

61. _____ Cyanosis is the cardinal symptom of pulmonary hypertension.

Questions

62. Write a nursing care plan for the patient with COPD. Use the following nursing diagnoses:

   1. Ineffective airway clearance related to excessive secretions

      Patient Outcome:

      Nursing Interventions:

   2. Ineffective breathing pattern related to increased work or breathing and need for oxygen

      Patient Outcome:

      Nursing Interventions:

Define

63. Bronchiectasis:

64. Atelectasis:

65. Pulmonary embolism:

66. Pneumothorax:

67. Hemothorax:

68. Subcutaneous emphysema:

69. Silicosis

70. Coal-miner's pneumoconiosis:

Questions

71. Which of the following individuals would be at the greatest risk for development of a pulmonary embolus?

   A. Male, 20 years old, admitted with pneumonia

   B. Female, 28 years old, admitted with asthma

   C. Female, 80 years old, with COPD, pneumonia, and stroke

   D. Male, 72 years old, in for a workup for possible lung cancer

72. The nurse should consider which intervention of primary importance in preventing the development of a pulmonary embolus?

   A. Bed rest with limited activity

   B. Early ambulation and leg exercises

   C. Administering antibiotics on time

   D. Administering oxygen therapy as ordered

73. Medical treatment for pulmonary embolus involves using heparin therapy. Which of the following is a desired effect of this treatment?

   A. PT level is 12 seconds

   B. PTT is 25–25 seconds

   C. PTT is 60–80 seconds

   D. Pulmonary function tests are normal

74. Which of the following is an adverse effect of thrombolytic therapy?

   A. Chest pain

   B. Cyanosis

   C. Hemoptysis

   D. Tachycardia

75. One of the main causes of pulmonary hypertension is:

   A. Pulmonary edema

   B. Cardiac arrhythmias

   C. Surgery

   D. Pulmonary embolism

76. A condition that may develop following the fracture of several ribs is known as flail chest. Symptoms which are present result from:

   A. Diminished movement of air

   B. Pulmonary hypertension

   C. Pain caused by the injury

   D. Hypoxia

77. Medical management for the patient with a flail chest following a serious traumatic injury might involve which of the following?

   A. Endotracheal intubation

   B. Surgical intervention

   C. Mechanical ventilation

   D. Any or all of the above

78. Problems which can occur as a result of chest trauma include which of the following? Check all that apply.

   A. Pulmonary congestion

   B. Atelectasis

   C. Lung abscess

   D. Pneumothorax

   E. Paralytic ileus

79. An open pneumothorax is often the result of which of the following? Check all that apply.

   A. Thoracentesis

   B. Stab wound

   C. Paracentesis

   D. Insertion of a Swan-Ganz catheter

   E. Insertion of a Dobbhoff tube

80. Medical management for the patient with a pneumothorax involves the insertion of a _____ to reestablish the _____ pressure.

Questions

81. You are caring for a patient with a spontaneous pneumothorax. Your primary nursing diagnosis is: Impaired gas exchange. Write a nursing care plan for this patient.

   Patient Outcome:

   Nursing Interventions:

82. Which type of bronchogenic carcinoma is the most common?

   A. Epidermoid (squamous cell) carcinoma

   B. Small-cell carcinoma

   C. Adenocarcinoma

   D. Large-cell carcinoma

83. The medical diagnosis of bronchogenic carcinoma is confirmed by which of the following?

   A. Chest x-ray and history

   B. Sputum cytology and bronchoscopy

   C. Chest x-ray and pulmonary function tests

   D. Open chest biopsy

84. Treatment for lung cancer involves which of the following forms of treatment?

   A. Chemotherapy

   B. Radiation therapy

   C. Surgical excision

   D. Any or all of the above

85. A finding of neck edema in the patient with adenocarcinoma suggests which of the following?

   A. Metastasis to the pleural space

   B. Metastasis to the brain

   C. Metastasis to the mediastinum

True or False

86. _____ Radiation is used as a definitive treatment for localized lesions.

87. _____ Metastasis occurs in 90% of the patients with lung cancer.

88. _____ Immunotherapy has been found to effect a cure in a large number of patients.

89. _____ Surgery is done when the tumor has metastasized.

Questions

90. A patient is admitted with a diagnosis of squamous cell cancer with possible metastasis.

    Nursing Diagnosis: Anxiety related to the diagnosis, treatment, and potential for recovery

    Write a nursing care plan for this patient.

    Patient Outcome:

    Nursing Interventions:

CLINICAL SITUATIONS

Situation ▪ 1

Mr. Stewart has had COPD for 20 years and has been hospitalized many times. Currently he is admitted with pneumonia. He shows signs of acute respiratory distress: dyspnea, cyanosis, and labored breathing. Orders include: O_2 at 2 L; cefoxitin 1 g every 6 hours; aminophylline drip, Solu-Cortef 100 mg every 6 hours.

1. On admission, a theophylline level is taken. The level is 5.5 mEq/ml. What is an appropriate nursing action?

    A. Stop the aminophylline drip and call the physician

    B. Do nothing; this is a therapeutic range.

    C. Call the physician; the aminophylline needs to be increased

2. The purpose of the aminophylline is to:

    A. Treat bronchospasm

    B. Treat the infection

    C. Prevent further complications

3. In assessing Mr. Stewart, which clinical manifestation would indicate a possible side effect of this therapy?

    A. Bradycardia

    B. Tachycardia

    C. Tachypnea

    D. Polycythemia

4. Mr. Stewart is coughing up sputum which is green in color. What organism is probably the cause of this?

    A. *Pseudomonas*

    B. *Klebsiella*

    C. *Candida*

    D. *Staphyloccus*

5. Mr. Stewart says, "I can't breathe, please turn up the oxygen." What is an appropriate action?

    A. Turn the oxygen up to 6 L

    B. Explain that too much oxygen will decrease his stimulus to breathe

    C. Call the physician, as Mr. Stewart needs a ventilator

    D. Check the results of the blood gases

6. An important nursing intervention with Mr. Stewart would be:

    A. Teach him to perform breathing exercises correctly

    B. Explain to him the reason to stay in bed: to increase his strength

    C. Restrict fluids to avoid complications

    D. Explain how to avoid irritation of the lungs

7. The rationale for teaching Mr. Stewart how to do diaphragmatic breathing is:

    A. To prolong the inspiratory phase of breathing

    B. To help conserve oxygen

    C. To help reduce expiration and exhale carbon dioxide

    D. To help control breathing and prolong expiration

Situation ▪ 2

Jim Baker was involved in a car accident 2 days ago. He suffered a concussion and fractured four ribs, which resulted in a flail chest. He was placed on mechanical ventilation, and two chest tubes were inserted.

1. What is the rationale for placing this patient on mechanical ventilation?

   A. To stabilize ventilation internally

   B. To prevent the patient from aspirating

   C. To prevent a hemothorax

2. The rationale for the placement of the chest tubes is:

   A. To prevent infection

   B. To remove air and fluid from the chest

   C. To administer oxygen

   D. All of the above

3. Which of the following medications might be ordered to keep the patient from bucking the ventilator?

   A. Morphine sulfate

   B. Demerol

   C. Pavulon

   D. Valium

4. The morning assessment of this patient reveals dyspnea, cough, fever, and chest discomfort. The nurse would suspect:

   A. Pneumothorax

   B. Atelectasis

   C. Pulmonary edema

   D. Pulmonary embolus

5. Jim is receiving heparin 5000 units subcutaneously every 12 hours. The nurse is aware that the reason for this is:

   A. To prevent embolus formation

   B. To prevent a stroke

   C. To increase clotting of the blood

   D. To help prevent pneumonia

Situation ■ 3

Mrs. Parsons is 65 years old. On a routine chest x-ray, a spot was noted on her lung. She is admitted for a bronchoscopy and biopsy. She has smoked for 45 years. She is found to have squamous cell carcinoma and is scheduled for a right pneumonectomy.

1. The nurse should include which of the following in the preoperative instructions? Star all that apply.

   A. A chest tube will be inserted during surgery

   B. An IV solution will be maintained

   C. A nasogastric tube will be inserted

   D. An order for pain will be left

2. Which of the following would the nurse demonstrate to the patient prior to surgery?

   A. Proper way to cough and deep breathe

   B. How to splint the incision

   C. How to use the call light

   D. All of the above

3. Which of the following symptoms are commonly seen following a pneumonectomy?

   A. Hypervolemia

   B. Bradycardia

   C. Cardiac arrhythmias

   D. Nausea

4. Mrs. Parsons asks you if her smoking had anything to do with her lung cancer. What do you reply?

   A. You'll have to speak with the doctor.

   B. Yes, smoking has been linked with this type of cancer.

   C. Definitely; didn't the doctor tell you not to smoke?

   D. No; you were just unlucky.

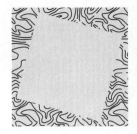

Unit Five

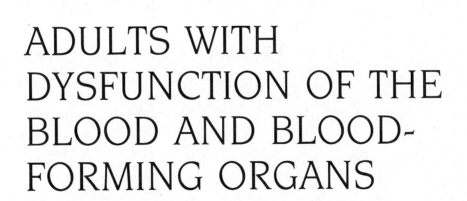

ADULTS WITH DYSFUNCTION OF THE BLOOD AND BLOOD-FORMING ORGANS

Chapter Fifteen

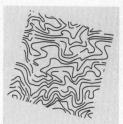

KNOWLEDGE BASIC TO THE NURSING CARE
of Adults with Dysfunction of the Blood and Blood-Forming Organs

Learning Objectives

1.0 Review the Anatomy and Physiology of the Hematologic System.

1.1 List the Components of the Hematologic System.
1.2 List the Functions of the Hematologic System.

2.0 Demonstrate an Understanding of Assessment Data Related to the Hematologic System.

2.1 Identify Clinical Manifestations of Disorders of the Blood and Blood-Forming Organs.
2.2 Review the Health History of an Adult with a Hematologic Disorder.
2.3 List Normal Laboratory Findings.
2.4 Identify Tests Used to Diagnose Hematologic Disorders.

3.0 Demonstrate an Understanding of Interventions Used to Treat Adults with a Hematologic Disorder.

3.1 Demonstrate an Understanding of Types of Nonsurgical Treatment of Hematologic Disorders.
3.2 Demonstrate an Understanding of the Use of Blood Transfusions in the Treatment of Hematologic Disorders.
3.3 Plan the Nursing Care for an Adult with a Disorder of the Hematologic System.

Learning Activities

Questions

1. List three of the main functions of blood.

   1.

   2.

   3.

2. List the five components of the hematologic system.

   1.

   2.

   3.

   4.

   5.

Matching

A. Red blood cells   D. Lymph nodes
B. White blood cells   E. Bone marrow
C. Platelets   F. Spleen

3. _____ Serve as filters

4. _____ Protect the body against microorganisms

5. _____ One of the larger organs of the body

6. _____ Carry oxygen to the cells

7. _____ Removes old or injured red blood cells and platelets

8. _____ Important in the blood-clotting process

9. _____ Composed of granulocytes and mononuclear cells

Questions

10. When a patient with a blood disorder exhibits symptoms of fatigue, weakness, and pallor, it often is due to:

    A. Decrease in erythrocytes

    B. Decrease in leukocytes

    C. Decrease in platelets

    D. All of the above

11. When a patient has a decrease in the platelet count, the nurse would assess for:

    A. Fatigue, weakness, pallor

    B. Temperature, infection

    C. Bruising, ecchymoses, petechiae

    D. All of the above

Fill In

Fill in the normal laboratory results for the following blood tests.

12. WBC _____ cu mm

13. RBC _____ million/cu mm (male)
    _____ million/cu mm (female)

14. Hematocrit _____ % (male)
    _____ % (female)

15. Hemoglobin _____ g/100 ml (male)
    _____ g/100 ml (female)

16. Platelet count _____ cu/mm

17. Prothrombin time _____ seconds

18. PTT _____ seconds

19. Serum iron _____ μg/dl (males)
    _____ μg/dl (females)

Matching

A. Leukocytosis   D. Leukopenia
B. Anemia   E. Thrombocytopenia
C. Polycythemia

20. _____ Low white blood cell count

21. _____ Increase in red blood cells

22. _____ Decrease in platelets

23. _____ Often seen with infections

24. _____ May occur with decreased cardiac output

25. _____ Occurs with aplastic anemia

26. _____ Can lead to shortness of breath

27. _____ May be seen with bone marrow failure

Questions

28. Symptoms of joint pain and deformities are often associated with:

    A. Leukemia

    B. Hemophilia

    C. Anemia

    D. Leukopenia

29. When a patient who has leukemia has symptoms of cough, dyspnea, and fever, the nurse would suspect:

    A. Respiratory infection

    B. Bleeding disorder

    C. Anemia

    D. Sepsis

30. Hemolysis of red blood cells in a patient with a hematologic disorder may lead to:

    A. Infection

    B. Bleeding tendency

    C. Nutritional deficit

    D. Jaundice and pruritus

31. A surgical patient who has developed a venous thrombosis has an increased risk of developing:

    A. Anemia

    B. Decrease in platelet aggregation

    C. Increase in platelet aggregation

    D. Increase in prothrombin time

32. A patient who has a decrease in intake and absorption of vitamin K has a risk of developing:

    A. Increase in prothrombin time

    B. Decrease in prothrombin time

C. Decrease in platelet aggregation

D. Decrease in bleeding time

33. A patient is receiving heparin therapy. The nurse would realize that the heparin is therapeutic if the PTT is:

    A. 35–45 seconds

    B. 45–55 seconds

    C. 55–70 seconds

    D. 60–90 seconds

34. A patient is admitted with a diagnosis of multiple myeloma. Which laboratory test would the nurse expect to be extremely elevated?

    A. WBC

    B. ESR

    C. RBC

    D. Platelet

35. A patient has an elevated reticulocyte count. The nurse interprets this as meaning:

    A. Increased rate of WBC production but low leukocyte count

    B. Increased rate of erythrocyte production with premature destruction of mature RBCs

    C. Decreased production of platelets and increased destruction of mature RBCs.

    D. Increase in production of WBCs, RBCs, and platelets

36. A patient is admitted with a diagnosis of possible leukemia. The test which would provide the best diagnostic information about this condition is:

    A. Shilling test

    B. Ultrasonography

    C. Complete blood count

    D. Bone marrow aspiration

37. The best explanation of a CT scan would be:

    A. A noninvasive procedure to visualize soft tissue structures

    B. A three-dimensional view of body tissue

    C. A radiation test which visualizes organs

    D. An invasive test in which tissue samples are taken

38. When a patient with anemia has a hemoglobin of 7.6 and slight fatigue, which therapy would the nurse expect to be ordered?

    A. Oxygen therapy

    B. Blood transfusions

    C. IV therapy

    D. Vitamin therapy

39. The type of transfusion which would be most appropriate for the patient who is hemorrhaging is:

    A. Whole blood

    B. Packed red cells

    C. Frozen red cells

    D. Platelets

40. To stop the bleeding in a patient with hemophilia, the type of transfusion which would be appropriate is:

    A. Whole blood

    B. Packed red cells

    C. Platelets

    D. Plasma

41. When a patient is very dehydrated, which of the following laboratory findings would be present?

    A. Rise in white count

    B. Rise in hematocrit

    C. Rise in BUN

    D. Rise in platelets

42. To help determine what type of anemia a patient has, the _____ would give the best information.

    A. Hemoglobin and hematocrit

    B. Red blood cell indices

    C. Platelet count

    D. Prothrombin test

Define

Define the following types of blood reactions.

43. Hemolytic reaction:

44. Non-hemolytic reaction:

45. Allergic reaction:

46. Anaphylactic reaction:

47. Septic reaction:

True or False

48. _____ Blood should be administered within 1 hour of receipt on the unit.

49. _____ The blood tubing should be primed with a dextrose solution.

50. _____ All blood should be administered on a pump.

51. _____ Blood should be warmed when given for massive blood loss.

52. _____ Tachycardia and dyspnea are signs of a transfusion reaction.

53. _____ A delayed transfusion reaction can occur days or weeks after the transfusion.

Questions

54. An appropriate nursing diagnosis for the patient with symptoms of fatigue, dyspnea, and weakness is: Activity intolerance.

    Write the nursing care plan.

    Patient Outcome:

    Nursing Interventions:

55. An appropriate nursing diagnosis for the patient with a bleeding disorder is: Alteration in tissue perfusion.

Write the nursing care plan.

Patient Outcome:

Nursing Interventions:

CLINICAL SITUATIONS

Situation ■ 1

A patient is admitted to the hospital with the following symptoms: fatigue, weakness, pallor, bruising, and swelling in the knees.

1. Which of the following laboratory studies would the nurse expect to be abnormal?

   A. WBC, RBC, platelets

   B. RBC, Hgb, Hct, platelets

   C. WBC, PTT, PT

   D. Leukocytes, CBC

2. Because of the patient's symptoms, an important nursing intervention would be aimed at:

   A. Preventing bleeding episodes

   B. Preventing infection

   C. Preventing fluid and electrolyte imbalance

   D. Preventing falls

3. If the patient were to exhibit signs of dyspnea and shortness of breath, the nurse would expect to administer:

   A. Antibiotics

   B. Anticoagulants

   C. Oxygen

   D. IV fluids

4. An important part of the nursing care of this patient is teaching, which would include:

   A. Staying in bed as much as possible

   B. Limiting fluid intake

   C. Taking antibiotics on a routine basis

   D. Carrying an identification card

Situation ■ 2

A patient has been receiving chemotherapy for leukemia. She is admitted to the hospital with short-ness of breath, loss of appetite, and weight loss of 20 pounds.

1. The reason for the shortness of breath in this patient is probably:

   A. Anemia

   B. Thrombocytopenia

   C. Leukopenia

   D. Leukocytosis

2. On assessment, the nurse notices that the patient has ulcerations of the mouth. An appropriate nursing diagnosis would be:

   A. Fluid volume deficit

   B. Alteration in nutrition: less than body requirements

   C. Alteration in urinary elimination

   D. Ineffective individual coping

3. Appropriate interventions to treat the mouth ulcers would be:

   A. Provide good mouth care and provide bland, soft foods

   B. Start the patient on tube feedings

   C. Have meals brought in from home

   D. Keep patient on NPO status until ulcers heal

4. Because the patient's condition worsens, the physician plans a bone marrow transplant. An important nursing diagnosis would be:

   A. Knowledge deficit

   B. Alteration in nutrition: less than body requirements

   C. High risk for infection

   D. Alteration in tissue perfusion

Situation ■ 3

A patient who has had recent surgery has a Hgb of 7.2 g/ml and a Hct of 27.9%. Because the patient has symptoms of hypoxia, the physician decides to order a blood transfusion.

1. The most appropriate type of transfusion for this patient would be:

   A. Whole blood

   B. Packed red cells

C. Plasma

D. Platelets

2. The morning after the transfusion, another Hgb and Hct is drawn. The nurse would expect to see:

A. Hgb up 1 g, Hct up 3%

B. Hgb up 2 g, Hct up 6%

C. Hgb up 3 g, Hct up 8%

D. Hgb up 4 g, Hct up 10%

3. The patient is still symptomatic, so another transfusion is ordered. If this patient were to develop a rash, itching, and a low grade fever, the nurse would suspect:

A. Hemolytic reaction

B. Non-hemolytic reaction

C. Circulatory overload

D. Septic reaction

4. The most appropriate nursing action would be:

A. Stop the infusion and notify the physician

B. Continue the infusion, but monitor the patient carefully

C. Slow down the infusion and notify the physician

Chapter Sixteen

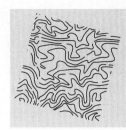

NURSING CARE
of Adults with
Disorders of the Blood
and Blood-Forming Organs

Learning Objectives

1.0 Demonstrate an Understanding of the Different Types of Hematologic Disorders of Adults.

1.1 Match Erythrocyte-Related Disorders to Their Defining Characteristics.
1.2 Identify the Clinical Manifestations of Several of the Hematologic Disorders.
1.3 Identify Nursing Interventions Appropriate for the Adult with a Hematologic Disorder.
1.4 Identify Medications Used for Adults with Hematologic Disorders.

2.0 Demonstrate an Understanding of the Neoplasms that Affect the Hematologic System.

2.1 Identify the Characteristics of Several Neoplasms of the Hematologic System.
2.2 Identify Types of Medical Treatment Used for Adults with Neoplasms of the Hematologic System.

3.0 Demonstrate an Understanding of Bleeding Disorders of the Hematologic System.

3.1 Matching Several of the Bleeding Disorders with Their Defining Characteristics.
3.2 Identify Medical Management of Bleeding Disorders.
3.3 Plan the Nursing Care for the Adult with a Bleeding Disorder.

Learning Activities

Matching

Match the following erythrocyte-related disorders with their defining characteristics.

A. Iron deficiency anemia
B. Aplastic anemia
C. Sickle cell anemia
D. Spherocytosis

E. Pernicious anemia
F. Thalassemia
G. G6PD deficiency
H. Immune hemolytic anemia

1. _____ Characterized by thin, fragile red blood cells known as target cells.

2. _____ Chronic hereditary hemolytic disorder found mainly in black Americans.

3. _____ Often related to poor nutrition.

4. _____ Characterized by small, sphere-shaped red blood cells which swell from accumulation of sodium and water.

5. _____ Inherited, sex-linked disorder involving a deficiency of an enzyme important in glucose metabolism.

6. _____ Caused by impaired red blood cell development within the bone marrow.

7. _____ Treatment involves taking vitamin B_{12}.

8. _____ Caused by the lysis of blood cells.

Questions

9. Anemia in an adult can result from:

   A. Blood loss

   B. Decreased RBC production

   C. RBC destruction

   D. All of the above

10. The adult with severe anemia may become confused and disoriented because of:

    A. Impaired gas exchange

    B. Ineffective breathing patterns

    C. Cerebral anoxia

    D. Hemorrhagic loss

11. The most common sign of anemia in adults is:

    A. Dyspnea

    B. Fatigue

    C. Anorexia

    D. Bruising

12. When a patient has anemia secondary to blood loss, the nurse would monitor carefully for signs of:

    A. Hypovolemia

    B. Diarrhea

    C. Vomiting

    D. Hypertension

13. If a patient with severe anemia and blood loss were to be hypotensive, have rapid deep respirations, low urine output, and disorientation, the nurse would realize this is due to:

    A. Low cardiac output

    B. Fluid shifts

    C. Increased plasma volume

    D. Dehydration

14. The management of the patient with hemorrhagic anemia is primarily aimed at:

    A. Arresting blood loss

    B. Replacing lost fluid

C. Preventing recurrence

D. All of the above

15. If a patient has fatigue, weakness, sensitivity to cold, dysphagia, mouth ulcers, and a red tongue, the nurse would suspect:

A. Hemorrhagic anemia

B. Iron deficiency anemia

C. Aplastic anemia

D. Pernicious anemia

16. Patients on iron therapy should be taught to take the medication with _____ to increase absorption.

A. Milk

B. Orange juice

C. Water

D. None of the above

17. The nurse would suggest that the patient with an iron deficiency eat food high in iron. The best sources would include:

A. Milk and dairy products

B. Bread and grains

C. Red meat, green vegetables

D. Chicken, fish, dried fruit

18. Impaired vitamin B_{12} absorption can lead to:

A. Iron deficiency anemia

B. Aplastic anemia

C. Pernicious anemia

D. Macrocytic anemia

19. An elderly individual with a history of past and current alcohol abuse is admitted to the hospital. The nurse is aware that this patient is at risk for developing:

A. Anemia

B. Folic acid deficiency

C. Sickle cell crisis

D. Aplastic anemia

20. Treatment for the individual with aplastic anemia may include:

A. Blood transfusions

B. Myelotoxic drugs

C. Bone marrow transplant

D. Any of the above

21. A side effect that may occur from excessive blood transfusions in individuals with certain anemias is:

A. Dehydration

B. Elevated iron levels

C. Sluggish circulation

D. Rise in hemoglobin

22. Symptoms which might be evident in the individual with polycythemia vera include:

A. Fatigue, shortness of breath

B. Increased blood pressure and pulse, headaches

C. Decreased blood pressure, weakness

D. Dizziness, cyanosis of extremities

23. Emergency management for the individual with polycythemia vera would include:

A. Oxygen therapy

B. Fluid replacement

C. Phlebotomies

D. Antiarrhythmics

24. The most appropriate diet for the individual with polycythemia vera would be:

A. Low sodium

B. Low cholesterol

C. Low potassium

D. High potassium

25. The most common hematologic found in the older adult is:

A. Anemia

B. Leukemia

C. Hemophilia

D. Multiple myeloma

26. A malignant disease that is characterized by the growth of plasma cells invading bone marrow, lymph nodes, liver, and spleen is:

A. Leukemia

B. Hodgkin's Disease

C. Non-Hodgkin's lymphoma

D. Multiple myeloma

27. Which type of leukemia is most common in individuals aged 40 to 60? Its primary symptoms include long bone pain, anemia, and splenomegaly.

A. Acute lymphocytic leukemia

B. Acute myelogenous leukemia

C. Chronic lymphocytic leukemia

D. Chronic myelogenous leukemia

28. The primary treatment for patients with acute leukemia would be:

A. Antibiotics

B. Analgesics

C. Chemotherapy

D. Radiation therapy

29. Which of the following statements best describes the prognosis of the adults with Hodgkin's disease?

A. Outcome is uncertain, with many remissions

B. Over 50% will be cured with chemotherapy

C. Over 95% will be cured if treated early

D. Approximately 25% will live 5 years

30. If a patient with Hodgkin's disease has respiratory changes, edema, and cyanosis, the nurse would realize that this results from:

A. Deficiency of the immune system

B. Pressure from enlarging lymph nodes

C. Red blood cell destruction

D. Overwhelming infection

31. For a patient with Stage III Hodgkin's disease, treatment would involve:

A. Chemotherapy

B. Radiation therapy

C. Radiation and chemotherapy

D. Bone marrow transplant

32. If a patient with a neoplasm of the hematologic system has thrombocytopenia, it would be important for the nurse to monitor for:

A. Signs of infection

B. Signs of bleeding

C. Signs of dehydration

D. Signs of confusion

33. A patient with multiple myeloma who has limited activity would be at risk for developing:

A. Kidney stones

B. Hypocalcemia

C. Polycythemia

D. Dehydration

34. Presence of Reed-Sternberg cells would indicate to the nurse that a patient might have:

A. Chronic leukemia

B. Hodgkin's disease

C. Aplastic anemia

D. Spirocytosis

35. Presence of Bence Jones protein in a patient's urine would indicate to the nurse that a patient might have:

A. Multiple myeloma

B. Hemophilia

C. Leukemia

D. Thalassemia

36. When a patient with a neoplasm is being treated with an alkylating agent such as Alkeran, the nurse would monitor for signs of:

A. Polycythemia

B. Leukocytosis

C. Iron deficiency anemia

D. Pancytopenia

Matching (Bleeding Disorders)

Match the following bleeding disorders with their defining characteristics.

A. Purpura   C. Hemophilia

B. Disseminated intravascular coagulation

37. _____ Hereditary coagulation disorder

38. _____ Bleeding into the tissue

39. _____ May result from thrombocytopenia

40. _____ A common acquired coagulation disorder

41. _____ Sex-linked recessive disorder

42. _____ Characterized by widespread coagulation in body

Questions

43. Write a nursing care plan for the adult with leukemia.

    Nursing Diagnosis: High risk for infection related to the compromised immune response

    Patient Outcome:

    Nursing Interventions:

44. Write a nursing care plan for the adult with Hodgkin's disease.

    Nursing Diagnosis: Ineffective breathing patterns related to obstruction from enlarged lymph nodes

    Patient Outcome:

    Nursing Interventions:

CLINICAL SITUATIONS

Situation ■ 1

Mary, age 24, is admitted to the hospital in sickle cell crisis. She has had the disease since age 2. She is complaining of severe pain in her knees and abdomen.

1. Which of the following statements best explains the etiology of sickle cell anemia?

    A. A fatal disease occurring after a blood transfusion

    B. A disease characterized by acute bleeding episodes

    C. A chronic hereditary disorder characterized by an abnormal hemoglobin

    D. An acute disease that is easily treatable

2. Which of the following events in Mary's past history may have precipitated the current crisis?

    A. Recent divorce

    B. Recent intestinal virus

    C. Promotion at work

    D. Change in medication

3. The reason for the pain in Mary's knees is:

    A. Occlusion of the circulatory system

    B. Bleeding into the joints

    C. Traumatic fall

    D. Lack of intrinsic factor

4. Medical management is primarily aimed at:

    A. Diet therapy

    B. Hydration and pain control

    C. Bed rest and immobilization of extremities

    D. Antibiotics and anti-inflammatories

5. The nurse is aware that a primary goal is to prevent complications such as:

    A. Cerebral hemorrhage

    B. Renal failure

    C. Cardiac disorders

    D. All of the above

Situation ■ 2

Mark Collins, age 18, has been recently diagnosed with acute myelocytic leukemia. He is admitted with an extremely low white count and signs of infection. He recently finished a course of chemotherapy.

1. Because of Mark's low white count and possible infection, he should be admitted to:

    A. Semiprivate room

    B. Private room

    C. Intensive care

2. Laboratory results showed that Mark also has anemia and thrombocytopenia. The nurse would monitor him closely for signs of:

   A. Bleeding

   B. Confusion

   C. Activity intolerance

   D. Visual impairment

3. Mark is complaining of a sore mouth. The nurse notices several mouth ulcers. An appropriate nursing intervention would be:

   A. Lemon-glycerin swabs

   B. Put him on NPO status

   C. Rinse with hydrogen peroxide and water

   D. Rinse with Cepacol mouthwash

4. Since Mark is receiving chemotherapy, he is anxious about his prognosis. Which statement by the nurse would be most appropriate?

   A. Average survival time with treatment is 5 years.

   B. With chemotherapy, complete remission occurs in 50–75% of all patients.

   C. Chemotherapy does not increase life span but does decrease symptoms.

   D. A complete remission is achieved in about 90% of all patients.

Situation ■ 3

Steven, age 21, has hemophilia A. He is in the hospital to control an acute bleeding episode.

1. Individuals with this type of hemophilia are known to be deficient in:

   A. Factor VI

   B. Factor VII

   C. Factor VIII

   D. Factor IX

2. Which statement best describes this disorder?

   A. It is a sex-linked recessive disorder transmitted by females.

   B. It is a sex-linked dominant disorder transmitted by males.

   C. It is a bleeding disorder occurring equally in males and females.

   D. It is an acquired coagulation disorder.

3. Medical management of Steven's bleeding episode would involve administration of:

   A. Plasma

   B. Cryoprecipitate

   C. Antihemophilic factor

   D. Any of the above

4. Steven has had several episodes of hemarthrosis. The most appropriate treatment for this would be:

   A. Apply direct pressure

   B. Pack the involved area in ice

   C. Administer analgesics

   D. Administer antibiotics

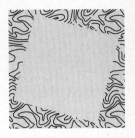

Unit Six

ADULTS WITH CIRCULATORY DYSFUNCTION

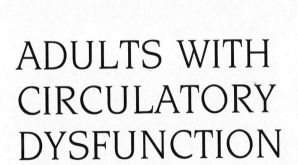

Chapter Seventeen

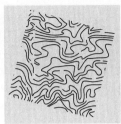

KNOWLEDGE BASIC TO THE NURSING CARE
of Adults with Cardiac Dysfunction

Learning Objectives

1.0 Review the Anatomy and Physiology of the Cardiac System.

1.1 Identify the Parts of the Heart.
1.2 Explain the Functions of the Heart.
1.3 Explain the Three Regulatory Mechanisms for Circulation.
1.4 Identify the Conduction System of the Heart.

2.0 Demonstrate an Understanding of Assessment Data Related to the Cardiac System.

2.1 Identify Symptoms of Cardiac Disorders.
2.2 Match the Heart Sounds with Their Specific Characteristics.
2.3 List the Cardiac Risk Factors.
2.4 Identify Tests Which are Used to Diagnose Cardiac Disorders.

3.0 Demonstrate an Understanding of Interventions Used to Treat Adults with a Cardiac Disorder.

3.1 Demonstrate an Understanding of the Types of Medical Treatment Used with Cardiac Disorders.
3.2 Demonstrate an Understanding of the Types of Surgical Interventions Used to Treat Cardiac Disorders.
3.3 Plan the Nursing Care for an Adult with a Disorder of the Cardiac System.

Learning Activities

Cardiac Anatomy

Identify

On the diagram below, identify the parts of the heart.

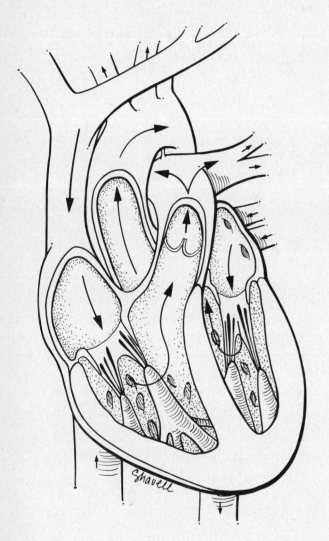

	Number
1. Superior vena cava	_____
2. Inferior vena cava	_____
3. Right atrium	_____
4. Left atrium	_____
5. Left ventricle	_____

6. Right ventricle	_____
7. Tricuspid valve	_____
8. Mitral valve	_____
9. Pulmonic valve	_____
10. Pulmonary arteries	_____
11. Pulmonary veins	_____
12. Aortic valve	_____
13. Ascending aorta	_____
14. Descending aorta	_____

Questions

15. Describe the functions of the heart:

16. Briefly explain how blood flows through the body:

Fill In

17. The _____ supply the cardiac muscle with blood, oxygen, and nutrients.

Questions

18. Explain the three regulatory mechanisms for circulation.

1.

2.

3.

Identify

19. Label and trace the conductive system through the heart.

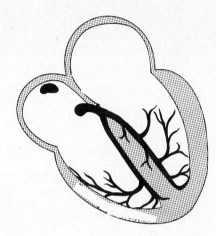

Questions

20. Explain what the following wave forms signify.
    1. P Wave:
    2. PR interval:
    3. QRS complex:
    4. T wave:

Matching

Match the following heart sounds with their specific characteristics.

A. S1   C. S3
B. S2   D. S4

21. _____ Normal in children, but pathologic after the age of 30.

22. _____ Produced by the simultaneous closure of the mitral and tricuspid valves.

23. _____ Produced by high-velocity blood flow during atrial contraction.

24. _____ Produced by the simultaneous closure of the aortic and pulmonic valves.

25. _____ Presence of this sound indicates a pathologic condition.

26. _____ Produced by the rapid, passive, atrial filling of a partially filled ventricle.

Define

27. Central venous pressure:

28. Pulmonary artery pressure:

29. Pulmonary wedge pressure:

30. Cardiac output:

Questions

31. List the cardiac risk factors:
    1. Nonmodifiable
       a.
       b.
       c.
    2. Modifiable
       a.
       b.
       c.
       d.

32. A test which records the individual's electrocardiogram during exercise is called a:
    A. Fluoroscopy
    B. Stress test
    C. Holter monitor
    D. Echocardiogram

33. The test that will give the best diagnostic information about the condition of the cardiac valves and the size of the cardiac chambers is:
    A. Holter monitor
    B. Radioactive imaging
    C. Stress test
    D. Echocardiogram

34. The type of test in which radiopaque contrast dye is injected into the cardiac chambers and coronary arteries in order to view blood flow is a:
    A. Cardiac catheterization

B. Cardiac stress test

C. Echocardiogram

D. Thallium stress test

35. When a cardiac patient has an acid-base imbalance, the nurse would monitor for:

    A. Hypoxia

    B. Dysrhythmias

    C. Pain

    D. Respiratory distress

36. If a cardiac patient has high BUN and creatinine levels, the nurse would realize that the patient has:

    A. High cardiac output

    B. Impaired gas exchange

    C. Fluid and electrolyte imbalance

    D. Decreased renal perfusion

37. When a patient has had myocardial damage, the first enzyme that will elevate is the:

    A. CPK

    B. LDH

    C. SGOT

    D. ESR

38. The blood test that would provide the best diagnostic information about whether a patient has had a myocardial infarction is the:

    A. CPK-MM

    B. CPK-MB

    C. LDH-2

    D. SGOT-BB

39. Cardiac patients often receive medications which slow the transmission of electrical impulses in the heart. An example of this is:

    A. Isordil

    B. Digoxin

    C. Lidocaine

    D. Lasix

40. When a patient is on a low-sodium diet, which of the following would NOT be permitted?

    A. Fresh fruit

    B. Cheese

    C. Fish

    D. Skim milk

41. In caring for a patient with angina, the nurse would instruct the patient to take nitroglycerin when chest pain occurs. An appropriate statement is:

    A. If you feel a burning sensation, the medication is no longer effective.

    B. Replace the medication at least every year.

    C. If relief of pain is not obtained after 3 nitroglycerin tablets, seek immediate medical attention.

    D. When pain occurs, take a tablet every 5 minutes until relief is obtained.

42. When a patient with a cardiac condition has a low cardiac output and is very symptomatic, an appropriate medication would be:

    A. Dopamine

    B. Lasix

    C. Apresoline

    D. Lidocaine

43. The drug of choice for the treatment of premature ventricular contractions is:

    A. Digoxin

    B. Verapamil

    C. Apresoline

    D. Lidocaine

44. Which nursing action has the highest priority when a patient is receiving thrombolytic therapy?

    A. Monitor for hypotension

    B. Monitor for arrhythmias

    C. Monitor for bleeding

    D. Monitor for pain

45. A serious complication that may occur whenever the heart-lung machine is used is:

   A. Respiratory arrest

   B. Embolus

   C. Arrhythmias

   D. Sepsis

46. When a patient develops cardiogenic shock, he or she may need intra-aortic balloon pump support. The two main goals of this therapy are:

   A. Reducing afterload and augmenting diastolic

   B. Increasing both preload and afterload

   C. Prevention of lethal arrhythmias

   D. Increasing the oxygen supply

47. Write a nursing care plan for the patient with an alteration in cardiac output related to mechanical failure.

   Nursing Diagnosis: Decreased cardiac output

   Patient Outcome:

   Nursing Interventions:

48. Write a nursing care plan for the patient with activity alterations secondary to a cardiac disorder.

   Nursing Diagnosis: Activity intolerance related to decreased oxygenation

   Patient Outcome:

   Nursing Interventions:

49. Write a nursing care plan for the patient who has had coronary artery bypass surgery.

   Nursing Diagnosis: Knowledge deficit: signs and symptoms of complication

   Patient Outcome:

   Nursing Interventions:

CLINICAL SITUATIONS

Situation ■ 1

Mike Brown is having a heart catheterization to determine if he is a candidate for open heart surgery. He has a history of angina, which has been worsening over the past 6 months.

1. Which of the following statements is NOT true about this procedure?

   A. It is painless

   B. It may produce a warm, tingling sensation

   C. An allergic reaction is possible

   D. It is done while the patient is awake

2. Mr. Brown had the catheter inserted in his right antecubital vein. He returns to the unit in stable condition. The nurse will assess:

   A. Fluid intake

   B. Peripheral pulses

   C. Insertion site

   D. All of the above

3. Because Mr. Brown is found to have extensive quadruple vessel disease, the most likely treatment will be:

   A. Oxygen and medication therapy

   B. Angioplasty

   C. Urokinase

   D. Bypass surgery

4. The goal of coronary artery bypass grafting is:

   A. Improve blood supply to the ischemic myocardium

   B. Decrease the oxygen demand

   C. Prevent pain

   D. Prolong life

Situation ■ 2

Melissa West, age 65, has severe coronary artery disease. She is 5'6" and weights 135 pounds. She has diabetes and hypertension and smokes a pack of cigarettes a day.

1. What change could Ms. West make that would bring about the most significant reduction in her cardiac risk factors?

   A. Lose weight

   B. Control her diabetes

   C. Stop smoking

   D. Reduce her stress

2. Ms. West is started on Lasix to help reduce fluid accumulation. She is told to eat a diet high in potassium. Which of the following foods would NOT be included?

   A. Green beans

   B. Bread and cereal

   C. Oranges

   D. Liver

3. Ms. West is also started on Isordil (a vasodilator). The nurse is aware that the purpose of this medication is:

   A. To help lessen pain

   B. To decrease fluid retention

   C. To lower cholesterol

   D. To increase oxygen supply

4. When a patient is receiving this medication, it would be important for the nurse to monitor:

   A. Blood pressure

   B. Pulse

   C. Respiratory rate

   D. Temperature

5. The physician decides to do a percutaneous transluminal coronary angioplasty (PTCA). Which of the statements is NOT true about this procedure?

   A. It is usually done when the atherosclerotic disease is limited to one vessel.

   B. Patient needs to sign a consent for coronary artery bypass surgery.

   C. It has a high rate of restenosis.

   D. Activity is limited for 4 weeks after discharge.

Chapter Eighteen

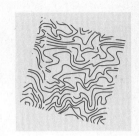

NURSING CARE
of Adults with
Cardiac Disorders

Learning Objectives

1.0 Demonstrate an Understanding of Infections and Inflammations of the Cardiac System.

1.1 Define Several of the Infections and Inflammations.
1.2 Identify the Clinical Manifestations of Several Cardiac Disorders.
1.3 Demonstrate an Understanding of the Medical Management of Infectious Cardiac Disorders.
1.4 Plan the Nursing Care for Adults with Infectious Cardiac Disorders.

2.0 Demonstrate an Understanding of Functional Disorders of the Cardiac System.

2.1 Identify the Etiology and Pathophysiology of Several Functional Cardiac Disorders.
2.2 Identify the Clinical Manifestations of Several Functional Cardiac Disorders.
2.3 Demonstrate an Understanding of the Medical Management of Functional Cardiac Disorders.
2.4 Plan the Nursing Care for Adults with Functional Cardiac Disorders.

3.0 Demonstrate an Understanding of Structural Disorders of the Cardiac System.

3.1 Identify the Etiology and Pathophysiology of Several Structural Cardiac Disorders.
3.2 Identify the Clinical Manifestations of Several Structural Cardiac Disorders.
3.3 Demonstrate an Understanding of the Medical Management of Structural Cardiac Disorders.
3.4 Demonstrate an Understanding of the Surgical Management of Structural Cardiac Disorders.
3.5 Plan the Nursing Care for Adults with Structural Cardiac Disorders.

Learning Activities

Define

1. Endocarditis:

2. Myocarditis:

3. Pericarditis:

4. Congestive heart failure:

5. Myocardial infarction:

6. Cardiomyopathy:

7. Cardiopulmonary resuscitation:

Questions

8. Adults who develop bacterial endocarditis may have had _____ as a child.
   A. Mononucleosis
   B. Rheumatic fever
   C. Scarlet fever
   D. Chicken pox

9. Assessment findings for the individual who has subacute bacterial endocarditis would include:
   A. Heart murmur
   B. S1, S2, S3
   C. Abnormal breath sounds
   D. Peripheral edema, weight gain

10. Medical management of bacterial endocarditis would be aimed at:
    A. Controlling the inflammatory process
    B. Preventing cardiac damage
    C. Preventing recurrence
    D. All of the above

11. Surgical management for the individual with subacute bacterial endocarditis and bacterial destruction would involve:
    A. Angioplasty
    B. Valve replacement
    C. Bypass graft
    D. Commissurotomy

12. If a patient with a cardiac condition were to become dyspneic and the nurse can auscultate rales and wheezes, the patient has developed:
    A. Cardiac tamponade
    B. Endocarditis
    C. Pleurisy
    D. Congestive heart failure

13. Which of the following rhythms, if seen on a cardiac monitor, would the nurse interpret as life threatening?
    A. Superventricular tachycardia
    B. Atrial fibrillation
    C. Premature ventricular complexes
    D. Ventricular tachycardia

14. If an individual has chest pain, a pericardial friction run, and ECG changes, the nurse would suspect:

    A. Myocardial infarction

    B. Subacute bacterial endocarditis

    C. Pericardial effusion

    D. Cardiac tamponade

15. Because elderly individuals have altered pain sensation, when they have cardiac pain, it is often:

    A. Atypical

    B. Severe

    C. Diffuse

    D. Radiating

16. The nurse is monitoring a patient's lab results and notes that the serum isoenzymes (CPK-MB) are greatly increased. This is due to:

    A. Extreme pain and anxiety

    B. Cellular membrane destruction

    C. Inadequate cardiac output

    D. Falling arterial pressure

17. The nurse administers nitroglycerin sublingually to a patient with angina. Which statement best explains the therapeutic action of this medication?

    A. Decreases the myocardial oxygen consumption

    B. Increases the filling pressure (preload)

    C. Causes vasoconstriction of the systemic bed

    D. Increases the systemic blood pressure

18. When a patient has left-sided heart failure, the nurse would consider which goal as primary?

    A. Maintaining adequate cardiac output

    B. Maintaining adequate tissue perfusion

    C. Maintaining adequate nutrition

    D. Maintaining effective coping skills

19. When a patient has cardiomyopathy, the nurse would monitor carefully for signs of:

    A. Infection

    B. Chest pain

    C. Low cardiac output

    D. Heart murmur

20. In a patient with life-threatening cardiomyopathy, the treatment that can offer the best chance of survival is:

    A. Bypass surgery

    B. Heart transplant

    C. Pacemaker insertion

    D. Implantable defibrillator

21. The best position for the patient in congestive heart failure would be:

    A. Prone

    B. Supine

    C. Semi-Fowler's

    D. Trendelenburg

22. A medication used to treat congestive heart failure by providing sedation and reduction of afterload is:

    A. Morphine sulfate

    B. Lasix

    C. Digoxin

    D. Verapamil

23. Treatment for the patient with a cardiac conduction block who is experiencing dizziness and confusion would probably include:

    A. Open heart surgery

    B. Pacemaker insertion

    C. Digoxin, Lasix

    D. Angioplasty

24. A cardiac patient is showing premature ventricular contractions (PVCs) on the monitor. Lidocaine is started. He then has a run of ventricular tachycardia followed by ventricular fibrillation. What is the proper nursing action?

    A. Set up for pacemaker insertion

    B. Prepare for surgery

    C. Increase the dose of lidocaine

    D. Prepare for defibrillation

25. Streptokinase is given to a patient who is having a myocardial infarction. The nurse is aware that it is a thrombolytic agent and that it:

    A. Causes serious allergic reactions

    B. Must be administered by the intracoronary route

    C. Has the potential to cause systemic bleeding

    D. Is a naturally occurring enzyme

26. The pain of a myocardial infarction differs from that of angina in that:

    A. It is retrosternal and radiating

    B. It is longer and not relieved by nitroglycerin

    C. It occurs with activity

    D. It is associated with epigastric distress

27. When a patient has had a myocardial infarction (MI), the nurse carefully monitors for complications. The most frequent complication is:

    A. Endocarditis

    B. Pulmonary embolism

    C. Congestive heart failure

    D. Cardiac arrhythmias

28. A patient who has had a myocardial infarction is usually treated with medications that:

    A. Increase blood pressure

    B. Increase preload and afterload

    C. Increase oxygen supply and demand

    D. Increase oxygen supply and decrease demand

29. The nurse is aware that the most common symptom experienced by patients with coronary artery disease is:

    A. Angina

    B. Intermittent claudication

    C. Hypoxia

    D. Confusion

30. When a patient has a diagnosis of left-sided heart failure, the nurse might expect the patient to relay which of the following symptoms?

    A. I am tired at the end of the day

    B. I have trouble breathing when I climb stairs

    C. My ankles are always swollen

    D. I feel bloated after I eat

31. The most appropriate diet for the patient with congestive heart failure is:

    A. Low sodium, high potassium

    B. Low potassium, low sodium

    C. Low fat, low calorie

    D. High calorie, low fat

32. The analgesic of choice for controlling chest pain associated with myocardial infarction is:

    A. Demerol

    B. Nitroglycerin

    C. Morphine sulfate

    D. Lidocaine

33. When lidocaine is not effective in treating ventricular arrhythmias, another drug which is often used is:

    A. Digoxin

    B. Procan

    C. Isordil

    D. Streptokinase

34. A disease that is the result of atherosclerosis is:

    A. Coronary artery disease

    B. Hypertension

    C. Peripheral vascular disease

    D. All of the above

35. A medication which will cause coronary and peripheral artery dilation as well as increase myocardial contractility is:

    A. Verapamil

    B. Lasix

    C. Inderal

    D. Digoxin

36. When a patient has aortic valve stenosis, the nurse would monitor for signs of:

    A. Angina

    B. Left ventricular failure

C. Peripheral edema

D. Cardiac dysrhythmias

37. When valvular problems develop following rheumatic endocarditis, the process involved is:

A. Valvular thickening, regurgitation

B. Stenosis, vegetation formation

C. Regurgitation, valvular thickening

D. Vegetation formation, stenosis

True or False

38. _____ Tamponade, if not relieved, will lead to cardiac arrest.

39. _____ Patients who have had an MI are kept on bed rest for 5 days.

40. _____ The exact cause of atherosclerosis is unknown.

41. _____ The best drug to treat PVCs is bretylium.

42. _____ Patients with mitral valve regurgitation are often asymptomatic.

43. _____ Maximum coronary blood flow at age 60 is about 35% less than that of a 30-year-old.

44. _____ It is often hard to diagnose an MI based on the type of chest pain the patient has.

Questions

45. Write a nursing care plan for the patient in congestive heart failure.

    Nursing Diagnosis: Decreased cardiac output related to altered myocardial contractility, alteration in cardiac rhythm

    Patient Outcome:

    Nursing Interventions:

46. Write a nursing care plan for the patient who has had an acute myocardial infarction.

Nursing Diagnosis: Knowledge deficit: nature of myocardial infarction, its treatment, and expected outcomes or lifestyle changes

Patient Outcome:

Nursing Interventions:

CLINICAL SITUATIONS

Situation ■ 1

A patient with a 10-year history of angina is admitted to the hospital with chest pain. He is admitted for a cardiac workup to rule out myocardial infarction.

1. The diagnosis of myocardial infarction will be based on:

A. History

B. Laboratory findings

C. Electrocardiogram

D. All of the above

2. The nurse notices a run of PVCs on the cardiac monitor. The physician would most likely order:

A. Digoxin

B. Lidocaine

C. Lasix

D. Morphine

3. The patient is determined to have had an acute anterior myocardial infarction. On the second hospital day, he becomes very short of breath. The nurse would suspect:

A. Heart failure

B. Angina

C. Cardiac arrhythmia

D. Extension of the MI

4. On the third day, he develops oliguria and edema. Which statement best explains why he has developed oliguria?

A. He has decreased renal perfusion due to reduced cardiac output.

B. His kidneys are conserving water because of increased cardiac volume.

C. He is in renal failure.

D. His fluid intake has been limited because of chest pain.

5. A cardiac catheterization is scheduled to:

A. Revascularize the myocardium

B. Study the action of the heart valves

C. Determine the extent of the MI

D. Administer medications

6. Findings from the heart catheterization show triple vessel disease with narrowing of greater than 60%. The most appropriate treatment would be:

A. Angioplasty

B. Medication

C. Exercise program

D. Bypass surgery

Situation ■ 2

Mr. Kellerman is on the open heart step-down unit. He had a coronary artery bypass surgery 2 days ago.

1. Mr. Kellerman suddenly becomes dyspneic and cyanotic and has a drop in cardiac output and a paradoxical pulse. These symptoms suggest:

A. Cardiac tamponade

B. Pulmonary hypertension

C. Rupture of the graft

D. Pericarditis

2. After calling the physician, the appropriate nursing action would be:

A. Set up a chest tube

B. Set up for pericardial tap

C. Call for a ventilator

D. Set up a dopamine drip

3. Mr. Kellerman recovers from this complication but still has some respiratory congestion. The nurse should:

A. Encourage the patient to cough and deep breathe every hour

B. Call for respiratory therapy to induce coughing

C. Use splinting when the patient coughs

D. All of the above

4. Ten days later, Mr. Kellerman is discharged. Discharge instructions would include telling him:

A. To follow a low-potassium diet

B. To avoid lifting

C. To avoid any activity

D. To return to the hospital in 1 week

Chapter Nineteen

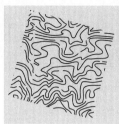

KNOWLEDGE BASIC TO THE NURSING CARE
of Adults with Vascular Dysfunction

Learning Objectives

1.0 Review the Anatomy and Physiology of the Vascular Structures.

1.1 Match the Vascular Structure with its Characteristics.
1.2 List Structural Factors which Affect Blood Flow.

2.0 Demonstrate an Understanding of the Assessment Data Related to Vascular Structures.

2.1 Identify the Clinical Manifestations of Peripheral Vascular Dysfunction.
2.2 Identify Tests Which are Used to Diagnose Vascular Dysfunction.
2.3 Interpret Assessment Findings that Relate to Vascular Dysfunction.

3.0 Demonstrate an Understanding of the Interventions Used to Treat Vascular Dysfunctions.

3.1 Demonstrate an Understanding of the Medical Management of the Patient with a Vascular Dysfunction.
3.2 Demonstrate an Understanding of the Surgical Management of the Patient with a Vascular Dysfunction.
3.3 Write a Nursing Care Plan for the Patient Undergoing Vascular Surgery.

Learning Activities

Matching

Match each vascular structure with its characteristics.

A. Arteries   D. Arterioles
B. Capillaries E. Venules
C. Veins   F. Lymphatics

1. _____ Thin-walled transit tubes which begin the conduit of blood returning to the heart.

2. _____ Blood flow here delivers nutrition and removes waste products.

3. _____ Begin the transport of oxygenated blood from the aorta.

4. _____ Serve as an accessory route for the transport of fluid and proteins away from interstitial space.

5. _____ High-resistance vessels which are innervated by the sympathetic nervous system.

6. _____ Low-pressure, unidirectional conduits that rely on muscle contraction to move blood.

Questions

7. List three of the structural factors that affect blood flow.

   1.

   2.

   3.

8. When pain is present in a patient with vascular dysfunction, it is usually related to:

   A. Decrease in blood flow

   B. Increase in blood flow

   C. Tissue hypoxia

   D. Tissue injury

9. Cramplike pain which is often felt in the calf muscles and is precipitated by walking is called _____ .

   A. Ischemia

   B. Arterial hypoxia

   C. Claudication

   D. Dysreflexia

10. Resting pain is a sign of acute _____ insufficiency.

    A. Arterial

    B. Venous

    C. Cerebral

    D. Coronary

11. If a patient with arterial insufficiency develops permanent dilatation of the arterioles, the extremities will:

    A. Appear cyanotic

    B. Appear pale

    C. Appear ruddy

    D. Appear brownish

12. When assessing a patient with arterial insufficiency, the nurse anticipates:

    A. Diminished or absent pulses

    B. Adequate capillary refill

    C. Peripheral edema and cyanosis

    D. Irregular pulses

13. During admission, a patient tells the nurse that he takes lovastatin. This would suggest that the patient has:

    A. High blood pressure

    B. Peripheral vascular disease

    C. High cholesterol

    D. Heart disease

14. An invasive test that is done to visualize the arteries and assess blood flow is known as:

A. Venogram

B. Arteriogram

C. Doppler ultrasound

D. Perthes' test

15. A noninvasive test that can detect auditory signs of blood flow to detect incompetent valves is known as:

A. Venography

B. Doppler ultrasound

C. Angiography

D. Impedance study

16. A test which is used to evaluate the presence of iliac or femoral veins by measuring resistance in veins as related to blood volume is:

A. Ultrasound

B. Perthes' test

C. Arteriography

D. Digital subtraction test

17. This test is done to detect early thrombi in leg veins in a patient too ill for a venogram. It is done in nuclear medicine.

A. Perthes' test

B. Arterial angiography

C. Radionuclide venography

D. Doppler studies

18. A medication that is used to treat peripheral vascular disease that works by making red blood cells more flexible is:

A. Vasodilan

B. Trental

C. Aspirin

D. Persantine

19. A medication that is often used by patients with peripheral vascular disease to help prevent platelet aggregation is:

A. Aspirin

B. Heparin

C. Coumadin

D. Trental

20. Peripheral angioplasty may be used to open up an arterial blockage by:

A. Vaporizing the plaque

B. Scraping the plaque from the artery

C. Compressing the plaque

D. Dissolving the plaque

21. Complications of angioplasty that the nurse would monitor for include:

A. Stenosis

B. Hemorrhage

C. Embolism

D. All of the above

22. The nurse would explain to a patient that surgical management of peripheral vascular disease is an option when:

A. The patient desires it

B. Medication doesn't work

C. Ischemic pain interferes with activity

D. All of the above

Fill In

23. A palliative surgical procedure that is done to help reduce pain is called a _____ .

24. The surgical removal of a clot in a vessel is called an _____ .

25. The surgical cleaning out of fatty plaque from the inner and middle layers of vessel walls is called a/an _____ .

26. The only therapeutic option when an extremities is ischemic, painful, and gangrenous is _____ .

Questions

27. Write a nursing care plan for the patient with peripheral vascular pain.

Nursing Diagnosis: Pain related to impaired peripheral circulation

Patient Outcome:

Nursing Interventions:

28. Write a nursing care plan for the patient who has had peripheral vascular surgery.

    Nursing Diagnosis: Alteration in peripheral tissue perfusion related to thrombus formation or re-occlusion

    Patient Outcome:

    Nursing Interventions:

CLINICAL SITUATIONS

Situation ■ 1

Ms. Yunger is admitted with severe leg pain. Her left foot is cold and no pulse is present. She is taken for an angiography. A clot is found in the artery and urokinase is started.

1. The nurse is aware that the purpose of this procedure is to:

    A. Remove the blood clot

    B. Stop formation of new clots

    C. Dissolve the clot

    D. Prevent an infection

2. Ms. Yunger is observed in the recovery room for 24 hours and then returned to the floor. She is now receiving heparin and Coumadin. Why would she be on both medications?

    A. They have a synergistic effect

    B. Heparin works faster, and Coumadin is slower

    C. Coumadin works faster, then heparin takes over

    D. Her condition is severe enough to warrant this

3. Ms. Yunger will probably be discharged when:

    A. Heparin is therapeutic

    B. Coumadin is therapeutic

    C. Both are therapeutic

4. Upon discharge, it is important for Ms. Yunger to:

    A. Have coagulation studies done frequently

    B. Check for any signs of unusual bleeding

    C. Practice safety measures to prevent cuts

    D. All of the above

Situation ■ 2

Mrs. Rossman is admitted with peripheral vascular disease which is not responding to medical treatment. She is having diagnostic testing and possible surgery.

1. If Mrs. Rossman has manifestations of arterial insufficiency, assessment findings would include:

    A. Brownish discoloration to skin, edema in feet

    B. Skin thick and rough, rosy color

    C. Feet warm with tissue edema

    D. Feet pale and cool, skin dry and smooth

2. She is scheduled for a Doppler ultrasound. The nurse explains that the purpose of this test is to:

    A. Detect disruption in blood flow in arteries or veins

    B. Measure ankle pressure during exercise

    C. Determine temperature changes with exercise

    D. Visualize the blood flow in veins and arteries

3. Results of the test are inconclusive and arterial angiography is ordered. What information would the nurse obtain prior to the test?

    A. Drug allergies

    B. History of renal problems

    C. Status of pulses

    D. All of the above

4. Results of the test indicate severe stenosis in the right femoral artery. She is scheduled for bypass surgery. Following surgery, the nurse would consider which of the following as a priority?

    A. Assessing respiratory status

    B. Assessing for cardiac arrhythmias

    C. Assessing peripheral pulses

    D. Assessing fluid status

5. Surgery goes well and Mrs. Rossman is preparing for discharge. She will be taking Persantine when she goes home. The nurse would explain that the action of this drug is to:

A. Provide pain relief

B. Promote blood clotting

C. Relax smooth muscle

D. Promote vasodilation

Chapter Twenty

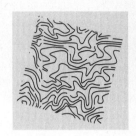

NURSING CARE
of Adults with Vascular Disorders

Learning Objectives

1.0 Demonstrate an Understanding of Common Arterial Vascular Disorders.

1.1 Review the Etiology and Pathophysiology of Several Common Vascular Disorders.
1.2 Match Common Arterial Disorders with Their Correct Definitions.
1.3 Demonstrate an Understanding of the Teaching Needs of the Patient with Arterial Vascular Disorders.
1.4 Identify Treatment Options Available for the Patients with Common Arterial Vascular Disorders.
1.5 Write a Nursing Care Plan for the Patient with an Arterial Vascular Disorder.

2.0 Demonstrate an Understanding of Common Venous Vascular Disorders.

2.1 Review the Etiology and Pathophysiology of Several Common Venous Vascular Disorders.
2.2 Identify the Characteristics of the Venous Vascular Disorders.
2.3 Write a Nursing Care Plan for the Patient with a Venous Vascular Disorder.

3.0 Demonstrate an Understanding of the Needs of the Patient with an Aneurysm.

3.1 Identify the Clinical Manifestations of Aneurysms.
3.2 Demonstrate an Understanding of the Medical and Surgical Interventions Used in Treating Aneurysms.
3.3 Plan Appropriate Nursing Interventions for the Patient with an Aneurysm.

4.0 Demonstrate an Understanding of the Needs of the Adult with Hypertensive Vascular Disease.

4.1 Identify the Risk Factors Associated with Hypertensive Vascular Disease.

4.2 Demonstrate an Understanding of the Medical Management of Hypertensive Vascular Disease.

5.0 Demonstrate an Understanding of Common Lymphatic Disorders.

5.1 Review the Etiology and Pathophysiology of Lymphatic Disorders.
5.2 Review Treatment Options Available for the Patient with a Lymphatic Disorder.

Learning Activities

Questions

1. List five risk factors that are related to the development of atherosclerosis and hypertension.

   1.

   2.

   3.

   4.

   5.

Matching

Match each disorder with its definition.

A. Atherosclerosis
B. Raynaud's disease
C. Buerger's disease
D. Takayasu's arteritis
E. Aneurysm
F. Arteriosclerosis obliterans
G. Thrombophlebitis
H. Varicose veins
I. Lymphangitis

2. _____ Abnormal dilation of the veins owing to venous insufficiency.

3. _____ An outpouching of a vessel wall or sac.

4. _____ Inflammation of the lymph system.

5. _____ Arterial walls become thick and rigid; called the pulseless disease.

6. _____ Walls of the arteries become calcified from fatty plaque.

7. _____ Characterized by paroxysmal, bilateral, digital ischemia induced by cold or emotional stress.

8. _____ Caused by atherosclerosis, which results in fatty plaque that blocks large vessels.

9. _____ Development of a clot in a vein.

10. _____ Chronic inflammatory process that involves medium-sized arteries and veins.

Questions

11. Intermittent claudication is a symptom that results from:

    A. Dorsiflexion of the foot when phlebitis is present

    B. Inadequate blood flow to the muscles after exercise

    C. Inadequate blood flow to the skin after exposure to cold

    D. Stenosis of the veins

12. During the admission history, a patient complains of burning and numbness in her hands. Her hands appear very red. A likely diagnosis is:

    A. Carpal tunnel syndrome

    B. Arterial occlusion

    C. Raynaud's disease

    D. Intermittent claudication

13. One of the most common and severe manifestations of thromboangiitis obliterans is:

    A. Cyanosis

    B. Inflammation

    C. Pain

    D. Fatigue

14. Which procedure might be recommended to promote vasodilation for the patient with Buerger's disease?

    A. Angioplasty

    B. Bypass surgery

    C. Sympathectomy

    D. Laser surgery

15. _____ would be contraindicated for patients who have vascular occlusive disease.

    A. Caffeine

    B. Smoking

C. Vigorous exercise

D. Alcohol intake

16. A patient with Raynaud's disease would exhibit which of the following clinical manifestations?

   A. Hands appear cool and cyanotic

   B. Numbness, edema, and decreased sensation

   C. Throbbing pain felt at the end of an episode

   D. Any of the above

17. The nurse would teach a patient with Raynaud's disease that it may be possible to end vasospastic episodes by:

   A. Taking antispasmodic medications

   B. Taking analgesics every day

   C. Following an exercise routine

   D. Placing the fingers in warm water

18. List five discharge instructions that the nurse would give to the patient with Raynaud's disease.

   1.

   2.

   3.

   4.

   5.

19. The medical treatment of choice for a patient with syphilitic aortitis would be:

   A. Procaine penicillin

   B. Tetracycline

   C. Hydrocortisone

   D. Acyclovir

20. A patient with a peripheral vascular disease and a history of rheumatic heart disease may be at risk for _____ .

   A. Pulmonary embolism

   B. Thrombus formation

   C. Cardiac failure

   D. Cerebral hypoxia

21. A patient is admitted to the hospital with a possible embolus in the brachial artery. The nurse would expect which of the following orders?

   A. Bed rest, heparin therapy

   B. Analgesic, force fluids, Coumadin therapy

   C. Radiology exam and possible angioplasty

   D. Narcotic analgesics and vasodilators

22. A patient is receiving a continuous heparin infusion for theraupeutic management of thrombophlebitis. Which lab value would the nurse monitor?

   A. Hemoglobin

   B. Prothrombin time

   C. Partial thromboplastin time

   D. Erythrocyte sedimentation rate

23. If a patient with atherosclerosis exhibits symptoms of dizziness, confusion, and transient ischemic attacks, the area affected is most likely the:

   A. Cerebral vein

   B. Carotid arteries

   C. Coronary arteries

   D. Peripheral vessels

24. When reviewing the lab results for a patient with hypertension and atherosclerosis, the nurse would expect to find:

   A. High potassium

   B. High sodium

   C. High cholesterol

   D. High BUN

25. Because adults with a vascular occlusive disorder should avoid factors that cause vasoconstriction, the nurse would recommend:

   A. Stop-smoking program

   B. Weight loss program

   C. Referral to psychologist

   D. Cardiac support group

26. If a patient with an abdominal aneurysm were to suddenly develop hypotension, mottled extremities, and absent pulses, the nurse would:

   A. Prepare the patient for surgery

   B. Elevate the legs

   C. Medicate the patient for pain

   D. Reassure the patient that this is normal

27. A patient with hypertension is to follow a low sodium diet. Which of the following foods should be avoided?

    A. Turkey breast

    B. Eggs

    C. Sausage

    D. Lowfat milk

28. In a patient with severe arterial occlusive disease, the following symptoms would be evident:

    A. Dependent rubor and pallor when the extremity is elevated

    B. Pallor and cyanosis in the extremity

    C. Peripheral edema, cyanosis, and numbness

    D. Brownish discoloration, edema

29. In caring for a patient with arterial occlusive disease, the nurse would position the patient with:

    A. Legs elevated above the heart

    B. Legs level with the heart

    C. Legs in a dependent position

    D. Legs in any comfortable position

30. Cerebrovascular manifestations of hypertension would include:

    A. Chest pain, dizziness when arising

    B. Vertigo, lightheadedness, blurred vision

    C. Peripheral edema, weight gain

    D. Fatigue, palpitations

31. Patients with hypertension might be treated with any of the following medications EXCEPT:

    A. Beta blockers

    B. Calcium channel blockers

    C. Anticoagulants

    D. Antispasmodics

32. A patient is admitted with mild back pain and a throbbing sensation in the abdomen. The nurse can auscultate a bruit over the abdomen. These symptoms suggest:

    A. Renal thrombosis

    B. Aortic aneurysm

C. Heart attack

D. Pulmonary embolism

33. In caring for a patient following resection of a thoracic aneurysm, the nurse would consider which goal as primary:

    A. Maintaining systolic blood pressure < 120

    B. Medicating the patient for pain

    C. Preventing infection

    D. Maintaining adequate nutrition

34. The nurse should use which action to prevent venous stasis in a patient with a history of varicose veins?

    A. Apply elastic stockings

    B. Increase fluid intake

    C. Maintain activity restrictions

    D. Keep legs in dependent position

35. In caring for a patient with a history of a vascular disorder who is on bed rest, the nurse would take appropriate precautions to:

    A. Avoid venous stasis

    B. Provide adequate nutrition

    C. Provide relaxation therapy

    D. Prevent infection

36. When a patient with thrombophlebitis develops sudden chest pain, dyspnea, diaphoresis, and cyanosis, the nurse suspects:

    A. Heart attack

    B. Cerebrovascular accident

    C. Pulmonary embolism

    D. Pneumonia

37. A nurse should teach a patient with chronic venous insufficiency to do all of the following EXCEPT:

    A. Sit with legs in a dependent position

    B. Sit with legs above the level of the heart

    C. Avoid constricting garments

    D. Sleep with the foot of the bed elevated

38. Treatment for the patient with venous stasis ulcers would most likely include:

    A. Betadine compresses, antibiotics

B. Bedrest, analgesics

C. Saline compresses, local corticosteroid

D. Narcotics, vasodilators

True or False

39. _____ The most common occlusive disorder of the arteries is atherosclerosis.

40. _____ Drug therapy is the treatment of choice for most aneurysms.

41. _____ Atherosclerosis has been found in adults as young as 20 years old.

42. _____ Aneurysms are most frequently located in the femoral artery.

43. _____ Primary hypertension is caused by smoking.

44. _____ A false aneurysm is often the result of trauma to the vessel wall.

45. _____ Most older adults have some degree of atherosclerosis.

Questions

46. Write a nursing care plan for the patient with an obstructive arterial vascular disorder.

    Nursing Diagnosis: Altered tissue perfusion, peripheral

    Patient Outcome:

    Nursing Interventions:

47. Write a nursing care plan for the patient with a thrombophlebitis.

    Nursing Diagnosis: Knowledge deficit: nature of the disease, its treatment, and measures to reduce risk

    Patient Outcome:

    Nursing Interventions:

CLINICAL SITUATIONS

Situation ■ 1

Mr. Young is admitted to the hospital with severe peripheral vascular disease. On admission he states that he has severe claudication in his left leg, which severely limits his activity. The nurse cannot palpate any pulse and sees that his extremities are pale and cool. The following questions relate to this situation.

1. Because the nurse is unable to palpate any pulses, the next step would be:

    A. Chart the findings

    B. Call the physician

    C. Use a Doppler probe

    D. Medicate for pain

2. The reason for claudication in a patient with peripheral vascular disease is:

    A. Too much exercise

    B. Tissue ischemia

    C. Lack of adherence to medications

    D. All of the above

3. Mr. Young will undergo a femoral-popliteal bypass operation with a graft inserted. The nurse would explain the procedure by stating:

    A. The diseased part of your artery will be removed and a graft inserted.

    B. A vein from your leg will be used to provide circulation.

    C. A synthetic graft will be inserted above and below the area of stenosis.

    D. The diseased part of your vein will be cleaned out and a graft placed around it.

4. The evening after surgery Mr. Young complains of numbness, pain, tingling, and burning pain in his leg. An appropriate nursing action would be:

    A. Assess pulses

    B. Medicate for pain

    C. Notify the physician

    D. Chart this information

5. Later in the evening, Mr. Young has severe pain in the leg and foot. The physician can no longer

find any pulses. A probable cause of these symptoms is:

A. Thrombus

B. Embolus

C. Vasospasm

D. Infection

6. The most likely intervention at this time would be:

A. Angioplasty

B. Medicate with narcotics

C. Embolectomy

D. X-ray of extremity

7. Following the procedure, Mr. Young is stabilized. Based on his history and postoperative complications, the nurse would anticipate that he would receive:

A. Narcotics

B. Anticoagulants

C. Vasodilators

D. Antibiotics

Situation ■ 2

Mrs. Raymond has been hospitalized for several weeks following a back injury. She has a history of hypertension, cardiac disease, and adult onset diabetes. The following questions relate to this situation.

1. Because the nurse recognizes problems that can result from immobility, she would be sure to assess _____ in this patient.

A. Trousseau's sign

B. Homans' sign

C. Pain response

D. Neurologic status

2. Late in the day, Mrs. Raymond complains of pain and warmth in her right calf. The following test is ordered:

A. Blood culture

B. Venogram

C. Arteriogram

D. Heart catheterization

3. A diagnosis of thrombophlebitis is confirmed. The patient is started on heparin therapy at 1000 units/hour. A nursing priority would be:

A. Monitor for bleeding

B. Monitor coagulation studies

C. Avoid the use of aspirin

D. All of the above

4. Since Mrs. Raymond is to be discharged on Coumadin, the nurse would provide the following instructions EXCEPT:

A. Take the medication until it is discontinued by the physician

B. Notify the dentist if any work is to be done

C. Continue to take all previous medications

D. Return to the medical laboratory for follow-up studies

Unit Seven

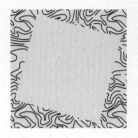

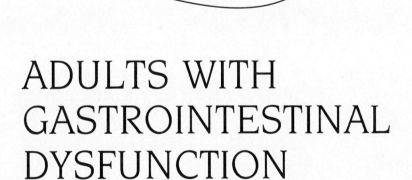

ADULTS WITH GASTROINTESTINAL DYSFUNCTION

Chapter Twenty-one

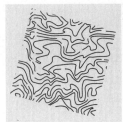

KNOWLEDGE BASIC TO THE NURSING CARE
of Adults with Gastrointestinal Dysfunction

Learning Objectives

1.0 Review the Anatomy and Physiology of the Gastrointestinal (GI) System.

1.1 Identify the Parts of the GI System.
1.2 Identify the Purposes of the Parts of the GI System.
1.3 Review the Process of Digestion.

2.0 Demonstrate an Understanding of the Assessment Data Related to the GI System.

2.1 Identify the Clinical Manifestations Which Indicate a GI Dysfunction.
2.2 Identify Specific Nursing Interventions Which are Appropriate for the Patient with Symptoms of GI Dysfunction.
2.3 Match Diagnostic Tests Used for GI Dysfunction with the Appropriate Description.
2.4 Demonstrate Application of the Nursing Process when Caring for the Patient Undergoing a Diagnostic Test.

3.0 Demonstrate an Understanding of the Medical Management of the Adult with a GI Alteration.

3.1 Identify the Rationale for Gastrointestinal Intubation.
3.2 Plan the Nursing Care for the Patient with a GI Tube.
3.3 Identify the Purposes of Enteral Hyperalimentation.
3.4 Demonstrate Application of the Nursing Process to the Care of the Patient on Enteral Feedings.

4.0 Demonstrate an Understanding of the Surgical Management of the Patient with a GI Alteration.

4.1 Identify Complications Associated with GI Surgery.
4.2 Plan the Postoperative Care of the Patient Having Gastric Surgery.
4.3 Demonstrate an Understanding of the Needs of the Patient with a Colostomy.
4.4 Write a Nursing Care Plan for the Patient Who Has Had Gastric Surgery.

Learning Activities

Fill In

1. The buccal glands, located in the oral cavity, secrete small amounts of _____ .

2. The organs of the GI tract below the esophagus are covered by the _____ .

3. Food and fluids are moved down the esophagus to the stomach by a process known as _____ .

4. The ringlike muscle which controls the opening between the stomach and the duodenum is known as the _____ .

5. The intrinsic factor, secreted in the stomach, is essential for the absorption of _____ in the terminal ileum.

6. Gastrin secretion is controlled by a _____ feedback mechanism based on the _____ of the stomach contents.

7. Food enters the stomach, is macerated and mixed with gastric secretions, then leaves in the form of a substance called _____ .

8. The three segments of the small intestine are the

_____ .

9. The principal organ of digestion and absorption is the _____ .

10. The adequate production of _____ is necessary to ensure the emulsification of fats into fatty acids and glycerides.

11. The _____ reabsorbs water and electrolytes and stores feces.

12. List three of the functions of the liver.
   1.
   2.
   3.

13. The major purpose of the gallbladder is to _____ bile.

14. The organ which is the primary producer of the digestive enzymes is the _____ .

Matching

A. Anorexia   C. Constipation
B. Nausea   D. Diarrhea

15. _____ Revulsion toward food
16. _____ Absence of a desire to eat
17. _____ Increased passage of liquid stool
18. _____ Infrequent passage of hard, dry stool

Questions

19. Susan is admitted with a diagnosis of anorexia, vomiting, and weight loss. Which of the following lab results would indicate she is in a state of malnutrition?

   A. WBC of 8500
   B. Hgb of 10.9
   C. Albumin of 3.0
   D. Potassium of 4.3

20. Before the nurse can establish a nursing care plan for Susan, what information should be obtained?

   A. Dietary history
   B. History and pattern of anorexia
   C. Factors which precipitate vomiting

D. General nutritional status

E. All of the above

21. Physical findings which indicate malnutrition include:

A. Heart rate of 100, respiratory rate of 22

B. Dull, thin, brittle nails

C. Dry skin, edema of the feet

D. Bruising of the forearms and trunk

22. If, during an abdominal assessment, the nurse finds the patient has a boardlike abdomen, she would notify the physician because this might mean:

A. Peritonitis

B. GI bleeding

C. Constipation

D. Aneurysm

23. The major complication of continuous vomiting is:

A. Weight loss

B. Cardiac dysrhythmias

C. Fluid and electrolyte imbalance

D. Aspiration of vomitus

24. The presence of coffee-ground material in vomitus is often indicative of:

A. Fresh gastrointestinal bleeding

B. Ingestion of excessive amounts of coffee

C. Old blood in the GI system

D. An obstruction in the biliary system

25. An appropriate nursing intervention to provide comfort for the patient who has severe diarrhea would be:

A. Give sitz baths several times daily

B. Administer analgesics

C. Administer antidiarrheal medication

D. Encourage bed rest

26. When a patient has several episodes of blood mixed with stool, the nurse would suspect:

A. Colon cancer

B. Inflammatory bowel disease

C. Malnutrition

D. Ulcer

Matching

Match the following diagnostic procedures with their descriptions.

A. Gastric analysis   E. Cholangiogram
B. Upper GI series   F. Esophagogastroduo-
C. Barium enema   denoscopy (EGD)
D. Oral cholecystogram   G. Ultrasonography

27. _____ Aids in the diagnosis of gallbladder disease

28. _____ Direct visualization of the esophagus, stomach, and duodenum

29. _____ X-ray examination of the esophagus, stomach, and duodenum

30. _____ Contrast medium is used to outline the hepatic, cystic, and common bile ducts

31. _____ Allows visualization of strictures as the patient swallows barium

32. _____ Radiologic examination of the rectum and colon

33. _____ Uses high-frequency sound waves to form images of internal structures

34. _____ Dependent on the absorption and excretion of orally ingested radiopaque dye tablets

35. _____ Done to determine if hydrochloric acid is present in the stomach

36. _____ Requires a bowel prep prior to the procedure

Questions

37. Absence of gastric acid in a gastric analysis may indicate:

A. Ulcer disease

B. Malignant disease

C. Occult bleeding

D. Pernicious anemia

38. A priority in the management of the patient with GI bleeding is:

A. Take vital signs and reassure patient

B. Transfer to ICU

C. Assess blood loss and return to hemodynamic stability

D. Replace blood loss with isotonic IV fluid

39. The nurse would recognize that a severe blood loss of over 40% of total volume has occurred in a person with a normal BP of 120/80 when:

A. Systolic pressure < 100 mm Hg and pulse > 100

B. Systolic pressure < 110 mm Hg and pulse > 120

C. Systolic pressure < 70 mm Hg and pulse > 130

D. Systolic pressure is 70–90 mm Hg and pulse 110–120

40. Which of the following conditions could not be detected through an upper GI series?

A. Esophageal tumor

B. Colon cancer

C. Diverticula

D. Gastric ulcer

41. Following the upper GI series, the nurse would:

A. Keep the patient flat for 4 hours

B. Force fluids

C. Administer a cathartic

D. Administer a diuretic

42. As the nurse prepares Mr. Martin for an oral cholecystogram, he says that he is allergic to shrimp. What is an appropriate nursing intervention at this time?

A. Call the physician and tell him of the allergy

B. Note the allergy but continue with the procedure

C. Call radiology and cancel the test

D. Administer the Telepaque tablets and keep the patient on NPO status

43. Mr. Martin is also scheduled for an EGD. The most serious complication following this procedure is:

A. Aspiration pneumonia

B. Perforation of the GI tract

C. Allergic reaction to dye

D. Fluid and electrolyte imbalance

44. Following the EGD procedure, how soon will Mr. Martin be allowed to resume his diet?

A. Eight hours after the procedure

B. As soon as he is alert

C. As soon as his gag reflex returns

D. As soon as he can talk

Matching

Match the following medications with their descriptions.

A. Laxatives   C. Antacids
B. Antidiarrheal

45. _____ Over-the-counter alkaline compounds that neutralize gastric acid.

46. _____ Drugs used to facilitate or stimulate passage of feces.

47. _____ Decrease fluidity of feces and the frequency of defecation.

48. _____ Can affect absorption of many drugs as a result of raising gastric pH.

49. _____ Side effects include dehydration and electrolyte imbalance.

Questions

50. List three reasons for gastrointestinal intubation.

1.

2.

3.

51. Which of the following nasogastric tubes has a double lumen and a small air vent?

A. Salem sump

B. Levin tube

C. Dobbhoff tube

D. Blakemore tube

52. What is the correct method of determining the distance to insert a nasogastric tube?

    A. Measure the distance from the tip of the nose to the earlobe to the xiphoid process

    B. Measure the distance from the tip of the nose to the earlobe to the xiphoid and add 5 cm

    C. Measure the distance from the tip of earlobe to the nose and then to the xiphoid

    D. Measure the distance from the nose to the area on the patient's left side just below the diaphragm

53. As the nurse slowly inserts an NG tube, the patient starts to cough. What is an appropriate intervention?

    A. Continue to advance the tube, but more slowly.

    B. Encourage the patient to take sips of water to facilitate passage and help him to stop coughing.

    C. Withdraw the tube and retry later.

    D. Withdraw the tube and call the physician.

54. A patient returns from surgery with an NG tube to intermittent suction. One of the nursing diagnoses is: altered oral mucous membrane. Which intervention will assist the nurse in reaching this goal?

    A. Have the patient take small sips of water or ice

    B. Have the patient use lemon and glycerin swabs

    C. Have the patient brush her teeth and rinse every 4 hours

    D. Have the patient gargle with Cepacol every 4 hours

55. Which of the following would NOT be an indication for enteral feedings (tube feeding)?

    A. Patient has anorexia and has lost 5 pounds.

    B. Patient has a GI obstruction.

    C. Patient has a decreased level of consciousness.

    D. Patient has malabsorption syndrome.

56. An unconscious patient is receiving a continuous tube feeding to provide needed nutrients. Which of the following feedings would not be appropriate for meeting his or her needs?

    A. Ensure

    B. Isocal

    C. Osmolite

    D. Vivonex

57. What is a rationale for using nasoenteric tubes for the administration of tube feedings?

    A. They are less likely to clog

    B. They help prevent reflux esophagitis

    C. They allow for rapid administration of feedings

    D. They don't have a weighted tip

58. An advantage of a percutaneous gastrostomy over a surgical gastrostomy is that:

    A. There is less risk since general anesthesia isn't used

    B. The procedure is less costly

    C. Recovery is faster

    D. All of the above

59. A patient with a jejunostomy tube is on continuous tube feeding. All of the following are important nursing interventions EXCEPT:

    A. Auscultate bowel sounds

    B. Check for placement of feeding tube

    C. Aspirate for residual

    D. Assess for tolerance of feeding

60. Which of the following symptoms, if present, would indicate that a patient cannot tolerate his tube feeding?

    A. Residual of 50 ml every 4 hours

    B. Patient is complaining of thirst and is confused

    C. Patient develops a respiratory infection

    D. Patient shows signs of dehydration

61. When would total parenteral nutrition (TPN) be the best choice to meet the individual's nutritional needs?

    A. When the patient is >75 years of age

    B. When the needs can't be met through the GI tract

    C. When the patient has a systemic infection

    D. When the patient is severely dehydrated

62. List three major complications which may occur during the administration of TPN.

    1.

    2.

    3.

63. A major complication which can occur during the insertion of the central venous catheter is:

    A. Pneumothorax

    B. Sepsis

    C. Hemorrhage

    D. All of the above

64. Why is TPN started at a slow rate and increased gradually?

    A. To prevent infection

    B. To allow the pancreas time to adjust

    C. To allow the liver time to adjust

    D. To prevent hypoglycemia

65. A patient is receiving TPN at 100 ml/hour. What is the rationale for having the patient perform a Valsalva maneuver during IV tubing changes?

    A. To prevent hemorrhage

    B. To prevent infection

    C. To prevent an air embolism

    D. To prevent speed shock

66. A patient is severely malnourished related to vomiting and anorexia. He is started on TPN. The nursing diagnosis is:altered nutrition. Pick an appropriate patient outcome.

    A. Patient describes the procedure involved with TPN

    B. Patient is afebrile during administration of TPN

    C. Patient is in positive nitrogen balance

    D. Patient states relief from anxiety

67. Patients having surgery of the GI tract are at risk for a number of complications. List four of these.

    1.

    2.

    3.

    4.

68. Why is a postoperative patient generally kept on NPO status until peristalsis returns?

    A. Because the surgery and anesthetic often result in some degree of paralytic ileus

    B. Because of the great risk of wound dehiscence

    C. Because of the high incidence of nausea and vomiting in the first 24 hours

    D. Because of the risk of developing an infection

69. From the list below, pick the appropriate preparation(s) of the patient prior to intestinal resection.

    A. Empty the bowel of all stool

    B. Give patient Go-Lytely or enemas

    C. Keep on low-residue diet

    D. Give oral anti-infectives

    E. Provide fluid and electrolytes

    F. Insert NG tube

70. Which of the following nursing interventions would be important to implement with the patient prior to gastric surgery?

    A. Teach patient how to cough and deep breathe

    B. Teach patient how to do incisional care

    C. Teach patient dietary restrictions

    D. All of the above

71. A surgical resection of the bowel has many potential complications. Which complication is more likely to occur about 1 week after surgery?

    A. Wound infection

    B. Wound dehiscence

    C. Paralytic ileus

    D. Pulmonary embolus

72. Following gastric surgery, what position would be best for the patient?

    A. Flat with the legs slightly elevated

    B. Left lateral Sims'

    C. Semi-Fowler's

    D. Prone

73. In a patient who has had a bowel resection, the nurse should take special precautions to prevent:

    A. Ineffective ventilation

B. Dehydration

C. Thrombophlebitis

D. All of the above

74. Following gastric surgery, there is an increased risk for an alteration in peripheral tissue perfusion. Choose an appropriate intervention to prevent this problem.

A. Have patient cough and deep breathe every 2 hours

B. Have patient do leg and foot exercises every 2 hours

C. Position patient with the head of the bed up and the knees gatched

D. Keep patient on bed rest for at least 72 hours

75. A patient undergoes an ascending colostomy. Which description is true about the fecal output?

A. The output is predominantly liquid

B. The output is tan and mushy

C. The output is soft and semiformed

D. The output is identical to normal stools

76. A temporary colostomy would not be performed for which of the following conditions?

A. Diverticulitis

B. Volvulus

C. Gunshot to the abdomen

D. Colorectal cancer

77. When a double-barreled colostomy is created on the abdominal wall, the functioning colon is the:

A. Proximal stoma

B. Distal stoma

C. Rectum

78. One of the potential complications of colostomy surgery is stomal necrosis. The cause of this condition is:

A. Infection

B. Hemorrhage

C. Impaired circulation

D. Bowel perforation

79. Which emotional response in the patient with a colostomy may indicate grieving because of altered body structure?

A. Anger

B. Depression

C. Denial

D. Withdrawal

E. All of the above

80. Which comment by the patient with a permanent colostomy would indicate to the nurse that the individual is NOT ready for learning?

A. Patient says, "This makes me anxious."

B. Patient says, "Why did this happen to me?"

C. Patient says, "I'm not going to look at that."

D. Patient says, "My father also had a colostomy."

81. When teaching a patient who has a sigmoid colostomy, the nurse is aware that:

A. Control over bowel elimination can never be totally regulated.

B. Control over bowel elimination may be gained in time by a regular diet.

C. Control over bowel elimination is gained through daily irrigations of the stoma.

D. Control is so difficult to achieve that it is usually a waste of time to try.

82. Individuals with a colostomy are generally taught to avoid foods that cause diarrhea, odor, and excessive flatus. From the foods listed below, which are likely to have these side effects?

A. Cheese, chocolate, milk

B. Fresh broccoli, mushrooms, cabbage

C. Nuts, cereal, pasta

D. Yogurt, buttermilk, parsley

83. A major problem for the patient with an ileostomy is:

A. High risk for fluid volume deficit

B. Potential for alteration in bowel elimination (constipation)

C. Potential for sexual dysfunction

D. Potential for ineffective breathing patterns

84. Teaching the patient about the care of the colostomy is an important nursing function. Write an appropriate nursing diagnosis, patient outcome, and several nursing interventions that address this.

    Nursing Diagnosis:

    Patient Outcome:

    Nursing Interventions:

85. Plan the nursing care for the patient scheduled for a subtotal gastrectomy.

    Write the appropriate patient outcomes and nursing interventions for each of the following nursing diagnoses.

    Nursing Diagnosis: Anxiety related to anesthesia and proposed surgery

    Patient Outcome:

    Nursing Interventions:

    Nursing Diagnosis: Knowledge deficit related to preoperative preparation and postoperative course.

    Patient Outcome:

    Nursing Interventions:

86. Plan the nursing care for the patient who has had a bowel resection.

    Write an appropriate patient outcome and several nursing interventions for each nursing diagnosis.

    Nursing Diagnosis: Pain related to surgical trauma to the abdomen

    Patient Outcome:

    Nursing Interventions:

    Nursing Diagnosis: Ineffective breathing pattern

    Patient Outcome:

    Nursing Interventions:

87. Write a nursing care plan for the patient with anorexia.

    Nursing Diagnosis: Altered nutrition: less than body requirements, related to lack of appetite.

    Patient Outcome:

    Nursing Interventions:

88. Write a nursing care plan for the patient with a gastrointestinal tube.

    Nursing Diagnosis: Altered oral mucous membrane related to mouth breathing

    Patient Outcome:

    Nursing Interventions:

CLINICAL SITUATIONS

Situation ■ 1

Paul Fitzpatrick is admitted with a history of intermittent vomiting for the past 2 weeks. He also states that he has had some diarrhea and black stools. He is to have diagnostic tests to determine the cause of his problem. The following questions relate to this situation.

1. Which nursing diagnosis would have a priority when you develop the nursing care plan?

    A. High risk for fluid volume deficit

    B. Decreased cardiac output

    C. Pain

    D. Activity intolerance

2. After being examined by the physician, Paul is told that he has gastrointestinal bleeding, possibly due to an ulcer. Which of the following data

would be consistent with a serious blood loss of 25–40%?

A. BP 100/60, Pulse 98

B. BP 88/50, Pulse 124

C. BP 70/40, Pulse 80

D. BP 90/44, Pulse 48

3. The results of the hemoglobin and hematocrit values are not truly reflective of the amount of blood loss until _____ after the onset of bleeding.

A. 4–6 hours

B. 6–12 hours

C. 12–24 hours

D. 24–36 hours

4. Outcomes which would indicate stabilization of the patient with acute bleeding would be:

A. Increase of BP by 20–30 systolic, decrease in pulse

B. Return of normal BP, disappearance of vasospasm, urine output of 30 ml/ hour

C. BP of 100/70, pulse > 50, improvement of cyanosis

D. BP returns to normal, pulse 60–120, RR 12–28

5. Results of which diagnostic test would determine the presence of an ulcer?

A. Arteriogram

B. Insertion of a nasogastric tube

C. Flexible endoscopy

D. Bronchoscopy

Situation ■ 2

Donna Perone is an 18-year-old who is admitted to the unit with severe anorexia nervosa. She has lost 30 pounds in the last 3 months. Her current weight is 90 pounds. She is admitted for evaluation and possible enteral feedings.

1. Which of the following statements is true in regard to nutritional needs of the normal adult?

A. Adults ordinarily need 1500–2000 calories and 0.5 g/kg of protein per day

B. Adults ordinarily need 1800–2500 calories and 1 g/kg of protein per day

C. Adults need 1500–2500 calories and 2 g/kg of protein per day

D. During illness, the calorie needs and protein needs will always decrease

2. Donna is started on Osmolite (1 calorie/ml). She is receiving a continuous feeding of 75 ml/hour per pump through a feeding tube. How many calories will this provide per day?

A. 1500 calories

B. 1800 calories

C. 2000 calories

D. 2400 calories

3. As the primary nurse, you choose a priority nursing goal for Donna. Which of the following would be most appropriate?

A. Altered nutrition: less than body requirements

B. Fluid volume deficit

C. Diarrhea related to formula intolerance

D. Potential for ineffective breathing pattern related to feeding tube

4. For the patient receiving enteral feedings, fluid status is always important. Knowing this, how much water would you give Donna, knowing her urine output was 2500 ml in the last 24 hours?

A. At least 200 ml in 24 hours

B. At least 800 ml in 24 hours

C. At least 1000 ml in 24 hours

D. At least 2000 ml in 24 hours

5. An important part of the nursing care for this patient is assessment of the tube for placement and residual. When you do the morning assessment, you obtain 100 ml of residual. What is an appropriate nursing action?

A. Stop the feeding for 60 minutes, then recheck

B. Stop the feeding for 4 hours, then recheck

C. Continue the feeding as ordered, but recheck in 1 hour

D. Continue the feeding, but tell the physician when he or she makes rounds

Situation ■ 3

Mrs. Wolf is very malnourished. She is having a central venous catheter inserted for the administration of TPN prior to having a surgical resection of the bowel. The following questions refer to this situation.

1. Following the insertion of the catheter, what would the physician order?

   A. CVC to be checked by a chest x-ray

   B. TPN to be administered at 25 ml/hour

   C. Dextrose and water to run at 50ml/hour

   D. To have a dressing applied to the CVC daily

2. The physician and the dietitian determine that it is best to start the TPN solution of 10% dextrose at 50 ml/hour. Which of the following complications can occur as a result of too rapid administration of the solution?

   A. Infection

   B. Hypoglycemic reaction

   C. Hyperglycemic reaction

   D. Overhydration

3. Which procedure should the nurse follow when changing the catheter tubing?

   A. With the patient lying flat, have her perform a Valsalva maneuver when the catheter is opened

   B. With the patient in Trendelenburg's position, have her breathe in and out slowly to change the catheter

   C. Have another nurse present; then always cross-clamp the tubing before changing it

   D. Change the tubing quickly, but proceed the same as with any other IV tubing change

4. Mrs. Wolf is also to receive 500 ml of 10% lipids twice a week. Which of the statements about lipid administration is NOT true?

   A. Keep at room temperature before administering

   B. Always administer through a filter

   C. Never leave the solutions hanging longer than 12 hours

   D. Run slowly initially and observe for adverse reactions

Chapter Twenty-two

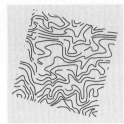

NURSING CARE
of Adults with
Disorders of the
Upper Gastrointestinal System

Learning Objectives

1.0 Demonstrate an Understanding of the Inflammatory Processes of the Upper Gastrointestinal (GI) System.

1.1 Identify Clinical Manifestations Associated with Esophagitis.
1.2 Identify Clinical Manifestations Associated with Gastritis.
1.3 Plan Nursing Interventions for the Patient with Gastritis.

2.0 Demonstrate an Understanding of the Structural and Functional Abnormalities of the Upper GI System.

2.1 Review the Etiology of Ulcer Disease.
2.2 Identify the Medical Treatment of the Patient with an Ulcer.
2.3 Identify Surgical Interventions Used in the Treatment of Ulcers.
2.4 Demonstrate Application of the Nursing Process when Caring for the Patient with a Functional Abnormality.
2.5 Identify the Learning Needs of the Patient with an Ulcer.
2.6 Plan the Nursing Care for the Patient Having a Surgical Resection of the Upper GI System.

3.0 Demonstrate an Understanding of the Types of Neoplasms That Affect the Upper GI System.

3.1 Identify the Clinical Manifestations Associated with Neoplasms of the Upper GI System.
3.2 Identify the Medical Management for the Patient with a Gastric Neoplasm.
3.3 Review the Surgical Management for the Patient with a Gastric Neoplasm.
3.4 Plan the Nursing Care for the Patient with a Gastric Neoplasm.

Learning Activities

Define

1. Esophagitis:

2. Gastritis:

3. Peptic ulcer:

4. Stress ulcer:

5. Hiatus hernia:

6. Achalasia:

7. Presbyesophagus:

8. Achlorhydria:

Questions

9. List three factors which may trigger an attack of esophagitis.

   1.

   2.

   3.

10. List three of the classic symptoms which have been associated with esophagitis.

    1.

    2.

    3.

Matching

A. Antacids
B. Histamine H_2 receptor

C. Proton pump inhibitors

11. _____ Decrease the basal secretion of gastric acid.

12. _____ Duration of action is 6–12 hours.

13. _____ Inhibit the enzyme that produces gastric acid.

14. _____ Neutralize acid present in the stomach.

15. _____ Can be taken orally once daily to suppress gastric acid secretion.

16. _____ Do not heal the ulcer but provide an environment conducive to healing.

Questions

17. Oral infections may be due to which of the following? Check all that apply.

    A. Poor oral hygiene

    B. Poor nutrition

    C. Stress

    D. Systemic disorders

18. Pain from ulcerated areas in the mouth may be relieved by which of the following? Check all that apply.

    A. Topical anesthetic agents

    B. Cepacol spray

    C. Soothing foods

    D. Viscous xylocaine

19. Which of the following medications has been found to irritate the gastric mucosa?

    A. Maalox

    B. Digoxin

    C. Tylenol

    D. Carafate

20. Medical management of esophagitis would include:

    A. Bland diet

    B. No smoking

    C. Antacids

    D. All of the above

21. For the patient with chronic esophagitis, surgical resection of the esophagus is indicated if _____ were to occur.

    A. Chronic reflux

    B. Perforation

    C. Stricture

    D. Bleeding

22. An undesirable side effect of over-the-counter (OTC) remedies for esophagitis is:

    A. Continued symptoms

    B. Hemorrhage

    C. Metabolic acidosis

    D. Diarrhea

23. Which statement made by Mr. Smith could indicate a precipitating factor in his current hospitalization for acute gastritis?

    A. I recently started drinking coffee

    B. I never touch alcohol

    C. I started going to Weight Watchers

    D. I walk 2 miles daily

24. Mr. Smith is placed on a medication to inhibit gastric acid secretion. This would most likely be:

    A. Carafate

    B. Aspirin

    C. Cimetidine

    D. Ampicillin

25. Mr. Smith is being discharged today. What is the best indicator that the nurse's teaching has been effective?

    A. Mr. Smith states that he will see the doctor in 6 weeks

    B. Mr. Smith lists foods which he should avoid

    C. Mr. Smith states that he won't eat after 5 PM

    D. Mr. Smith says that he has no questions

True or False

26. _____ Calcium-based antacids cause diarrhea.

27. _____ The etiology of chronic gastritis is unknown.

28. _____ Chronic gastritis is often asymptomatic.

29. _____ Chronic gastritis is treated with Zantac or Tagamet.

30. _____ Gastric cancer occurs more often in patients with chronic gastritis.

31. _____ Antacids can heal an ulcer.

32. _____ Histamine H_2-receptor antagonists facilitate ulcer healing.

33. _____ A vagotomy is done to promote parasympathetic stimulation.

34. _____ Surgery is recommended for the patient with a bleeding ulcer.

35. _____ Adenocarcinomas are the most common forms of oral cancers.

36. _____ Malignant lesions of the lip tend to rise in areas of leukoplakia.

37. _____ Nonmetastasized lesions of the lip are treated with chemotherapy.

38. _____ Esophageal cancer has a good prognosis with surgery.

Questions

39. The presence of stomatitis in the patient with chronic gastritis indicates which of the following?

    A. Deficiency of calcium

    B. Deficiency of vitamin K

C. Deficiency of vitamin B_{12}

D. Deficiency of histamine

40. Ulcers are a common disorder. They account for approximately what percentage of hospital admissions?

A. 10%

B. 20%

C. 30%

41. The major symptom(s) of uncomplicated peptic ulcer is:

A. Hemorrhage

B. Change in appetite

C. Nausea and vomiting

D. Pain

42. Gastric ulcers are thought to result from:

A. Decreased mucosal resistance to the effects of gastric acid

B. Increased exposure of the mucosa to highly acidic materials

C. Increase in the amount of gastric secretion

D. Stress and overactive acid production

43. In the individual with a gastric ulcer, what are two potential complications if it is left untreated?

A. Infection, stricture

B. Obstruction, bleeding

C. Hemorrhage, perforation

D. Sepsis, obstruction

44. When is the pain of a gastric ulcer most likely to occur?

A. Immediately before meals

B. Immediately after eating

C. Several hours after eating

D. Anytime during the day

45. A diagnosis of a peptic ulcer would be confirmed by which of the following diagnostic tests?

A. Endoscopy

B. Sigmoidoscopy

C. Barium studies

D. Angiogram

46. Which particular diet has been found to be effective in the treatment of ulcers?

A. Sippy diet

B. Bland, soft diet

C. Diet low in fiber and roughage

D. Diet which avoids irritating foods

47. Which of the following symptoms indicates a possible obstructive process in the individual with a peptic ulcer?

A. Vomiting of partially digested food

B. Flat, rigid, boardlike abdomen

C. Sudden loss of consciousness

D. Projectile vomiting of blood

48. If, when assessing a patient, the nurse notices _____ , these symptoms indicate a possible perforated ulcer.

A. Tachycardia, hypertension, cyanosis

B. Rigid abdomen, severe pain, symptoms of shock

C. High fever, lethargy, sudden vomiting

D. Mid-epigastric pain, diarrhea, vomiting

49. Medical treatment of a perforated ulcer would include which of the following interventions? Check all that apply.

A. Nasogastric or gastric suction

B. Fluid and electrolyte replacement

C. Antibiotic therapy

D. Ventilator support

E. Surgical intervention

50. The type of ulcer which might develop in the patient who has experienced a severe burn is known as:

A. Cushing's ulcer

B. Peptic ulcer

C. Curling's ulcer

D. Duodenal ulcer

51. When assessing the patient admitted with a stress ulcer, the nurse would expect to find:

    A. History of chronic pain

    B. History of nausea and vomiting

    C. History of hematemesis or melena

    D. History of acute sharp pain and reflux

52. Treatment of an acute stress ulcer would involve which of the following medical regimens?

    A. Antacids every hour, histamine antagonists every 2 hours

    B. Antacids every 4 hours by mouth

    C. Parenteral histamine antagonists; antacids by nasogastric tube every hour

    D. Analgesics, antibiotics every 4 hours, Maalox PRN for pain

53. Medical management of an acute bleeding ulcer would include which of the following? Check all that apply.

    A. Preparation for surgery

    B. Gastric lavage and vasoconstrictive medication

    C. Electrocoagulation during endoscopy

    D. Histamine H_2 receptors given IV

54. What is the major contributing factor which has been found to lead to the development of a hiatus hernia?

    A. Recurrent attacks of stress ulcers

    B. Prolonged use of steroids

    C. Repeated abdominal surgeries

    D. Increase in intra-abdominal pressure

55. When a patient has a hiatus hernia, the nurse would expect the patient to have _____ as the main symptom.

    A. Pain when swallowing

    B. Heartburn

    C. Belching

    D. Vomiting

56. The diagnosis of a hiatus hernia is confirmed by which of the following diagnostic tests?

    A. Barium swallow

    B. Sigmoidoscopy

    C. Bronchoscopy

    D. Chest x ray

57. The nurse is doing discharge planning for a patient with a hiatus hernia. Which of the following statements would indicate that the patient has a clear understanding of the nurse's instructions?

    A. I must eat three regular meals daily

    B. I should remain sitting after my meals

    C. I should lie down and rest for 30 minutes after meals

    D. I can eat anything I want, as long as I take my medicine

58. In the patient who has had a fundoplication for the treatment of a hiatus hernia, which of the following would be your choice for the nursing diagnosis?

    A. High risk for fluid volume deficit

    B. High risk for aspiration

    C. Ineffective airway clearance

    D. Alteration in tissue perfusion

59. Symptoms associated with achalasia are:

    A. Difficulty swallowing, pain radiating to the jaw

    B. Heartburn, vomiting

    C. Nausea, vomiting, diarrhea

    D. None of the above

60. Medical management of achalasia aimed at alleviating the obstruction in the esophagus might include:

    A. Esophageal dilatation

    B. Drug therapy

    C. Surgery

    D. Any of the above

61. Factors which have been identified as being causes of oral cancer are:

    A. Use of tobacco and alcohol

    B. Stress and smoking

C. Low residue diet

D. OTC drugs such as aspirin and antacids

62. In caring for a patient who has had intermaxillary fixation, the nurse would consider which nursing diagnosis as primary?

A. High risk for infection

B. Ineffective airway clearance

C. Ineffective individual coping

D. Altered nutrition: potential for more than body requirements

63. Which equipment should the nurse keep at the bedside of the patient having an intermaxillary fixation?

A. Tracheotomy set

B. Large hemostats

C. Wire cutters

D. Ambu bag

64. In caring for a patient having a total glossectomy, the nurse would be chiefly concerned with which patient outcome?

A. Patient socializes with other patients.

B. Patient asks to eat meals in private.

C. Patient tells friends not to visit yet.

D. Patient watches television for distraction.

65. Which of the following factors have been implicated in the development of esophageal cancer? Check all that apply.

A. Smoking

B. Alcohol abuse

C. Poor nutrition

D. Poor hygiene

66. Diagnosis of esophageal cancer is usually made by

A. Chest x-ray

B. CT scan

C. X-ray of the esophagram with a barium swallow

D. Angiogram

67. The treatment of choice for the individual with cancer of the esophagus would most likely be:

A. Chemotherapy

B. Surgery

C. Radiation

68. A frequently fatal development that can result from esophagogastrectomy is:

A. Septic shock

B. Hemorrhage

C. Leaking of the anastomosis

D. Pulmonary emboli

69. You are caring for a patient who has had radiation treatment for esophageal cancer. Which symptom is most indicative of a side effect of radiation therapy?

A. Continuous vomiting

B. Alopecia

C. Diarrhea

D. Pain on swallowing

70. Which of the following symptoms has been found to be related to gastric cancer?

A. Abdominal pain

B. Vague epigastric distress after eating

C. Sharp midsternal pain 2 hours after eating

D. Inability to swallow

71. For the elderly person who suffers from dysphagia, which foods would you instruct him or her to avoid?

A. Bananas, peanut butter

B. Apples, raisins

C. Oatmeal, whole wheat

D. Lettuce, tomatoes

72. Write a nursing care plan for the patient who has acute esophagitis.

Nursing Diagnosis: Pain related to esophageal inflammation

Patient Outcome:

Nursing Interventions:

73. Write a nursing care plan for the patient who has acute mid-epigastric pain and a possible ulcer.

Nursing Diagnosis:

Patient Outcome:

Nursing Interventions:

74. Write a nursing care plan for the patient with oral cancer who has had a total glossectomy and removal of the mandible. What is the most important aspect of your nursing care? Write this as a nursing diagnosis.

Nursing Diagnosis:

Patient Outcome:

Nursing Interventions:

CLINICAL SITUATIONS

Situation ■ 1

Mr. Wilson is a 44-year-old carpenter who is admitted with an episode of acute GI bleeding. He has a history of a peptic ulcer for 10 years.

1. Which of the following assessment data would indicate that the patient is bleeding internally?

   A. Hypotension, tachycardia, tachypnea

   B. Cyanosis, respiratory distress

   C. Hypertension, bradycardia, dyspnea

   D. Diaphoresis, abdominal pain

2. How would the nurse explain to Mr. Wilson what an ulcer is?

   A. Breaks along the intestinal tract

   B. Broken areas throughout the system caused by stress

   C. Ulceration of the gastric mucosa resulting from excessive amount of gastric secretions

   D. Opening in the stomach and intestine

3. Which observation on the part of the nurse is most indicative of this particular condition?

   A. Patient is pale and diaphoretic

   B. Patient is grimacing in pain

   C. Patient is vomiting

   D. Patient is lethargic

4. In a review of the patient's past medical history, which of the following medications would have been used in treatment for his peptic ulcer?

   A. Maalox and Zantac

   B. Cimetidine and Diuril

   C. Ampicillin and Lasix

   D. Maalox and Reglan

Situation ■ 2

Mr. Wilson does not respond to traditional medical treatment and is scheduled for a gastric resection in the morning. The nurse's responsibility involves preoperative teaching.

1. Mr. Wilson asks you what his surgery involves. You know that he is scheduled for a subtotal gastrectomy. You explain:

   A. The entire stomach is removed and the esophagus is attached to the duodenum

   B. The distal portion of the stomach, including the antrum and pylorus, is removed and attached to the duodenum

   C. The pylorus is incised and resutured

   D. The stomach is resected and the vagus nerve severed

2. Nursing care of a patient having this surgery should include observation for postoperative complications. These would include:

   A. Hemorrhage, projectile vomiting, ileus

   B. GI obstruction, infection

   C. Peritonitis, GI bleeding, GI obstruction

   D. Nausea, vomiting, infection

3. Mr. Wilson has been doing well when suddenly he complains of sudden, sharp, mid-epigastric pain which spreads across the abdomen. Based on your understanding of postoperative complications, what is a possible explanation for these symptoms?

   A. Mr. Wilson is hemorrhaging

   B. Mr. Wilson has developed peritonitis

C. Mr. Wilson is overreacting to normal pain

D. Mr. Wilson has a GI perforation

4. Mr. Wilson spends several days in ICU but is finally ready for discharge. Which of the following would you include in your discharge instructions? Check all that apply.

A. Instruct patient on ways to cope with stress

B. Instruct patient on foods which should be avoided

C. Instruct patient to drink 1 quart of water per day

D. Instruct patient to change jobs to avoid stress

Situation ■ 3

Mr. Baily is a 60-year-old plumber who has been having difficulty swallowing for 2 months. He has been diagnosed as having squamous cell carcinoma of the esophagus and is scheduled for surgery.

1. Mr. Baily is having an esophagogastrostomy. How would the nurse explain this procedure?

A. The tumor is resected and the esophagus reanastamosed

B. The tumor is removed and the stomach attached to the remaining esophagus

C. The tumor is removed and a segment of colon is attached in the esophagus

2. What would the nurse tell Mr. Baily to prepare him for the postoperative course?

A. You will have a nasogastric tube and not be allowed to take anything in by mouth for 5 days

B. You will be in intensive care and on a ventilator

C. You will be started on clear liquid in 48 hours

D. You will have chest tubes for 7 days

3. Nursing care in the postoperative period is directed toward preventing:

A. Cardiac arrhythmias

B. Respiratory infections

C. Fluid volume overload

D. Diarrhea

Situation ■ 4

Mrs. Norris is 48 years old and has a history of chronic gastritis. She has lost 20 pounds and has had indigestion for the past 6 weeks. She is admitted for testing.

1. Mrs. Norris is scheduled for a barium study and gastroscopy in the morning. What information would you give to the patient?

A. You will have a liquid diet tonight, then nothing by mouth

B. You can have a regular diet tonight and liquid in the morning

C. You will have an enema in the morning

D. You don't have any special preparation for the test

2. Mrs. Norris has had a gastric resection. She is still in intensive care on the 3rd postoperative day. Which of the following findings is abnormal?

A. NG tube is draining a small amount of bloody drainage

B. Chest tube output of 50 ml serosanguineous drainage every 8 hours

C. Urinary output is 240 ml in 6 hours

D. Chest dressing is still draining pink fluid

3. Once Mrs. Norris is permitted to take fluids, what would the nurse do to prevent any problems associated with oral intake?

A. Give liquids only for 1 week

B. Give six small feedings daily

C. Maintain the NG tube for tube feedings

D. Maintain TPN until caloric intake is adequate

4. Instruct Mrs. Norris to lie down for 30 minutes after eating to prevent which of the following problems?

A. Postural hypotension

B. Gastric spasm

C. Dumping syndrome

D. Gastric reflux

Chapter Twenty-three

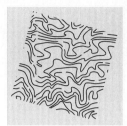

NURSING CARE
of Adults with Disorders of the Lower Gastrointestinal System

Learning Objectives

1.0 Demonstrate an Understanding of the Inflammatory Processes of the Lower Gastrointestinal System.

1.1 Define Several Lower Gastrointestinal (GI) Disorders.
1.2 Identify the Clinical Manifestations Associated with Lower GI Disorders.
1.3 Identify Medical Interventions Used to Treat Inflammatory Processes of the Lower GI System.
1.4 Identify Nursing Interventions Appropriate for Patients with an Inflammatory Bowel Disorder.
1.5 Identify Surgical Procedures Used for the Patient with an Inflammatory Bowel Disorder.

2.0 Demonstrate an Understanding of the Functional Disorders of the Lower GI System.

2.1 Define Several of the Functional Disorders.
2.2 Identify the Pathophysiology Involved with Several of the Functional Disorders.
2.3 Identify the Medical Management of Several Functional Disorders of the Lower GI System.
2.4 Identify Several of the Functional Disorders of the Lower GI Tract which Affect Nutrition.
2.5 Write a Nursing Care Plan for the Patient with a Functional Disorder of the Lower GI System.

3.0 Demonstrate an Understanding of the Structural Disorders of the Lower GI System.

3.1 Identify the Pathophysiology Involved with Several of the Structural Disorders.
3.2 Demonstrate an Understanding of the Medical Interventions Used to Treat Structural Disorders.

3.3 Demonstrate an Understanding of the Surgical Procedures Used to Treat the Structural Disorders.
3.4 Write a Nursing Care Plan for the Patient with a Structural Disorder of the Lower GI System.

4.0 Demonstrate an Understanding of the Types of Neoplasms that Affect the Lower GI System.

4.1 Identify the Clinical Manifestations of the Neoplasms which Affect the Lower GI System.
4.2 Review the Medical Management of the Patient with Cancer of the Colon.
4.3 Review the Surgical Management of the Patient with Colorectal Cancer.
4.4 Write a Nursing Care Plan for the Patient with a Neoplasm of the Lower GI System.

Learning Activities

Define

1. Peritonitis:

2. Appendicitis:

3. Ileus:

4. Diverticulitis:

5. Intestinal hernia:

6. Intestinal adhesions:

7. Hemorrhoids:

Fill In

8. In the pathology of appendicitis, an obstruction often results in an increased _____ pressure, which predisposes to _____ invasion.

9. List three of the predisposing factors which can lead to the development of hemorrhoids.

   1.

   2.

   3.

10. A paralytic ileus is due to reduced or absent _____ , whereas a mechanical ileus is a result of an _____ .

11. A simple diagnostic test which can be performed to make a diagnosis of lactase deficiency is _____

Questions

12. The individual with an inguinal hernia should be taught to avoid doing anything which could increase the intraabdominal pressure and result in actual herniation. List three instructions:

    1.

    2.

    3.

13. The most common cause of peritonitis is:

    A. Bacterial infection

    B. Viral infection

    C. Chemical irritation

    D. Environmental factors

14. Of the following conditions, which is NOT likely to lead to peritonitis?

    A. Perforated peptic ulcer

    B. Acute salpingitis

    C. Peritoneal dialysis

    D. Meningitis

15. The primary symptom of peritonitis is:

    A. Projectile vomiting

    B. Severe abdominal pain

    C. High temperature

    D. Anorexia, weight loss

16. When a patient develops peritonitis, the nurse would anticipate treatment with:

    A. Antiviral drugs

B. Antibiotics

C. Antipyretics

D. Analgesics

17. As a result of fluid loss from both the bowel lumen and the peritoneal cavity, the individual with peritonitis can develop:

A. Hypovolemia

B. Hemoconcentration

C. Acute tubular necrosis

D. All of the above

18. Which of the following would be indications that the treatment for peritonitis is effective?

A. Vital signs, including temperature, are normal

B. Active bowel sounds, passing stool, temperature normal

C. Patient is pain free, appetite returns, dressing is dry and intact

D. Patient is asymptomatic

19. One of the complications of appendicitis, perforation, can lead to:

A. Peritonitis

B. Hemorrhagic

C. Urosepsis

D. Diverticulitis

20. Which of the following clinical manifestations indicates a possible condition of appendicitis in a patient?

A. Rebound tenderness

B. Pain at McBurney's point

C. Anorexia and nausea

D. Any of the above

21. Medical management for the patient with appendicitis might include all of the following except:

A. Clear liquid diet

B. Intravenous fluids

C. Intravenous antibiotics

D. Diagnostic studies

22. Treatment of choice for acute appendicitis is:

A. Antibiotic therapy

B. Analgesics

C. Surgery

D. Laser surgery

23. When checking a patient following an appendectomy, the nurse notices abdominal distention and an absence of bowel sounds. This suggests:

A. Peritonitis

B. Diverticulitis

C. Paralytic ileus

D. Septicemia

True or False

24. _____ Crohn's disease can affect any part of the GI tract.

25. _____ Ulcerative colitis is caused by a viral infection.

26. _____ The GI tract has a cobblestone appearance in the patient with Crohn's disease.

27. _____ Severe diarrhea and rectal bleeding are common with ulcerative colitis.

28. _____ Ulcerative colitis often begins in the ileum and spreads distally.

Questions

29. The area of the colon that is most often involved when a patient has Crohn's disease is the:

A. Terminal ileum

B. Duodenum

C. Distal part of the jejunum

D. Sigmoid colon

30. Which assessment data would suggest Crohn's disease in a patient?

A. Nausea, vomiting, frequent bloody diarrhea

B. Pain after eating, fever, non-bloody diarrhea

C. Fever, chills, anorexia, constipation

D. Chronic pain, alternating constipation and diarrhea

31. Nursing care of the patient who has Crohn's disease is aimed at preventing complications such as

    A. Bowel obstruction

    B. Bowel perforation

    C. Fistula formation

    D. All of the above

32. When a patient has an acute exacerbation of Crohn's disease, the pharmacologic treatment that takes priority would include:

    A. Analgesics

    B. Antibiotics

    C. Antidiarrheals

    D. Corticosteroids

33. When a patient with an inflammatory bowel disorder is admitted with severe diarrhea and vomiting, which nursing action receives priority?

    A. Administer analgesics

    B. Maintain bed rest

    C. Maintain fluid and electrolyte balance

    D. Encourage patient to discuss feelings

34. Discharge instructions for the patient with an inflammatory bowel disease would include diet information. Which of the following foods should be avoided?

    A. Eggs, skim milk, cheese

    B. Coffee, beans, raw vegetables

    C. Meat, green vegetables

    D. Cereal products, chicken

35. A patient with ulcerative colitis needs to understand medications. The nurse explains that the effect of the anticholinergic drugs is to:

    A. Reduce the frequency of bowel movements

    B. Reduce inflammation and infections

    C. Decrease peristalsis and gastrointestinal secretions

    D. Decrease pain and control diarrhea

36. A patient had just had an excision of an anorectal abscess. The nursing diagnosis that would have priority is:

    A. Alteration in nutrition: less than body requirements

    B. High risk for infection

    C. Ineffective individual coping

    D. Ineffective breathing pattern

37. Which of the following conditions can cause a mechanical ileus?

    A. Adhesions

    B. Hernia

    C. Foreign bodies

    D. Volvulus

    E. Any of the above

38. Which symptoms in the postoperative patient indicate a mechanical ileus?

    A. Nausea and anorexia

    B. Sharp, knifelike pain at the umbilicus

    C. Absence of bowel sounds

    D. Distention and inability to pass stool

39. Diagnosis of a mechanical ileus is based on patient medical history and physical and x-ray findings, which would show:

    A. Tortuous narrowing of the bowel

    B. Air and fluid levels in the obstructed bowel

    C. Cobblestone ulcers throughout the lumen

    D. Dilatation of bowel from the duodenum to the rectum

40. Initial treatment of a bowel obstruction would include insertion of a nasogastric tube. The rationale for the insertion of the NG tube is:

    A. To provide a route for medication

    B. To allow for tube feedings

    C. To decompress the intestine

    D. To remove liquid stool

41. Which nursing diagnosis would be a priority in the patient with a mechanical ileus?

    A. High risk for fluid volume deficit

    B. Pain related to increased pressure

    C. Altered health maintenance

D. Knowledge deficit related to unknown outcome of treatment

42. Which of the following conditions is the most likely cause of a paralytic ileus?

A. Volvulus

B. Neoplasm

C. Abdominal surgery

D. Third degree burns

43. The underlying cause of the events leading to a paralytic ileus is thought to be:

A. Excessive sympathetic nervous system activity

B. Excessive parasympathetic nervous system activity

C. Changes in intraluminal pressure

D. Severe fluid shifts and electrolyte changes

44. The nurse is assessing a postoperative patient. Which of the following findings would be indicative of a paralytic ileus?

A. Hyperactive bowel sounds, nausea

B. Hypoactive bowel sounds, increased gastric drainage

C. Abdominal pain, projectile vomiting

D. Increased temperature, hypotension, abdominal pain

Matching

Match the following disorders with their descriptions.

A. Gluten-induced enteropathy
B. Lactase deficiency
C. Malabsorption syndrome

45. _____ A disorder also referred to as celiac sprue.

46. _____ A syndrome which results from impaired passage of nutrients across the intestine and into the circulation.

47. _____ A condition in which there are low levels of lactase in the intestine.

48. _____ A disorder which is due to immunologic sensitivity to gluten.

Questions

49. The nurse would instruct the patient with a gluten sensitivity to eliminate:

A. Yogurt

B. Wheat bread

C. Green vegetables

D. Red meats

50. The nurse would instruct the patient with a lactase deficiency to eat foods high in calcium such as:

A. Milk and red meats

B. Green and yellow vegetables

C. Salmon and sardines

D. Wheat and oat cereal

51. If, when assessing a patient, the nurse identifies the symptoms of _____ , it would be suggestive of malabsorption syndrome.

A. Weight loss, anorexia, bloating, bulky stools

B. Nausea, vomiting, abdominal pain

C. Cramping, passage of clay-colored stool

D. Fatigue, weakness, confusion, diarrhea

52. Diagnostic testing for the patient with malabsorption syndrome would reveal all of the following EXCEPT:

A. Decreased serum albumin

B. Decreased potassium

C. Decreased prothrombin time

D. Increase in stool fat

53. A person with a lactase deficiency is most likely to exhibit these symptoms.

A. Anorexia, vomiting, weight loss

B. Abdominal pain, bloating, diarrhea

C. Nausea, vomiting, abdominal cramps

D. Intermittent cramps, constipation, lethargy

54. Dietary teaching for the patient with gluten-induced enteropathy requires avoiding all cereal grain EXCEPT:

A. Wheat

B. Rice

C. Oat

D. Rye

55. Which of the following data obtained by the nurse in the health history would indicate a predisposition to the development of diverticular disease? Check all the apply.

A. History of chronic diarrhea, vomiting

B. History of passing small, scant stools

C. Eats a diet low in fiber

D. Eats a diet high in fiber

E. History of frequent use of laxatives

56. Which of the following findings would NOT be indicative of diverticular disease?

A. Left quadrant pain, which may radiate to the back

B. Constipation alternating with diarrhea

C. Chronic watery stool, constant crampy pain

D. Fever and leukocytosis

57. Medical management of diverticulosis is aimed at:

A. Decreasing stool; antidiarrheal drugs

B. Antispasmodic drugs; liquid diet

C. Low-fiber diet; anticholinergic drugs

D. High-fiber diet; bulk-forming laxatives

58. The nurse would instruct the patient with diverticular disease to avoid foods such as:

A. Apples

B. Popcorn

C. Whole wheat bread

D. Raw vegetables

59. The nurse should suspect incarceration of a hernia when which of the following symptoms are present?

A. Severe pain, nausea, vomiting

B. Left quadrant pain, diarrhea

C. Fever, hypoactive bowel sounds, anorexia

D. Rebound tenderness, hyperactive bowel sounds

60. The treatment of choice for an incisional or inguinal hernia is:

A. Diet and exercise

B. Surgical repair

C. Analgesics and antispasmodic medications

D. Antibiotics and use of a truss

61. A patient returns to the unit after an inguinal herniorrhaphy. Which of the following observations is most indicative of a problem following surgery?

A. Patient complains of pain

B. Patient is nauseated

C. Patient has difficulty voiding

D. Patient is anxious about getting out of bed

62. Medical management is often possible for uncomplicated hemorrhoids. Which of the following would not be used?

A. Sitz baths

B. Witch hazel preparations

C. Low-fiber diet

D. Stool softeners

63. Hemorrhoidectomy is the treatment of choice for which of the following?

A. Patient with internal hemorrhoids

B. Patient with prolapsed hemorrhoids

C. Patient with occasional rectal bleeding

D. Patient with external hemorrhoids who has no symptoms

64. When doing discharge planning for a patient following herniorrhaphy, the nurse would stress:

A. Pain can last up to 7 days

B. Resume activity after 2 weeks

C. Avoid heavy lifting and sexual activities for 6 weeks

D. Follow a low-residue diet and avoid laxatives

65. What is the rationale for having rectal polyps surgically removed?

A. They often rupture and bleed

B. They are potentially malignant

C. They often become infected

D. They predispose to diverticulosis

True or False

66. _____ Colon cancer is seen more in men than women.

67. _____ Most cancers of the GI tract occur in the colon or rectum.

68. _____ The cause of colorectal cancer is unknown.

69. _____ There is a poor prognosis with colorectal cancer.

70. _____ Colorectal cancers are primarily adenomas.

71. _____ Changes in bowel habits are often the first symptoms of colorectal cancer.

72. _____ Inflammatory bowel disorders are not a problem with the elderly.

73. _____ Occlusion of the mesenteric vessels can lead to bowel ischemia.

74. _____ Chronic constipation in the elderly can lead to hemorrhoids.

75. _____ Appendicitis is more serious in the elderly.

Questions

76. Which of the following would NOT be an expected clinical finding 24 hours after a colostomy is performed?

    A. Stoma is bright red and oozing.

    B. NG tube puts out 200 ml of green drainage in 8 hours.

    C. Abdomen is slightly distended, with absent bowel sounds.

    D. Catheter is in place with urine output of 150 ml in 8 hours.

77. After abdominal surgery, penrose drains are often inserted. The nurse explains to the patient that they will be removed when:

    A. The patient can tolerate a liquid diet

    B. Bowel function returns

    C. Drainage is less than 50 ml in 24 hours

    D. They fall out naturally

78. Which of the following signs, when present, should the nurse report immediately to the physician?

    A. Positive Homans' sign

    B. Hyperactive bowel sounds

    C. Scattered rhonchi in the lung fields

    D. Ankle edema

79. Colostomy care is important to prevent impairment to skin integrity. List several interventions which are important.

80. Write a nursing care plan for the patient who has had an incision and drainage of a rectal abscess.

    Nursing Diagnosis: Pain related to surgical trauma

    Patient Outcome:

    Nursing Interventions:

81. Plan the nursing care for the patient with an ileus.

    Nursing Diagnosis: High risk for fluid volume deficit related to fluid shifts and vomiting

    Patient Outcome:

    Nursing Interventions:

82. The nurse is aware that the patient with diverticulitis may have a problem with constipation. Write a nursing diagnosis, patient outcome, and several interventions which relate to this problem.

    Nursing Diagnosis:

    Patient Outcome:

    Nursing Interventions:

83. A patient is scheduled for an abdominal-perineal resection for colorectal cancer. This patient is

exhibiting signs of extreme anxiety. Write a nursing diagnosis, patient outcome, and several interventions that address this need.

Nursing Diagnosis:

Patient Outcome:

Nursing Interventions:

84. Following a hemorrhoidectomy, pain control is important. Write a nursing diagnosis, patient outcome, and several nursing interventions that address this problem.

Nursing Diagnosis:

Patient Outcome:

Nursing Interventions:

CLINICAL SITUATIONS

Situation ■ 1

Molly is a 28-year-old legal secretary who has been diagnosed as having Crohn's disease. She is admitted to the hospital with anorexia and malnutrition related to inability to eat and frequent diarrhea.

1. All of the following are treatment goals EXCEPT:

   A. Restoring normal nutritional status

   B. Suppressing inflammation

   C. Minimizing pain and diarrhea

   D. Providing education about surgery

2. The nurse reviews the medication record. She sees that the patient is receiving a medication which is an anti-infective and anti-inflammatory. This is:

   A. Azulfidine

   B. Prednisone

   C. Cefazolin

   D. Valium

3. The nurse performs a thorough assessment, keeping in mind to look for signs of a _____ problem.

   A. Skin and hygiene

   B. Bowel and bladder

   C. Fluid and electrolyte

   D. Diet and elimination

4. The nurse should consider which responsibility of primary importance when preparing this patient for a colonoscopy?

   A. Keep patient on NPO status

   B. Medicate prior to procedure

   C. Start IV therapy as ordered

   D. Ask about allergies to dye

5. Following the colonoscopy, the nurse would expect to administer which medication to Molly?

   A. A laxative

   B. A stool softener

   C. An antacid

   D. An analgesic

6. Which goal for Molly will take priority during the initial portion of the hospitalization?

   A. Promotion of positive self-image

   B. Promotion of rest and comfort

   C. Maintenance of adequate nutrition

   D. Prevention of injury

Situation ■ 2

Mrs. Nevil is admitted to the health care facility because of left-sided pain, abdominal pain, and intermittent diarrhea. She also noted blood in her stools. The physician orders diagnostic tests to determine the cause of her symptoms.

1. The nurse is preparing Mrs. Nevil for a barium enema. The nurse realizes that a colonoscopy is usually contraindicated during an acute stage because of the risk of _____ .

   A. Hemorrhage

   B. Infection

   C. Perforation

   D. Obstruction

2. The test confirms a diagnosis of diverticulitis. The physician opts for medical management first. All of the following medications would be appropriate EXCEPT:

A. Narcotic analgesics

B. Stool softeners

C. Antibiotics

D. Antispasmodics

3. Mrs. Nevil does not respond to the medical management, and a decision is made to do a surgical resection of the bowel with a temporary colostomy. The nurse realizes that the patient needs more information when she states:

A. I don't think I can cope with having a colostomy for the rest of my life.

B. I realize that I am going to have to make some diet changes.

C. I never realized how important it was to watch my diet and fluid intake.

D. I am anxious about the outcome of the surgery.

4. When Mrs. Nevil is ready for discharge, the nurse will review the diet recommendations. The diet is based on the knowledge that:

A. All food high in fiber and roughage should be eliminated.

B. Liquids and fluid intake are limited to prevent diarrhea.

C. Taking laxatives and prune juice regularly will ensure proper functioning of the colostomy.

D. Diet restrictions are often determined individually, knowing to avoid gas-forming foods and irritants.

Situation ■ 3

Mr. Powers has been admitted for diagnostic testing. His symptoms include weakness, anorexia, weight loss, and occasional bleeding with defecation. He also has a chronic cough and back pain.

1. Mr. Powers is diagnosed as having a large tumor in the sigmoid colon. He is scheduled for surgery. The surgical procedure which will be performed is most likely:

A. Right colectomy with ileotransverse anastomosis

B. Left colectomy with transverse anastomosis

C. Temporary transverse colostomy

D. Abdominal perineal resection

2. Nursing care in the preoperative period is directed toward which of the following?

A. Control of pain

B. Improvement of nutritional status

C. Correction of bowel habits

D. Increasing mobility

3. To reduce the risk of contamination at the time of surgery, the nurse will probably administer which of the following medications to Mr. Powers?

A. Laxatives and anti-infectives

B. Analgesics, antispasmodics

C. Anticholinergics, antispasmodics

D. Analgesics, antibiotics

4. Nursing care in the postoperative period is directed toward preventing:

A. Problems related to inactivity

B. Ineffective breathing patterns

C. Imbalances of food and fluids

D. Injury related to weakness

5. Mr. Powers is also scheduled for a course of chemotherapy. Which symptom indicates a possible side effect of this therapy?

A. Mucositis

B. Abdominal pain

C. Hiccupping

D. Leg cramps

6. The nurse is teaching Mr. Powers how to care for the colostomy. Which of the following statements is most accurate in terms of regulation of bowel habits?

A. Daily irrigation will keep elimination regular

B. Regular bowel elimination is almost impossible

C. Control of bowel elimination is often possible by following a dietary regimen and regular habits

D. None of the above

7. Disturbance in body image may be a serious problem following a colostomy. Which of the following interventions would be inappropriate?

A. Recognize that rejection is a common reaction

B. Permit denial while promoting acceptance

C. Avoid looking at the stoma or calling it by name

D. Encourage good hygiene and grooming

8. Mr. Powers says he is ready to learn to care for his colostomy. Which of the following nursing interventions is most likely to be effective in preparing him to look at his colostomy?

A. Encourage him to verbalize his concerns about the colostomy.

B. Have a friend with a colostomy visit.

C. Use prepared materials with illustration for the first session.

D. Explain that he will have no problems adjusting.

Chapter Twenty-four

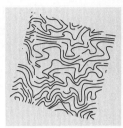

NURSING CARE
of Adults with Disorders of the Accessory Organs of Digestion

Learning Objectives

1.0 Demonstrate an Understanding of the Inflammatory or Infectious Disorders of the Accessory Organs of Digestion.

1.1 Identify the Clinical Manifestations of Cholecystitis.
1.2 Review the Medical and Surgical Management of Cholecystitis.
1.3 Review the Nursing Care of the Patient having a Cholecystectomy.
1.4 Review the Pathophysiology Involved in Pancreatitis.
1.5 Plan the Nursing Care for the Patient with Acute and Chronic Pancreatitis.

2.0 Demonstrate an Understanding of a Structural Abnormality of the Accessory Organs of Digestion.

2.1 Identify the Clinical Manifestations of a Structural Abnormality.
2.2 Identify an Inflammatory Disorder that can Lead to the Development of a Structural Abnormality.

3.0 Demonstrate an Understanding of the Type of Neoplasm that Affects the Accessory Organs of Digestion.

3.1 Identify the Clinical Manifestations of Pancreatic Cancer.
3.2 Review the Medical Interventions used to Treat Cancer of the Pancreas.
3.3 Review the Surgical Management of Cancer of the Pancreas.
3.4 Write a Nursing Care Plan for the Patient who has Undergone a Whipple Procedure.

Learning Activities

Define

1. Cholecystitis:

2. Pancreatitis:

Fill In

3. One symptom of cholecystitis which is unique to this condition is _____ .

4. Stasis of _____ , imbalances in _____ , and _____ seem to precipitate the development of cholecystitis.

5. The basic factor in the onset of acute pancreatitis is the presence of activated _____ .

Questions

6. Vascular congestion, edema, and distention of the gallbladder occurs within how many hours after injury?

    A. 4–6 hours

    B. 6–12 hours

    C. 12–24 hours

    D. 24–48 hours

7. Elevations in which of the following laboratory data would be suggestive of acute cholecystitis?

    A. CBC, SGOT, LDH

    B. WBC, SGOT, CPK

    C. WBC, alkaline phosphatase, SGOT, LDH

    D. BUN, creatinine, bilirubin

8. Symptoms associated with cholecystitis that the nurse would expect the patient to relate include which of the following? Check all that apply.

    A. Nausea

    B. Vomiting

    C. Flatulence

    D. Elevated temperature

    E. Generalized abdominal pain

9. What is one of the drawbacks of use of gallstone-dissolving drugs such as chenodeoxycholic acid?

    A. They have serious side effects

    B. They are very expensive

    C. They may take up to 6 months to work

    D. All of the above

10. A patient is scheduled for a cholecystectomy and choledochotomy. This means that the surgeon will remove the gallbladder and:

    A. Drain the pancreatic duct

    B. Explore the common bile duct

    C. Explore the pancreatic duct

    D. Remove part of the colon

11. When a patient is scheduled for an endoscopic sphincterotomy, the nurse would give the patient the following information:

    A. A spinal or general anesthetic is used

    B. You will be in the recovery room for 2 hours

    C. Valium is used for sedation and oral intake is resumed when the gag reflex returns

    D. Normal activities can be resumed immediately

12. Discharge instructions for the patient who has had extracorporeal lithotripsy would include:

    A. Continue taking oral bile acids

    B. Continue taking antibiotics

    C. Avoid lifting for 6 weeks

    D. Return to physician in 6 months

13. If a patient has an obstruction of the common bile duct, the nurse would observe for signs of:

A. Respiratory distress

B. Gastric pain

C. Urinary stasis

D. Prolonged bleeding time

14. After a choledocholithotomy is performed, what is the reason for the placement of a T-tube?

A. To facilitate drainage

B. To prevent infection

C. To maintain patency

D. To prevent stone recurrence

15. How much bile would the nurse expect the T-tube to drain during the first 24 hours after surgery?

A. 50–100 ml

B. 150–250 ml

C. 300–500 ml

D. 500–1000 ml

16. Which of the following findings indicates a possible surgical complication following a cholecystectomy?

A. T-tube has stopped draining

B. NG tube drains 100 ml in 4 hours

C. Penrose drain falls out

D. Respirations are 20 and shallow

17. When would laparoscopic cholecystectomy be contraindicated for a patient?

A. When the patient is over age 65

B. When the patient has diabetes

C. When the patient has multiple adhesions

D. All of the above

18. When the patient has had a laparoscopic cholecystectomy, a nursing intervention that is unique to this procedure would be:

A. Administer narcotics as needed

B. Place patient in semi-Fowler's position and apply heat to the shoulder

C. Keep patient in prone position with an abdominal binder

D. Instruct patient to gradually resume normal activities

19. Following removal of the gallbladder, it is still possible to have an intolerance to fatty foods. What is the reason for this?

A. Bile is no longer being produced adequately

B. Bile flows into the duodenum constantly

C. Bile can no longer be absorbed in the duodenum

D. Bile supply cannot keep up with demand

20. Which of the following foods would be most appropriate for the patient who is to follow a low-fat diet?

A. Cheese omelette and vanilla pudding

B. Egg salad sandwich and fruit

C. Ham salad and custard

D. Turkey sandwich with tomato

21. All of the following have been indicated in the development of pancreatitis EXCEPT:

A. Excessive use of alcohol

B. Use of antibiotics

C. Biliary tract disease

D. Metabolic disorders

22. Because of the systemic vasodilation and increased vascular permeability, the individual with pancreatitis is predisposed to:

A. Hypovolemic shock

B. Sepsis

C. Adult respiratory distress syndrome

D. Hypertensive crises

23. Which of the following laboratory results would be consistent with acute pancreatitis?

A. WBC of 15,000

B. BUN of 32 Creatinine 1.2

C. LDH of 40, CPK of 100

D. Serum amylase of 520

24. During the critical stage, medical management of acute pancreatitis would include all of the following EXCEPT:

A. Nasogastric tube to suction

B. Clear liquid diet

C. Narcotics for pain control

D. IV therapy

25. During the critical stage, in caring for the patient with acute pancreatitis, which nursing action would have the highest priority?

    A. Have patient turn every 2 hours

    B. Assess hemodynamic status and urine output every hour

    C. Maintain patency of the NG tube

    D. Medicate for pain every 3 hours

26. Presence of muscle twitching and tremors can be indicative of which condition in a patient?

    A. Hypokalemia

    B. Hypocalcemia

    C. Dehydration

    D. Acidosis

27. An order for which of the following pain medications should be questioned by the nurse?

    A. Demerol 25 mg IVP, Q3H

    B. Talwin 30 mg IM, Q3H

    C. Codeine 30 mg IM, Q4H

    D. Morphine Sulfate 10 mg, Q3H

28. Individuals with chronic pancreatitis will generally seek medical attention when:

    A. They notice blood in their stools

    B. They experience pain

    C. They are unable to tolerate food

    D. They begin to vomit

29. Laboratory findings consistent with chronic pancreatitis would include:

    A. Increased alkaline phosphate; decreased serum glucose

    B. Increased serum glucose; increased pancreatic juices

    C. Decreased alkaline phosphate; decreased pancreatic juices

    D. Increased alkaline phosphate; decreased pancreatic juices

30. Because of the vitamin deficiencies associated with chronic pancreatitis, the nurse is aware

that a patient with this condition is at risk for developing:

    A. Duodenal ulcer

    B. GI bleeding

    C. Pernicious anemia

    D. Lactase deficiency

31. In the patient with chronic pancreatitis, it is not uncommon for the stools to appear:

    A. Black and liquid

    B. White and chalky

    C. Tan, oily, and foul-smelling

    D. Frothy, bulky, and foul-smelling

True or False

32. _____ Lithotripsy is a painless procedure.

33. _____ Laparoscopic cholecystectomy is done under general anesthesia.

34. _____ The patient with acute pancreatitis will need oral pancreatic enzymes.

35. _____ The patient with chronic pancreatitis may need to take insulin.

36. _____ Pancreatic fistulas are most often a result of pancreatic abscesses.

37. _____ Surgery is not recommended for treatment of chronic pancreatitis.

38. _____ Cancer of the pancreas is rare in the U.S.

39. _____ Pancreatic cancers are generally adenocarcinomas.

Questions

40. A nursing intervention which would be appropriate for the patient with a pancreatic fistula would be:

    A. Saline wet-to-dry dressings

    B. Betadine wet-to-dry dressings

    C. Sterile, dry occlusive dressing

    D. Irrigate the area with saline and then leave it open to the air

41. When a patient with pancreatic cancer has a jaundiced appearance, the nurse would suspect:

A. Chronic pancreatitis

B. Biliary obstruction

C. Gastritis

D. Nutritional deficiency

42. The purpose of performing the Whipple procedure as a treatment for cancer of the pancreas is:

A. To stop the spread of the disease

B. To prevent a reoccurrence of the disease

C. To allow enzymes to empty in the jejunum to allow normal digestion to take place

D. To remove the pancreas and allow its functions to be taken over by the other accessory organs of digestion

43. A patient is scheduled for a Whipple's operation. The lab results show: WBC 7.8; PTT 24.5; K 3.8 What treatment would be ordered?

A. Administration of antibiotics

B. Administration of vitamin B_{12}

C. Administration of KCl 40 mEq

D. Administration of vitamin K

44. One of the major complications of the Whipple's operation is:

A. Hemorrhage

B. Necrosis

C. Fistula formation

D. All of the above

45. The nurse is caring for the patient with acute pancreatitis. Write a patient outcome and interventions that relate to this nursing diagnosis.

Nursing Diagnosis: High risk for fluid volume deficit

Patient Outcome:

Nursing Interventions:

46. Write a nursing care plan for the individual with chronic pancreatitis who will need to take medications and follow diet restrictions.

Nursing Diagnosis:

Patient Outcome:

Nursing Interventions:

47. A major problem for the individual who has had a Whipple procedure will be a nutritional alteration. Write a care plan using this as a diagnosis.

Nursing Diagnosis:

Patient Outcome:

Nursing Interventions:

CLINICAL SITUATIONS

Situation ■ 1

Mr. Tillman is admitted to the hospital with acute pain in his side, as well as nausea and vomiting. After examination, the physician diagnoses acute pancreatitis.

1. After obtaining a patient history, the nurse identifies which of the following behaviors as related to the diagnosis?

A. Smokes 2 packs of cigarettes a day

B. Takes Tylenol 10 grain four times a day for arthritis

C. Follows a low-sodium, low-cholesterol diet

D. Takes Bactrim for urinary stasis

2. The initial diagnosis of pancreatitis would be confirmed if Mr. Tillman has a significant elevation in serum:

A. Glucose

B. Amylase

C. Creatinine

D. Calcium

3. Because Mr. Tillman has a strong religious aversion to drinking, he becomes very upset when the physician asks him several times if he has a problem with alcohol intake. The nurse would explain to the family that the reason for these questions is:

A. There is a strong link between alcohol use and this disease.

B. Use of alcohol will cause inaccurate results in the lab test.

C. All patients admitted to the hospital are asked these questions.

D. The physician is new and not very sensitive.

4. During the initial assessment, the nurse notices that Mr. Tillman has muscle twitching in his forearms. The nurse should report this finding immediately because patients with this condition are at serious risk for:

A. Hypoglycemia

B. Hypocalcemia

C. Hyperkalemia

D. Hyponatremia

5. During the acute period of his illness, Mr. Tillman's diet will most likely be:

A. NPO

B. Clear liquids

C. Bland, no stimulants

D. Low-fat, high-carbohydrate

6. The nurse assesses Mr. Tillman and finds his abdomen has a small reddened area that is warm to the touch. He has a temperature of 101.2°F. What is a likely cause of this finding?

A. The patient has developed an abscess

B. The patient has developed a fistula

C. The patient has an internal bleed

D. The patient has developed an ulcer

Situation ■ 2

Mr. Barry is admitted with a diagnosis of chronic pancreatitis. He has a history of alcohol abuse and has been admitted twice in the past 5 years for the same problem. He is complaining of severe abdominal pain. He has lost 20 pounds in the last 6 months.

1. The nurse is reviewing the chart to determine Mr. Barry's nutrition status. Malnutrition would be a probable diagnosis if there is a significantly low level in serum:

A. Glucose

B. Total protein

C. Potassium

D. Calcium

2. What is the probable reason for the weight loss by Mr. Barry?

A. Drinking causes him to forget to eat

B. Malabsorption and vitamin deficiencies

C. Hyperactivity of pancreas uses up the calories

D. Increase in digestive enzymes

3. The nurse is aware that the goal of medical therapy is to decrease stimulation of pancreatic function. One of the drugs which would be useful is:

A. Cimetidine

B. Morphine sulfate

C. Motrin

D. Inderal

4. Once Mr. Barry is stabilized, he will be given information about his diet. An appropriate diet for the individual with chronic pancreatitis would be:

A. Low-protein, high-fiber diet with 5 feedings

B. Low-fat, bland diet with 5 feedings

C. High-calcium, soft diet with 3 meals

D. Low-residue, high-protein, high-fat diet

5. Mr. Barry will also be taking pancreatic enzymes. How would the nurse teach him to monitor for the effectiveness of the therapy?

A. Monitor fluid intake

B. Do daily finger sticks for blood sugar

C. Observe stools for steatorrhea

D. Monitor urine for sediment

Situation ■ 3

Mrs. Milles, 56, is admitted for a cholecystectomy. She has a history of cholelithiasis for several years and has been having attacks more and more frequently. She is 5' 6", weighs 190 pounds, and currently has right quadrant pain.

1. Based on the patient history, the nurse is aware that all of the following factors would predispose Mrs. Milles to cholelithiasis EXCEPT:

A. Age

B. Weight

C. Sex

D. Diet

2. In caring for Mrs. Milles, the nurse realizes that her diagnosis means that she has:

A. An infection in her gallbladder

B. An obstruction in the bile duct

C. Presence of stones in the gallbladder

D. All of the above

3. Following the surgery, Mrs Milles returns to the unit with an IV of dextrose/.45 normal saline at 100 ml/hour and a nasogastric tube to low wall suction. Her abdominal dressing is dry and intact and her vital signs are stable. When Mrs. Milles complains of nausea and distention, what should the nurse do first?

A. Increase the IV rate

B. Give the patient an antiemetic

C. Medicate the patient for pain

D. Assess the NG tube for patency

4. Based on the above information, what would be an important nursing diagnosis at this time?

A. High risk for fluid volume deficit

B. Constipation

C. High risk for activity intolerance

D. Altered role performance

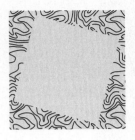

Unit Eight

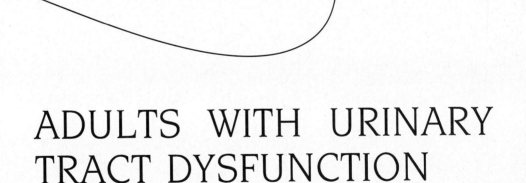

ADULTS WITH URINARY TRACT DYSFUNCTION

Chapter Twenty-five

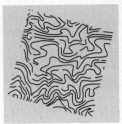

KNOWLEDGE BASIC TO THE NURSING CARE
of Adults with
Urinary Tract Dysfunction

Learning Objectives

1.0 Review the Anatomy and Physiology of the Urinary System.

1.1 Identify the Parts of the Kidney.
1.2 List the Functions of the Renal System.
1.3 Explain the Physiology of the Urinary System.
1.4 Explain the Physiology of Micturition.

2.0 Demonstrate an Understanding of the Assessment Data Related to the Urinary System.

2.1 Define Several Symptoms of a Urinary Tract Disorder.
2.2 Identify Clinical Manifestations of Urinary Tract Dysfunctions.
2.3 Identify Diagnostic Procedures Used to Identify Abnormalities of the Urinary System.
2.4 Plan Nursing Care for the Patient Having a Cystoscopy.

3.0 Demonstrate an Understanding of the Interventions Used to Treat Adults with Urinary Tract Dysfunction.

3.1 Review the Types of Bladder Catheterization.
3.2 Plan Teaching Measures for the Patient who is Performing Self-catheterization.
3.3 Plan Nursing Measures for the Patient who has a Problem with Urinary Incontinence.

Learning Activities

Identify

1. Label the kidney anatomy on the following diagram.

   A. Cortex   D. Glomeruli
   B. Nephron   E. Tubules
   C. Medulla   F. Pelvis

Questions

2. List the five main functions of the renal system.

   1.

   2.

   3.

   4.

   5.

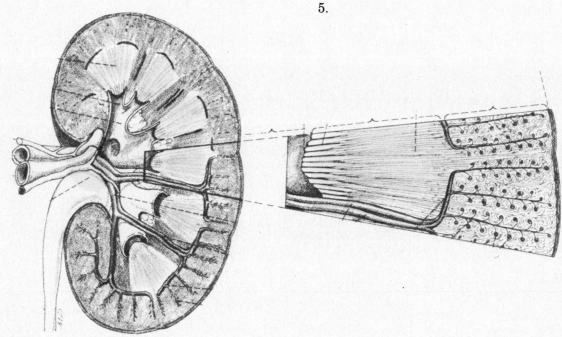

Fill In

3. The functional unit of the kidney is the

   _____.

Questions

4. What are the three factors which are responsible for the glomerular filtration rate in the kidney?

   1.

   2.

   3.

5. List three factors which contribute to normal micturition.

   1.

   2.

   3.

Define

6. Frequency:

7. Urgency:

8. Dysuria:

9. Nocturnal enuresis:

10. Incontinence:

Fill In

11. _____ is an end product of muscle metabolism that is excreted through the glomeruli in constant amounts in the body.

12. The kidneys regulate blood pressure through regulation of plasma volume and the _____ system.

Matching

Match the following diagnostic tests with their descriptions.

A. KUB x-ray
B. Voiding urogram
C. Cystogram
D. Ultrasound
E. MRI
F. Cystometrogram

13. _____ Study based on the reaction of protons and electrons in living tissue to a magnetic field.

14. _____ Radiologic study in which the patient is catheterized, contrast dye is instilled, and films are taken.

15. _____ Radiographic film of the major organs of the urinary tract.

16. _____ Measures bladder pressure during the filling and storage phases of micturition.

17. _____ A transducer is passed over the kidney to evaluate it for abnormalities.

18. _____ Radiographic study using contrast dye, which is observed as it passes through the urinary tract.

Questions

19. Which part of the renal system is responsible for most of the process of reabsorption?

A. Glomerulus

B. Proximal tubule

C. Loop of Henle

D. Distal tubule

20. The kidneys receive _____% of the total cardiac output.

A. 10

B. 25

C. 40

D. 60

21. The normal creatinine clearance in an adult with normal kidneys is:

A. 40–60 ml/min

B. 60–80 ml/min

C. 80–100 ml/min

D. 100–120 ml/min

22. The normal response of the kidney when acidosis occurs is to:

A. Secrete excess hydrogen ions

B. Reabsorb excessive hydrogen

C. Retain potassium

D. Excrete chloride

23. The production of _____ in the renal parenchyma is necessary for RBC production.

A. Creatinine

B. Erythropoietin

C. Calcitonin

D. Hemoglobin

24. Which of the following would not be a cause of urinary frequency?

A. Anxiety

B. Increased volume of urine

C. Decreased volume of urine

D. Inflammation of the bladder

25. Which of the following would lead to nocturia in an elderly patient?

A. Fluid retention during the day

B. Consumption of 2 cups of coffee at 2 P.M.

C. Consumption of 4 cups of water daily

D. Medication for angina

26. Which statement best explains the process of bladder emptying?

A. It occurs by parasympathetic facilitation and sympathetic inhibition.

B. It occurs by sympathetic facilitation and parasympathetic inhibition.

27. A definition of urinary retention is:

A. Voiding frequently during the day

B. Residual urine of 50% of total bladder content

C. Residual urine of 80% of total bladder content

D. Voiding less than 200 ml of urine daily

28. The primary reason that the patient will seek a urologic consultation is usually:

A. Bleeding with urination

B. Inability to urinate

C. Pain within the urinary tract

D. Inability to control urination

29. The presence of blood in the urine is a situation which requires evaluation. Which of the following is NOT a cause of hematuria?

A. Presence of a tumor

B. Urinary infection

C. Benign prostatic hypertrophy

D. Hydronephrosis

30. Urinary output of between 100–400 ml in a 24-hour period is defined as:

A. Anuria

B. Oliguria

C. Nonuria

D. Polyuria

31. The phenolsulfonphthalein (PSP) test is a simple way to:

A. Determine the presence of bacteria in the urine

B. Determine the presence of renal dysfunction

C. Determine presence of obstructive processes

D. Determine presence of a neoplasm

32. Two tests which are most commonly used to measure glomerular filtration are:

A. PSP and WBC

B. WBC and BUN

C. BUN and creatinine

D. Creatinine and CPK

33. As the nurse caring for a patient who is having a workup for possible renal disease, what is the most important information to obtain?

A. History of cardiac dysfunction

B. Family history of diabetes and hypertension

C. Allergy to contrast dye

D. Presence of gastrointestinal problems

34. An excretory urogram would be contraindicated for which type of patient?

A. Patient with diabetes

B. Patient with heart disease

C. Patient with renal failure

D. Patient with hypertension

35. You are caring for a patient who has just returned from an intravenous pyelogram. Which nursing intervention would you implement following the test?

A. Assessment of vital signs every 10 minutes for 2 hours

B. Maintain patient on bed rest for 48 hours

C. Encourage fluid intake and monitor intake and output

D. Maintain patency of the urinary drainage system

36. Which of the following diagnostic tests are most informative in terms of the urological evaluation?

    A. PSP and IVP

    B. Cystoscopy and IVP

    C. Ultrasound and CT scan

    D. BUN and IVP

37. Which of the following conditions can be diagnosed using cystoscopic examination?

    A. Recurrent urinary infections

    B. Congenital defects

    C. Prostatism

    D. All of the above

38. The nurse is doing discharge instruction for a patient who has had a cystoscopy that morning. Which information would the nurse explain to the patient?

    A. Urine may be slightly blood tinged for 24–48 hours

    B. Urine should be clear after the first urination

    C. Burning with urination is common after this test

    D. Fluids should be limited for the first 24 hours

39. Ms. Madison calls the clinic at 10 A.M. She reports that since her cystoscopy test yesterday at 11 A.M. she has not been able to urinate. What should the nurse tell her?

    A. Have her drink fluids and call back at 6 P.M.

    B. Have her come to the clinic as soon as possible

    C. Have her go to the emergency room

    D. Have her call back when she has urinated

40. A patient who is predisposed to urinary calculus formation would be on what type of diet?

    A. Low sodium

    B. Fluid restriction

    C. Low calcium

    D. Low protein

41. What diagnostic procedure would you expect the physician to perform on the patient who has been having hematuria and is suspected to have adenocarcinoma of the bladder?

    A. Voiding cystogram

    B. Intravenous pyelogram

    C. Cystoscopy with biopsy

    D. CT scan of abdomen

42. A bladder biopsy would be contraindicated when a patient is taking which of the following medications?

    A. Coumadin

    B. Indocin

    C. Lasix

    D. Ampicillin

43. Mr. Close has just returned to the unit following a closed renal biopsy. The nurse is aware that the most common complication of this procedure is:

    A. Infection

    B. Bleeding

    C. Obstruction

    D. Incontinence

44. The nurse would suspect a problem if Mr. Close exhibited which of the following symptoms?

    A. Drop in blood pressure

    B. Presence of pink-tinged urine

    C. Tenderness in the flank area

    D. Anxiety after the procedure

45. The explanation of urodynamics testing that the nurse would give to the patient is:

    A. A test that measures the ability to concentrate urine

    B. A test to visualize the urinary system

    C. A test to look for kidney stones

    D. A procedure to measure the urinary function

46. Which of the following symptoms would probably result in a delay of urodynamic testing?

    A. Temperature of 98.9°F

    B. Presence of sugar in the urine

C. Presence of bacteria in the urine

D. Blood pressure of 150/90, pulse of 92

47. Which of the following medications is contraindicated during urodynamic testing?

A. Cholinergic agents

B. Anticholinergic agents

C. Analgesics

D. All of the above

48. When would a patient be a candidate for a suprapubic catheter rather than an indwelling catheter?

A. When he or she has recurrent bladder infections

B. When there is a urethral obstruction

C. When there is hydronephrosis of the kidney

D. When he or she has a kidney stone

49. Which is an appropriate nursing intervention used in the care of the patient with a suprapubic catheter?

A. Change catheter every week

B. Irrigate to maintain patency

C. Limit fluid intake

D. Change dressing twice daily

50. What is the purpose of the Credé maneuver?

A. To aid in the passage of urine from the bladder

B. To avoid having to catheterize the patient

C. To prevent recurrent bladder infections

D. To minimize trauma to the urethra

51. Management of the patient with a urinary tract disorder may involve diet therapy. The nurse would teach the patient all of the following EXCEPT:

A. Increase intake of acidic foods

B. Increase fluids to 3000 ml per day

C. Increase intake of dairy products

D. Decrease intake of caffeine and alcohol

52. A nurse is teaching her patient with a urinary dysfunction Kegel exercises. The purpose for this is:

A. To regain voluntary bladder control

B. To control involuntary loss of urine

C. To prevent hematuria

D. To prevent recurrent bladder infections

True or False

53. _____ Painless hematuria is a serious symptom.

54. _____ Incontinence is a problem that is related to the aging process.

55. _____ Both men and women can use external catheters.

56. _____ Reusable undergarments are preferable to disposable adult diapers.

57. _____ To obtain a culture from an indwelling catheter, disconnect the catheter and obtain 10 ml of urine for analysis.

58. _____ Time-voiding may assist an elderly patient to obtain a safe pattern of urination.

59. _____ To reduce the bacteria count in an indwelling catheter, the catheter should be changed weekly.

Questions

60. The nurse who has a patient with an indwelling catheter is responsible for preventing complications related to this procedure. List five nursing interventions that should be implemented.

1.

2.

3.

4.

5.

61. Write a nursing care plan for the patient with urinary retention.

Nursing Diagnosis: Urinary retention related to postoperative complications

Patient Outcome:

Nursing Interventions:

62. Write a nursing care plan for the patient with an indwelling Foley catheter.

    Nursing Diagnosis: Alteration in urinary elimination related to irritation of the mucosa due to catheterization.

    Patient Outcome:

    Nursing Interventions:

CLINICAL SITUATIONS

Situation ■ 1

Ms. Norris is seen in the emergency room of her local hospital. She is complaining of a sudden onset of severe colicky pain which radiates from the left side to the groin.

1. Based on the above information, what is the most likely cause of her problem?
   A. Urinary tract infection
   B. Urinary tract obstruction
   C. Severe menstrual cramps
   D. Pelvic inflammatory disease

2. Ms. Norris is to obtain urine for culture and sensitivity. The nurse explains that the purpose of this test is:
   A. To rule out an obstruction
   B. To determine the presence of a neoplasm
   C. To identify any bacteria
   D. To determine if she has diabetes

3. A diagnostic procedure that will probably be ordered for this patient is:
   A. Intravenous pyelogram
   B. Sonogram
   C. Doppler studies
   D. Angiogram

4. Following this procedure, what is an important nursing intervention?
   A. Increase fluid intake
   B. Limit fluid intake

C. Keep patient on bed rest for 24 hours
D. Maintain patency of the drainage catheter

5. Ms. Norris is able to pass her kidney stone during the hospitalization. She is discharged on a low-calcium diet. Which food should she avoid?
   A. Green leafy vegetables
   B. Rice and pasta
   C. Fish
   D. Soft drinks

Situation ■ 2

Marcia Wells has a neurogenic bladder condition and upon discharge from the hospital will be doing self-catheterization. She will need discharge instructions.

1. The first step in your teaching plan would be to:
   A. Emphasize that this is a sterile procedure
   B. Review the female anatomy with Marcia
   C. Gather all the appropriate equipment
   D. Provide a sedative before you begin the procedure

2. To instruct Marcia in this procedure, the nurse would tell her to:
   A. Look for the meatus in a mirror; insert catheter straight in and insert 2 inches
   B. After locating the meatus, clean it with betadine and insert the catheter 4 inches
   C. Palpate the meatus; insert catheter in an upward direction for 3 inches
   D. View the meatus, clean it with soap and antiseptic solution; insert catheter 6 inches

3. To further instruct Marcia in the care of the catheter, the nurse would tell her to:
   A. Clean it after each use, soak it once a week to remove exudate, and discard it after 4–6 weeks of use
   B. Use a clean, sterile catheter each time
   C. Sterilize it with alcohol after each use and discard it after using it three times
   D. Clean it as recommended by the physician after using the catheter for 24 hours; discard it after 1 week

Chapter Twenty-six

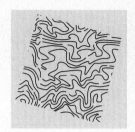

NURSING CARE
of Adults with
Urinary Tract Disorders

Learning Objectives

1.0 Demonstrate an Understanding of the Infections and Inflammations of the Urinary Tract.

1.1 Identify Several Inflammatory Disorders of the Urinary Tract.
1.2 Recognize the Clinical Manifestations of Several Inflammatory Disorders of the Urinary Tract.
1.3 Plan the Nursing Care for the Patient with Glomerulonephritis.
1.4 Plan the Nursing Care for the Patient with Cystitis.

2.0 Demonstrate an Understanding of Renal Failure.

2.1 Identify Clinical Manifestations of Acute and Chronic Renal Failure.
2.2 Demonstrate an Understanding of the Pathology Involved in Chronic Renal Failure.
2.3 Review the Medical Management of the Patient with Renal Failure.
2.4 Demonstrate an Understanding of Treatment Options for the Patient with Renal Failure.
2.5 Plan the Nursing Care for the Patient with Renal Failure.

3.0 Demonstrate an Understanding of Obstructive Disorders of the Renal System.

3.1 Identify the Clinical Manifestations of the Patient with an Obstructive Disorder.
3.2 Plan the Nursing Care for the Patient with a Renal Calculi.
3.3 Review the Medical and Surgical Treatment Options for the Patient with an Obstructive Disorder.
3.4 Plan Appropriate Nursing Interventions for the Patient with an Obstructive Disorder.

4.0 Demonstrate an Understanding of the Types of Traumatic Injuries that can Affect the Renal System.

4.1 Identify the Clinical Manifestations of Renal Trauma.
4.2 Review the Medical and Surgical Treatments used for Patients with Traumatic Injuries.
4.3 Plan Nursing Interventions for the Patient with a Traumatic Injury.

5.0 Demonstrate an Understanding of the Neoplasms which can Affect the Renal System.

5.1 Identify the Clinical Manifestations of Several Types of Renal Neoplasms.

5.2 Review the Surgical Interventions Used in the Treatment of Renal Neoplasms.

5.3 Plan the Nursing Care for the Patient with a Neoplasm of the Renal System.

Learning Activities

Define

1. Pyelonephritis:

2. Cystitis:

3. Urethritis:

4. Glomerulonephritis:

5. Acute renal failure:

6. Chronic renal failure:

7. Tubular necrosis:

8. Azotemia:

Questions

9. When reviewing the laboratory results for a patient, the nurse is aware that a urinary tract infection is present if there are more than _____ organisms per mm in the clean-catch specimen.

A. 10,000

B. 30,000

C. 50,000

D. 100,000

10. In females, the most common way that cystitis occurs is:

A. Develops secondary to a strep infection

B. Develops after exposure to a bacteria or virus

C. Develops after bacteria from the rectum or vagina ascend to the bladder

D. Develops as a result of an existing problem in the urinary tract

11. Discharge planning for the patient who has had cystitis should include which of the following instructions?

A. Inform patient to take antibiotics for 6 more weeks

B. Inform patient to maintain restricted activity

C. Inform patient to refrain from sexual activity

D. Inform patient on proper hygienic methods

12. Which of the following nursing interventions would be used to alleviate bladder spasm for the patient with cystitis?

A. Administer antispasmodics or analgesics as ordered

B. Encourage fluid intake

C. Encourage the patient to urinate frequently

D. All of the above

13. In males, the most common cause of gonorrhea is:

A. Cystitis

B. Urethritis

C. Pyelonephritis

D. Prostatitis

14. The most common cause of pyelonephritis is:

    A. Invasion of bacteria into the bladder

    B. Reflux of infected urine

    C. Contamination from GI tract

    D. Sepsis

15. A medical diagnosis of pyelonephritis is confirmed by which of the following tests?

    A. Urine culture, WBC, KUB

    B. Urinalysis, CBC, WBC

    C. Urine culture, IVP, BUN

    D. CT of abdomen

16. Mr. Hill has been admitted with a diagnosis of acute pyelonephritis. The nurse assigned is to obtain a urine specimen for culture and sensitivity. When should the specimen be obtained?

    A. Immediately upon admission

    B. Immediately after starting his antibiotic

    C. As soon as he urinates 100 ml of urine

    D. Within the first 24 hours of admission

17. Mr. Hill has been treated with antibiotics for the past week. He continues to have a persistent fever and edema over the area of his right kidney. What is a possible explanation for his symptoms?

    A. He may be resistant to antibiotic therapy

    B. He may have developed an abscess

    C. He may have developed a neoplasm

    D. He may have a hematoma

18. What type of diet would probably be ordered for a patient with acute glomerulonephritis who is edematous?

    A. Low fat, low protein

    B. Low salt, high protein

    C. High carbohydrate, low salt

    D. High fat, high calorie

19. Which of the following statements is MOST accurate about the cause of glomerulonephritis?

    A. It is caused by *Staphylococcus*

    B. It develops secondary to a streptococcal infection

C. It is caused by an immunologic reaction

D. It usually leads to renal failure

20. Renal failure will occur when there is functional loss of what portion of the kidney's nephrons?

    A. 20%

    B. 40%

    C. 60%

    D. 75%

21. Prerenal failure is thought to be caused by:

    A. Hypovolemia

    B. Low cardiac output

    C. Renal artery obstruction

    D. All of the above

22. For the patient in acute renal failure, which of the following laboratory findings is most serious?

    A. Hgb 10.8

    B. BUN 28

    C. Creatinine 1.8

    D. Potassium 6.2

23. The management of patients with acute renal failure is primarily directed toward decreasing _____ .

    A. Sodium and chloride levels

    B. BUN and creatinine levels

    C. Hgb and Hct levels

    D. CO_2 levels

24. Which assessment data indicates the presence of acute renal failure?

    A. Urine excretion of 500 ml/day, hypertension, nausea

    B. Urine excretion of 200 ml/day, edema, mental changes

    C. Urine excretion of 600 ml/day, BUN 30, creatinine 1.8

    D. Urine excretion of 500 ml/day, fever, flank pain

25. The nursing assessment of a renal patient reveals a fever, nausea, pleuritic pain, and an audi-

ble friction rub. The nurse suspects the patient has developed:

A. Chronic renal failure

B. Uremia

C. Pericarditis

D. Pneumonia

26. The nurse's responsibility in caring for the patient with renal failure would be centered around:

A. Controlling fluid and electrolyte balances

B. Controlling pain and anxiety

C. Controlling altered level of consciousness

D. Controlling altered breathing patterns

27. In the individual with chronic renal failure, which symptoms would always be present?

A. Oliguria, hypokalemia, alkalosis

B. Polycythemia, hypovolemia, acidosis

C. Uremia, anemia, acidosis

D. Dehydration, anemia, hypercalcemia

28. Nursing care of the patient with chronic renal failure would include information on a _____ diet.

A. Low-fat, low-protein, low-sodium

B. High-carbohydrate, high-fat, low-protein

C. High-calorie, high-carbohydrate, low-protein, low-sodium

D. Low-carbohydrate, no simple sugars, moderate sodium

29. Which condition, if present in a patient with chronic renal failure, would be a reason to institute dialysis?

A. Severe dehydration

B. Uremia

C. Hypokalemia

D. Hypertension

30. The type of dialysis that involves dialyzing for 40 hours per week with 3–7 dialysis runs is _____ . It involves a cycling machine, and the abdomen is dry between runs.

A. Hemodialysis

B. Intermittent peritoneal dialysis

C. Continuous ambulatory dialysis

D. Continuous cycle peritoneal dialysis

31. List five of the advantages of using peritoneal dialysis for the patient.

1.
2.
3.
4.
5.

32. What are the four main goals of hemodialysis?

1.
2.
3.
4.

33. Why would peritoneal dialysis be chosen as the treatment of choice over hemodialysis?

A. It provides for less chance of infection

B. It provides for more patient independence

C. It allows for more rapid removal of waste products

D. It is appropriate for all patients

34. A patient is scheduled for peritoneal dialysis. Presence of which condition would contraindicate this procedure?

A. Cardiac disease

B. Diabetes

C. Neurologic impairment

D. Inflammatory bowel disease

35. What is the most appropriate action for the nurse to take if, during the peritoneal dialysis procedure, the patient becomes short of breath and diaphoretic?

A. Call for respiratory treatment

B. Stop procedure for this time

C. Continue infusion but notify physician

D. Elevate the bed, assess respiratory status

36. What is the main difference between hemodialysis and peritoneal dialysis?

    A. Peritoneal dialysis is more effective

    B. Hemodialysis requires vascular access

    C. Hemodialysis takes longer to complete

    D. Peritoneal dialysis has fewer complications

True or False

37. _____ Hemodialysis can be used for both acute and chronic renal failure.

38. _____ Hemodialysis can be done at home.

39. _____ Dietary protein is severely restricted during hemodialysis.

40. _____ Weight stays the same before and after dialysis.

41. _____ Peritoneal dialysis is a clean procedure.

42. _____ The amount of hematuria after renal trauma is a good indication of the severity of the injury.

43. _____ Most patients with penetrating renal trauma need surgery.

Questions

44. When checking the patient who returns from dialysis, the nurse notices periods of confusion and altered perception. This is most likely due to:

    A. Rapid removal of fluid

    B. Rapid removal of urea

    C. Sudden drop in blood pressure

    D. Sudden onset of infection

45. In the patient who has had a renal transplant, the most common infection which can result in graft loss is:

    A. Cytomegalovirus

    B. HIV

    C. Fungal

    D. Herpes

46. The management of patients who have had a renal transplant involves administering immunosuppressive agents to prevent what complication?

    A. Rejection of the transplanted organ

    B. Systemic infection

    C. Fungal infection

    D. Clotting of the graft

47. For the patient who is receiving immunosuppressive agents, the nurse would be concerned if she finds which symptom during her assessment?

    A. Weight loss of 2 pounds

    B. Temperature of 98.8°F

    C. Productive cough

    D. Hyperactive bowel sounds

48. In a large portion of the individuals who develop urinary calculus, what is the causative factor?

    A. Fluid restrictions

    B. Dietary habits

    C. Geographic location

    D. Heredity

49. In caring for the patient who is admitted with a calculus in the urinary tract, the primary nursing goal would be:

    A. Alleviation of pain

    B. Maintain fluid balance

    C. Promote mobility

    D. Prevent respiratory complications

50. The treatment of choice for large renal or ureteral calculi which don't pass spontaneously is:

    A. Surgical removal of the stone

    B. Pain control and fluid therapy

    C. Extracorporeal lithotripsy

    D. Renal angioplasty

51. A patient with a kidney stone is being managed conservatively. Knowing the usual medical treatment, what instruction would the nurse give to this patient?

    A. Stay on complete bed rest

    B. Strain all urine

    C. Avoid pain medication because it masks symptoms

    D. Limit fluid to 1000 ml daily

52. Following extracorporeal lithotripsy, the nurse should consider which goal as primary?

    A. Control of pain

    B. Maintain patency of urinary system

    C. Maintain electrolyte status

    D. Prevent infection of suture line

53. Diagnosis of a stricture of the urinary system is most likely to be made by:

    A. Angiogram

    B. Excretory urogram

    C. KUB

    D. CT scan

54. The nurse is aware that obstructive disorders of the urinary system, if untreated, will eventually lead to:

    A. Renal neoplasm

    B. Tubular osmosis

    C. Hydronephrosis

    D. Renal calculi

55. In a patient who had acute renal failure in the past, which of the following conditions will increase his or her risk for developing further renal problems?

    A. Cholecystitis

    B. Abdominal aneurysm

    C. Angina

    D. Rheumatic fever

56. Mr. Perry had surgery for an obstructive disorder. The surgeon inserted two ureteral stints. What is an important nursing intervention postoperatively?

    A. Prevent skin breakdown

    B. Promote oral hygiene

    C. Maintain bed rest

    D. Teach patient self-care

57. Which clinical manifestation is a sign of an obstruction of a urethral stricture?

    A. Hematuria and burning with urination

    B. Hesitancy, urinary retention

    C. Flank pain, dysuria

    D. Frequency, pain with intercourse

58. The most common therapy for a urethral stricture would involve:

    A. Extracorporeal lithotripsy

    B. Balloon angioplasty

    C. Mechanical dilatation

    D. Intravenous pyelogram

59. Which of the following patients would be at the greatest risk for the development of an extrinsic urethral obstruction?

    A. Patient receiving chemotherapy for lung cancer

    B. Patient who is undergoing popliteal revascularization

    C. Patient who is receiving pelvic radiation therapy

    D. Patient with diabetes on insulin therapy

Fill In

60. Traumatic injuries to the genitourinary tract are usually the result of _____ _____ injuries.

Questions

61. Assessment of which system would take priority over assessment for renal trauma?

    A. Respiratory

    B. Cardiovascular

    C. Central nervous system

    D. All of the above

62. Urethral trauma is generally treated by:

    A. Drug therapy

    B. Bed rest and fluids

    C. Surgical repair

    D. Antibiotics

63. Mr. Flowers is admitted following a crushing injury. Presence of which of the following symptoms might indicate a ruptured bladder?

A. Flank pain, hematuria, frequency

B. Lower abdominal pain, inability to void

C. Abdominal rigidity, sharp, knifelike pain

D. Bladder spasm, urinary retention

64. Since Mr. Flowers has not yet urinated, it would be important for the nurse to do which of the following interventions first?

A. Catheterize the patient

B. Assess the type of injury sustained

C. Encourage fluid intake

D. Medicate for pain

65. In the patient who has a urethral tear without extravasation, the nurse would expect that treatment would involve:

A. Insertion of a Foley catheter for 7–10 days

B. Surgical repair as soon as possible

C. Surgical repair after the bleeding has ceased

D. Analgesics and anti-inflammatory medications

True or False

66. _____ The presenting symptoms of renal cancer are usually hematuria and pain.

67. _____ Metastasis of a renal cell carcinoma occurs in about one fourth of cases.

68. _____ Chemotherapy is the treatment of choice for renal cell carcinoma.

69. _____ Malignant tumors of the bladder are the most frequently occurring tumors within the urinary system.

70. _____ The most common symptom of bladder cancer is painless hematuria.

Questions

71. In caring for the patient who has had a radical nephrectomy, the nurse should be chiefly concerned with which goal during the immediate postoperative period?

A. Maintaining stable fluid and electrolyte status

B. Maintaining effective breathing patterns

C. Maintaining adequate nutrition

D. Preventing problems related to immobility

72. Which of the following therapies is used MOST often in the treatment for superficial bladder cancer?

A. Transurethral resection

B. Intravesical chemotherapy

C. Laser therapy

D. Radical surgery

73. Which form of therapy has been successful in curing some patients with nonpapillary bladder cancer?

A. Transurethral resection

B. Intravesical chemotherapy

C. Intravesical immunotherapy

D. Radical cystectomy

74. Which of the following patients would be a candidate for external radiation therapy to treat a malignant bladder tumor?

A. Young adult with papillary bladder cancer

B. Middle-aged female with a nonpapillary bladder neck tumor

C. Elderly female with invasive bladder cancer

D. Any of the above

75. Write a nursing care plan for the patient with cystitis.

Nursing Diagnosis: Altered urinary elimination related to inflammation

Patient Outcome:

Nursing Interventions:

76. Write a nursing care plan for the renal patient.

Nursing Diagnosis: Alteration in renal tissue perfusion related to chronic renal failure

Patient Outcome:

Nursing Interventions:

CLINICAL SITUATIONS

Situation ■ 1

Ms. Reiny is admitted with a sore throat, fever, flank pain, and peripheral edema. The diagnosis is possible glomerulonephritis.

1. The nurse reviews Ms. Reiny's lab results. Which of the following findings would tend to confirm this diagnosis?

   A. Presence of protein and blood in the urine, high BUN

   B. Elevated white count, low hemoglobin

   C. Presence of *E. Coli* in the urine

   D. High sedimentation rate, low platelet count

2. A renal biopsy is performed and the diagnosis is confirmed. Ms. Reiny wonders if this is a serious condition. What information would the nurse give her?

   A. Explain that this is a mild inflammation that is easily treated

   B. Explain that this is a serious condition which needs aggressive treatment

   C. Explain that this is a chronic condition that often leads to end-stage renal disease

   D. Explain that everyone you have seen with the condition does well with treatment

3. What is the reason that Ms. Reiny is ordered to be placed on bed rest?

   A. To prevent any further damage to the renal tubules

   B. To prevent the spread of infection

   C. To conserve energy

   D. To prevent injury from falls

Situation ■ 2

Mr. Prince has been gradually losing renal function. A decision is made to start hemodialysis. He is admitted for the placement of an AV graft (Gore-Tex) in the right forearm.

1. Mr. Prince asks the nurse to explain to him what this procedure involves. The nurse would explain:

   A. A vein and artery are surgically joined together.

   B. A bridge is made between an artery and vein using a synthetic material.

   C. A graft of teflon is implanted outside the femoral artery.

2. Mr. Prince returns to the unit after the graft insertion. Which is the method by which the nurse can assess for patency of the graft?

   A. Perform circulation check every hour

   B. Check vital signs every 30 minutes

   C. Assess graft for presence of thrill and bruit

   D. Keep compression dressing in place for 24 hours

3. Which of the following would be a priority to prevent complications related to the dialysis procedure?

   A. Assess vital signs every 4 hours

   B. Assess respiratory status

   C. Assess the fluid status before and after the procedure

   D. Draw blood from the graft before starting the procedure

4. Mr. Prince wonders if he can have a kidney transplant. You tell him that the two major factors in donor and recipient determination are:

   A. Age and blood type of donor

   B. Blood type and histocompatibility

   C. Blood type and sex of donor

   D. Blood crossmatch and donor desire to participate

Situation ■ 3

Ken Brown was injured when he hit a tree on his motorcycle. In addition to a concussion and fractured ribs, he received a laceration of the right kidney. After stabilization, he was taken to surgery for repair of the laceration.

1. Which information would be important for the floor nurse to obtain from the recovery room nurse?

A. Vital signs

B. Level of consciousness

C. Presence of drainage tubes

D. All of the above

2. Ken has a nephrostomy tube as well as an indwelling catheter. Which information is true about this type of drainage?

A. Most of the urinary drainage occurs through the stent

B. Most of the urinary drainage occurs through the catheter

C. All drainage occurs through the stent

D. All drainage occurs through the catheter

3. As part of his discharge instructions, what would be important for Ken to know?

A. How to handle the urinary drainage system

B. How to change his abdominal dressing

C. How to irrigate the catheter

D. How to prevent problems related to immobility

Situation ■ 4

Mrs. Watkins, age 50, is admitted with bladder cancer which has not responded to conservative methods of treatment. She is scheduled for a radical cystectomy. The physician is planning on constructing an ileal conduit.

1. Mrs. Watkins does well for the first 48 hours, but today she is withdrawn. She always turns away when you assess her urinary drainage system. Which nursing diagnosis might be applicable at this time?

A. Ineffective breathing pattern

B. Fluid volume deficit

C. Body image disturbance

D. Alteration in nutrition: less than body requirements

2. Which would be an appropriate referral for the primary nurse to implement?

A. Consultation with the enterostomal therapist

B. Referral to social services for home care

C. Referral for a psychiatric evaluation

D. Referral to the physician about the condition

3. The nurse would realize that teaching had been effective when Mrs. Watkins says which of the following?

A. I'm glad everything is back to normal

B. I didn't realize how the diversion would really look

C. I didn't realize that I couldn't have sex again

D. I'm just glad to be alive

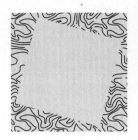

Unit Nine

ADULTS WITH
HEPATIC DYSFUNCTION

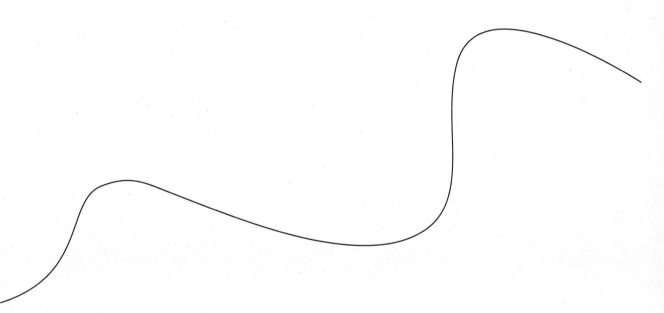

Chapter Twenty-seven

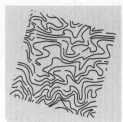

KNOWLEDGE BASIC TO THE NURSING CARE
of Adults with Hepatic Dysfunction

Learning Objectives

1.0 Review the Anatomy and Physiology of the Hepatic System.

1.1 Identify the Parts of the Hepatic System.
1.2 Demonstrate an Understanding of the Metabolic Processes of the Hepatic System.
1.3 List Five of the Functions of the Liver.
1.4 Identify the Underlying Pathology Associated with Certain Clinical Manifestations.

2.0 Demonstrate an Understanding of the Assessment Data Related to the Hepatic Dysfunction.

2.1 List Clinical Manifestations Associated with Hepatic Disorders.
2.2 Match Specific Diagnostic Tests with Their Descriptions.
2.3 Fill in the Correct Value for Laboratory Tests.
2.4 Identify the Results of Specific Diagnostic Tests as they Relate to the Hepatic Disorders.
2.5 Plan the Nursing Care for the Patient Undergoing Diagnostic Studies.

3.0 Demonstrate an Understanding of the Interventions Appropriate for the Adult with Hepatic Dysfunction.

3.1 Identify the Medical Treatment of Patients with Hepatic Disorders.
3.2 Plan the Nursing Care for the Patient with Hepatic Encephalopathy.
3.3 Write Appropriate Nursing Interventions for the Patient who has had a Paracentesis.
3.4 Write a Nursing Care Plan for the Patient with Ascites.
3.5 Identify the Nursing Interventions Appropriate for the Patient with a LeVeen shunt.

Learning Activities

Identify

1. On the drawing below, identify the following parts of the hepatic system:

   A. Right lobe of liver

   B. Left lobe of liver

   C. Inferior vena cava

   D. Gallbladder

   E. Hepatic ducts

   F. Cystic duct

   G. Gallbladder

   H. Common bile duct

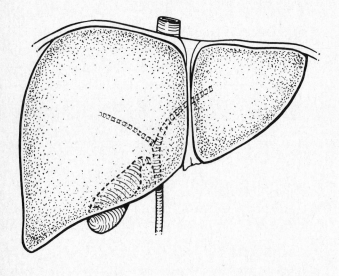

Questions

2. List five of the functions of the liver.

   1.

   2.

   3.

   4.

   5.

3. List five major clinical manifestations associated with hepatic disorders.

   1.

   2.

   3.

   4.

   5.

Matching

Match each of the following diagnostic tests with its description.

A. Liver scan   C. Esophagoscopy

B. Abdominal   D. Peritoneoscopy
   ultrasound

4. _____ Permits the direct visualization of the liver.

5. _____ Determines the size, shape, position, and functioning capability of the liver.

6. _____ Can be used to identify esophageal varices.

7. _____ Uses sound waves to differentiate tissues within the abdominal cavity.

Fill In

Fill in the normal value, then indicate if the value will increase or decrease with liver dysfunction.

	Value	Increase	Decrease
8. Urine urobilinogen	_____ mg/24 hr		
9. Total serum protein	_____ g/dl		
10. Serum albumin	_____ g/dl		
11. Blood ammonia	_____ μg/dl		
12. Total cholesterol	_____ mg/dl		
13. Prothrombin time	_____ sec		
14. Alpha-fetoprotein	_____ ng/ml		
15. AST (or SGOT)	_____ U/L men		
	_____ U/L women		

Questions

16. The functional units of the liver are the:

    A. Nephrotic capsules

    B. Sinusoids

    C. Hepatic lobules

    D. Capsules of Glisson

17. The blood supply to the liver is transported via the:

    A. Hepatic artery

    B. Hepatic portal vein

    C. Inferior vena cava

    D. Mesenteric artery

18. The process by which the liver converts glycogen to glucose to meet energy needs is known as:

    A. Glycogenesis

    B. Glycogenolysis

    C. Glucolysis

    D. Glyconeogenesis

19. An important function of the liver which aids the body in the digestion of fats is:

    A. Production of cholesterol

    B. Production of ketones

    C. Production of bile

    D. Production of amino acids

20. Ammonia, an end product of protein metabolism, is removed from the body by:

    A. Destruction in the liver

    B. Filtration in the hemopoietic system

    C. Destruction to amino acids and excretion in urine

    D. Conversion to urea and excretion in urine

21. Which of the following clinical manifestations would indicate to the nurse that a patient has a deficiency in bile production?

    A. Steatorrhea

    B. Dermatitis

    C. Glossitis

    D. Osteomalacia

22. If a patient has a hepatic disorder and a deficiency in vitamin K, the nurse would assess for:

    A. Clotting disorders

B. Hypoglycemic reactions

C. Anemia

D. Fluid volume changes

23. A nurse is assessing a patient with jaundice. The nurse realizes that this is caused by:

A. Rapid increase in by-products of protein metabolism

B. Elevated levels of bilirubin

C. Increase in red blood cells

D. Excessive excretion of bile salts

24. In caring for the patient with jaundice, an appropriate nursing intervention would be:

A. Bathe the patient in cool water and apply lotion

B. Massage the skin every 4 hours

C. Monitor intake and output frequently

D. Encourage fluid intake

25. A patient is admitted with a diagnosis of intrahepatic obstruction. In reviewing the medical history, which problem is most likely related to this condition?

A. History of bowel obstruction

B. History of congestive heart failure

C. History of hepatitis

D. History of diabetes

26. When assessing a patient with liver failure, what would be an appropriate nursing intervention to detect portal hypertension?

A. Assess heart sounds every shift

B. Assess abdominal girth daily

C. Assess for change in level of consciousness

D. Assess patient weight weekly

27. A patient is admitted with ascites. The nurse probably will be administering _____ to help remove excessive sodium.

A. Nifedipine

B. Catapres

C. Digoxin

D. Aldactone

28. Assuming all these patients have ascites, which one would be most likely to have a paracentesis?

A. Patient with 10-pound weight gain

B. Patient with irregular heart rhythm

C. Patient with respiratory difficulty

D. Patient with recent change in mental status

29. A patient has a LeVeen shunt inserted to control ascites. What is the best indication that the treatment is effective?

A. Improved cardiac output and urine output

B. Improved breathing patterns

C. Improvement in ability to ambulate

D. Improvement in appetite

30. Which of the following is considered an adverse effect of a LeVeen shunt insertion?

A. Weight loss of 10 pounds in 1 week

B. Abdominal girth decreasing by 1 inch

C. Hematuria and bleeding at IV site

D. Nausea and vomiting

31. Following insertion of a LeVeen shunt, which intervention by the nurse will prevent fluid from being removed too rapidly from the peritoneal cavity?

A. Ambulate the patient for 100 feet twice a day

B. Restrict fluids to 1000 ml daily

C. Place the patient in a sitting position

D. Monitor abdominal girth daily

32. When checking a patient with liver failure, the nurse notices petechia and bruising on the forearms. This suggests:

A. A clotting disorder exists

B. The LeVeen shunt has malfunctioned

C. A nutritional deficiency exists

D. A fluid imbalance is present

33. The nurse observes hematuria in a patient with a liver disorder. An appropriate nursing intervention would be:

A. Instruct patient to avoid all activities that can precipitate bleeding

B. Apply pressure at all venipuncture sites for 5 minutes

C. Have patient shave with an electric razor

D. All of the above

34. The nurse is aware that hepatic encephalopathy can occur in a patient with cirrhosis as a result of:

   A. Excessive intake of fluids

   B. Excessive ingestion of protein, and gastric bleeding

   C. Excessive restriction of proteins and fats

   D. Exposure to stressors

35. When a patient with a liver disorder exhibits restlessness, slurred speech, and tremors, the nurse would suspect:

   A. Clotting disorder

   B. Portal hypertension

   C. Nutritional deficiency

   D. Hepatic encephalopathy

36. A patient with a hepatic disorder is on a diet to restrict ammonia production. The nurse should instruct the patient to restrict:

   A. Fruit and fruit juice

   B. Cheese and daily products

   C. Bread and cereal

   D. Green and yellow vegetables

37. In caring for the patient with signs of hepatic encephalopathy, the nurse would probably administer:

   A. Lasix or diazide

   B. Neosporin

   C. Penicillin

   D. Neomycin

38. The nurse is administering lactulose to a patient. _____ is likely to occur as a result of this treatment.

   A. Fluid diuresis

   B. Hypokalemia

   C. Diarrhea

   D. Hematuria

39. In caring for a patient with hepatic encephalopathy, the nurse would expect to see improvement when there is a decrease in the serum level of:

   A. Amylase

   B. Ammonia

   C. Potassium

   D. Glucose

40. A nurse is assessing a patient with hepatic encephalopathy. Which assessment data is a sign of impending coma?

   A. Refusal to answer questions

   B. Presence of asterixis, liver flap

   C. Presence of ecchymosis on abdomen

   D. Increase in abdominal girth

41. Write a nursing care plan for the patient who has had a paracentesis.

   Nursing Diagnosis: Fluid volume excess

   Patient Outcome:

   Nursing Interventions:

42. A patient with alcoholism and a hepatic disorder is admitted with a nutritional deficiency. The reason for this condition is most likely:

   A. Inadequate nutrient intake

   B. Excessive carbohydrate intake

   C. Insufficient finances

   D. Unilateral neglect

43. The chronic alcoholic is often at risk for developing malabsorption of certain vitamins because of:

   A. Insufficient fluid intake

   B. Excessive intake of nonessential nutrients

   C. Inflammation of the gastrointestinal tract

   D. Lack of a balanced diet

44. The nurse is aware that the alcoholic patient often exhibits signs of impaired carbohydrate metabolism. Findings would include:

   A. Hyperglycemia

   B. Hypoglycemia

C. Albuminuria

D. Proteinemia

45. A patient would likely be ordered to receive vitamin K if which of the following lab tests are abnormal?

A. Prothrombin time is prolonged

B. Prothrombin time is decreased

C. Thromboplastin time is decreased

D. SGOT is elevated

46. Write a nursing care plan for the patient with advanced hepatic encephalopathy.

Nursing Diagnosis: High risk for injury

Patient Outcome:

Nursing Interventions:

47. Write a nursing care plan that will address the nutritional needs of a patient with cirrhoses and alcoholism.

Nursing Diagnosis:

Patient Outcome:

Nursing Interventions:

CLINICAL SITUATIONS

Situation ■ 1

Mark Harvey, age 55, is admitted for diagnostic testing for possible liver disease. He has a history of drug and alcohol abuse.

1. The nurse is reviewing the records. Liver damage would be indicated by an increase in serum:

A. AST (or SGOT)

B. CK or CPK

C. BUN and creatinine

D. WBC, platelets

2. When checking the patient, the nurse finds Mr. Harvey has rapid, shallow respirations and a large firm abdomen. These findings would suggest the presence of:

A. Jaundice

B. Dehydration

C. Ascites

D. Encephalopathy

3. Mr. Harvey is scheduled for a paracentesis. An important nursing intervention would include:

A. Position patient in prone position

B. Have patient void immediately before procedure

C. Administering preoperative medication

D. Administering oxygen

4. Following the procedure, which of the following symptoms, when present, would indicate a complication?

A. Increase in pulse and decrease in blood pressure

B. Discomfort in the area of needle insertion

C. Abdominal girth decreased by 3 inches

D. Rise in blood pressure and pulse rate

Situation ■ 2

Mr. Billmore is being treated for cirrhosis. He is exhibiting symptoms of hepatic encephalopathy. He has been admitted many times in the past with gastrointestinal bleeding and respiratory distress.

1. The nurse is assessing the patient. Findings include rapid respirations, distant heart sounds, enlarged abdomen, altered thought process with confusion, and tremors. The patient is at risk for:

A. Gastrointestinal bleeding

B. Impending coma

C. Fluid deficit

D. Impaired tissue perfusion

2. The nurse would anticipate that this patient would exhibit an increase in serum levels of _____ as a result of his advanced cirrhosis.

A. Albumin

B. Globulin

C. Total cholesterol

D. Glucose

3. Medical management of Mr. Billmore will include preventing clotting disorders. The nurse would anticipate administering:

   A. Vitamin B_{12}

   B. Vitamin C

   C. Vitamin K

   D. Potassium

4. In order to determine the source of Mr. Billmore's bleeding, the nurse will prepare him for a/an:

A. MRI

B. CT scan

C. Abdominal ultrasound

D. Esophagoscopy

5. Mr. Billmore is receiving neomycin by mouth four times a day. The nurse is aware that the rationale for this treatment is:

   A. Removal of by-products of carbohydrate metabolism

   B. Reduction of the bacteria in the bloodstream

   C. Reduction in fluid retention in the abdomen

   D. Reduction of ammonia-producing organisms in the intestine

Chapter Twenty-eight

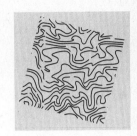

NURSING CARE
of Adults with
Hepatic Disorders

Learning Objectives

1.0 Demonstrate an Understanding of the Infectious and Inflammatory Disorders of the Hepatic System.

1.1 Identify the Clinical Manifestations of Infectious and Inflammatory Disorders of the Hepatic System.
1.2 Identify Complications Associated with Hepatitis.
1.3 Identify and Differentiate the Different Types of Hepatitis.
1.4 Recognize the Medical Management of the Infectious and Inflammatory Disorders.
1.5 Identify Ways to Prevent Hepatitis.
1.6 Write a Nursing Care Plan for the Patient with Hepatitis.

2.0 Demonstrate an Understanding of the Structural Abnormalities of the Hepatic System.

2.1 Demonstrate an Understanding of the Etiology of Several Types of Cirrhosis.
2.2 Recognize the Medical Management of the Patient with Cirrhosis.
2.3 Identify Complications Associated with Cirrhosis.
2.4 Plan Nursing Interventions Appropriate for the Patient with Cirrhosis.
2.5 Write a Nursing Care Plan for the Patient with Cirrhosis.

3.0 Identify Types of Traumatic Injuries Which can Affect the Liver.

3.1 Identify Clinical Manifestations Associated with Liver Trauma.
3.2 Identify the Medical Management for the Patient with Liver Trauma.

4.0 Demonstrate an Understanding of the Neoplasms Which can Affect The Hepatic System.

4.1 Identify Clinical Manifestations of Hepatic Tumors.
4.2 Recognize the Types of Medical Management for Individuals with Hepatic Tumors.
4.3 Recognize the Surgical Management of the Patient with Hepatic Abnormalities.

Learning Activities

Questions

1. The type of hepatitis which is related to poor sanitation and can be spread by contaminated food is:

   A. Hepatitis A

   B. Hepatitis B

   C. Hepatitis D

   D. Non-A, non-B hepatitis

2. The type of hepatitis which is related to an increase in IV drug use and is spread via the parenteral route is:

   A. Hepatitis A

   B. Hepatitis B

   C. Hepatitis D

   D. All of the above

3. The best way to characterize the process of hepatitis is:

   A. Liver cell necrosis, inflammation, and cell regeneration

   B. Liver cell necrosis, degeneration, and chronicity

   C. Liver cell hypoxia, obstruction

   D. Liver cell destruction, scarring, infiltration

4. A nurse has been exposed to hepatitis B. The incubation for this disease can be as long as:

   A. 20 days

   B. 45 days

   C. 90 days

   D. 180 days

5. Clinical manifestations associated with the pre-icteric phase of hepatitis include:

   A. Anorexia and jaundice

   B. Fatigue, nausea, anorexia

   C. Right upper quadrant pain, fatigue

   D. Vomiting, diarrhea, dark urine, dark stool

6. The nurse would explain to a patient with hepatitis who has obstruction of bile flow that he or she will have:

   A. Urine which is light in color

   B. Stool which is dark and tarry

   C. Urine which is dark in color

   D. Skin which is pale

7. A patient is admitted with acute viral hepatitis. The nurse would expect to see a rise in serum _____.

   A. PT, PTT

   B. SGOT, ESR

   C. Potassium

   D. BUN, creatinine

8. Assessment findings which would demonstrate to the nurse that the patient with hepatitis is in the recovery phase include:

   A. Weight returns to normal, ascites disappears

   B. Jaundice disappears, normal energy levels return

   C. Normal heart and breath sounds, active bowel sounds

   D. Stool and urine normal in color, appetite improves

9. When an individual with hepatitis has an obstruction in bile flow, this is due to:

   A. Hepatocyte inflammation

   B. Liver cell necrosis

   C. Leukopenia

   D. Biliary obstruction

10. A health care institute is testing its staff for the presence of hepatitis markers. The best explanation of what the presence of this marker in the serum indicates is:

A. Exposure to a hepatitis virus with antibody formation

B. Active hepatitis currently in the system

C. Past infection with the hepatitis virus

D. Immunity to the hepatitis A virus

11. One of the nurses is found to have the hepatitis marker HBeAg in her serum. This would indicate:

A. Current infection of hepatitis A

B. Current infection of hepatitis B

C. Past infection of hepatitis B

D. Present infection of hepatitis C

12. Medical management for the patient with acute viral hepatitis would include:

A. Hospitalization, antibiotic therapy

B. Bedrest, hydration, antibiotics

C. Rest, avoid fatigue, well-balanced diet

D. Bedrest, low-calorie diet, force fluids

13. Once an individual has had an episode of hepatitis, the nurse would be sure to include the following instructions:

A. Avoid all foods high in protein

B. Avoid alcohol

C. Don't donate blood

D. Stop smoking

True or False

14. _____ Previously healthy individuals who develop hepatitis usually recover completely.

15. _____ The major complication associated with a hepatitis infection is chronic hepatitis.

16. _____ In chronic hepatitis, there is liver cell necrosis and portal tract obstruction.

17. _____ Chronic active hepatitis can progress to cirrhosis.

18. _____ Individuals who develop fulminant hepatitis will recover completely.

19. _____ Individuals who are traveling to the

tropics should receive immune serum globulin.

Questions

20. The administration of hepatitis B immunoglobin is indicated in which of the following instances?

A. A nurse has received a needle stick injury

B. A person has tested positive for HB_S Ag

C. A person is splashed in the face with HB_S Ag material

D. A patient is traveling to an area where hepatitis B is endemic

21. There is an increase in the number of cases of both hepatitis A and B in health care institutes. Nurses are at the highest risk of developing hepatitis B in which area?

A. Emergency room

B. Intensive care unit

C. Dialysis unit

D. Cardiac unit

22. Approximately 75% of post-transfusion hepatitis is _____.

A. Hepatitis A virus

B. Hepatitis B virus

C. Non-A, non-B hepatitis

D. Hepatitis D virus

23. Which group of hospital patients is particularly at risk for acquiring non-A, non-B hepatitis?

A. Cardiac patients

B. Renal patients

C. Cancer patients

D. Surgical patients

24. The administration of hepatitis B vaccine would be recommended for which of the following individuals?

A. Hemodialysis patients

B. Homosexually active males

C. Sexual contacts of hepatitis B carriers

D. All of the above

25. Write a nursing care plan for the patient with hepatitis A.

    Nursing Diagnosis: High risk for altered health maintenance related to insufficient knowledge of disease process and mode of transmission

    Patient Outcome:

    Nursing Interventions:

26. When a patient is admitted with a possible liver abscess, which test would be most diagnostic?

    A. Chest x-ray

    B. Ultrasonography

    C. VQ scan

    D. MRI scan

27. Which nursing action has the highest priority when caring for the patient with multiple liver abscesses?

    A. Maintain strict bedrest

    B. Administer antibiotics on time

    C. Maintain fluid restrictions

    D. Administer pain medications as needed

28. A patient is admitted to the hospital with toxic hepatitis. On review of the chart, the nurse identifies which information as having a possible relationship to the current problem?

    A. Recent travel to Haiti

    B. Recent discharge from the Army

    C. Employed by dry cleaning company

    D. Ingestion of 2 glasses of wine daily

29. In caring for the patient with toxic hepatitis, the nurse's responsibility would include:

    A. Prevention of reexposure to hepatotoxin

    B. Administration of analgesics frequently

    C. Prevention of skin breakdown

    D. Administering antibiotics

30. Elderly individuals are at risk for the development of toxic hepatitis because of:

    A. Poor dietary habits

    B. Decrease in level of activity

    C. Increased susceptibility to infection

    D. Use of multiple medications

31. The type of cirrhosis which has been linked to alcohol consumption is known as:

    A. Primary biliary cirrhosis

    B. Necrotic cirrhosis

    C. Laënnec's cirrhosis

    D. Secondary obstructive cirrhosis

32. One of the first manifestations of liver damage which results from alcoholism is:

    A. Fatty cirrhosis

    B. Muscle wasting

    C. Alcoholic hepatitis

    D. Biliary obstruction

33. When working with individuals with cirrhosis, the nurse is aware that regardless of the cause of the problem, the end result will be:

    A. Fatty nodules and liver abscess formation

    B. Biliary tract obstruction

    C. Destruction and regeneration of liver cells

    D. Destruction of hepatocytes and impaired liver function

34. The nurse should consider which nursing diagnosis a priority when caring for a patient with newly diagnosed Laënnec's cirrhosis?

    A. Ineffective breathing pattern

    B. Ineffective individual coping related to chronic disease

    C. Alteration in nutrition: more than body requirements

    D. Knowledge deficit related to disease cause and prognosis.

35. The nurse's responsibility in preventing complications associated with cirrhosis includes:

    A. Monitor for signs of bleeding

    B. Monitor for fluid and electrolyte imbalance

    C. Monitor for signs of skin breakdown

    D. Monitor for signs of malnutrition

36. Medical management of a patient who has esophageal varices would include the administration of:

    A. Corticosteroids

    B. Antibiotic therapy

    C. Vasopressin

    D. Streptokinase

37. The physician orders oral neomycin four times a day for a patient with cirrhosis. The nurse explains to the patient that the purpose of this therapy is to:

    A. Reduce edema and abdominal swelling

    B. Remove intestinal contents and block ammonia formation

    C. Prevent esophageal and rectal bleeding

    D. Prevent infection from spreading throughout the system

38. The nurse will carefully observe the patient with cirrhosis for signs of portal systemic encephalopathy. The nurse would be alerted to a change in condition if there is a change in the patient's:

    A. Blood pressure and pulse

    B. Level of consciousness

    C. Urine output

    D. Level of mobility

39. Write a nursing care plan for the patient with cirrhosis and encephalopathy.

    Nursing Diagnosis: High risk for injury related to altered thought process

    Patient Outcome:

    Nursing Interventions:

40. A patient is admitted to the emergency room following a car accident. Which of the following signs, if present, would indicate liver trauma?

    A. Restlessness, signs of shock, absent bowel sounds

    B. Anxiety, rise in blood pressure and heart rate

    C. Vomiting, sharp abdominal pain

    D. Agitation, altered level of consciousness

41. Management of a suspected liver laceration in an unstable patient would involve:

    A. Monitor vital signs every hour

    B. Surgical intervention

    C. Administer blood products

    D. Stabilization and transfer to a trauma unit

42. A patient is admitted with a possible neoplasm of the liver. The nurse is aware that a definitive diagnosis can be made by:

    A. Scanning techniques

    B. Results of lab work

    C. Liver biopsy

    D. Abdominal x-ray

43. A patient with liver cancer is to receive chemotherapy via a hepatic catheter. An important nursing responsibility would be:

    A. Prepare patient for a lengthy hospitalization

    B. Instruct patient to perform wet-to-dry dressing changes

    C. Provide dietary instructions and limitations

    D. Instruct patient in aseptic care of the catheter and pump

44. A primary nursing responsibility when caring for the patient who has received a liver transplant involves

    A. Checking the vital signs and neurologic status frequently

    B. Monitoring for signs of infection or rejection

    C. Monitoring continuous feedings

    D. Preventing ventilator malfunction

45. The nurse is caring for a patient who has received a liver transplant. Which of the following is a positive sign indicating liver function?

    A. Thick, green bile drainage from the T-tube

    B. Decrease in abdominal girth

    C. Increased output with a decrease in edema

    D. Stable vital signs, normal urine and stools

46. When assessing the patient who has had a liver transplant, the nurse finds the patient has a low-grade fever and joint pain. This can indicate:

A. Infection

B. Rejection

C. Suppression

D. Either A or B

CLINICAL SITUATIONS

Situation ■ 1

Alice is admitted with fatigue, anorexia, and jaundice. She is homeless and was brought to the hospital by police. A tentative diagnosis of hepatitis is made.

1. Because of the symptoms that Alice currently has, the nurse would expect to see an increase in serum:

    A. WBC

    B. BUN

    C. Ammonia

    D. Bilirubin

2. A diagnosis of hepatitis A is made. This is confirmed by the presence of which hepatitis marker?

    A. HAV-Ab/IgM

    B. HAV-Ab/IgG

    C. HB_E Ag

    D. Antihepatitis C virus

3. Which of the following information provided by Alice is a clue as to how she contracted the disease?

    A. I sleep in the shelters

    B. I don't have warm clothes

    C. I eat out of garbage cans

    D. I have a friend who uses drugs

4. An important nursing intervention for the acute phase of Alice's illness would be:

    A. Provide rest periods frequently throughout the day

    B. Increase fluid intake, especially water

    C. Measure abdominal girth daily

    D. Increase activity as tolerated

5. The nurse is aware that the virus which causes hepatitis A will be excreted from Alice's system mainly through:

    A. Skin

    B. Feces

    C. Urine

    D. Saliva

Situation ■ 2

Mr. Black is admitted with cirrhosis. He states that he drinks heavily and has been admitted several times for bleeding. He has jaundice and a protruding abdomen. He is complaining of right upper quadrant pain.

1. During the initial assessment, the nurse gathers enough data to indicate that Mr. Black may have portal hypertension. Assuming all these findings are present, which one would lead to that conclusion?

    A. Jaundiced appearance

    B. Low-grade fever

    C. Ascites and edema

    D. Palpable liver

2. Mr. Black begins to hemorrhage. The physician inserts a Sengstaken-Blakemore tube to control the bleeding. The rationale for this treatment is:

    A. The suction removes the bleeding

    B. It provides a route for administering medications

    C. The inflated balloon exerts pressure on the bleeding site

    D. It provides a route for rapid blood administration

3. To prevent any complications associated with the use of the Sengstaken-Blakemore tube, the nurse will carefully assess:

    A. Cardiac function

    B. Respiratory status

    C. Fluid status

    D. Neurologic status

4. The physician is able to stop the bleeding and

stabilize the patient. He decides that Mr. Black may benefit from sclerotherapy. The nursing care would include:

A. Preparing the patient for endoscopy procedure

B. Preparing the patient for surgery

C. Administering vasopressors

D. Administering antibiotics

5. Mr. Black is complaining of dry and itchy skin. The nurse is aware that this problem is a result of which problem associated with cirrhosis?

A. Elevated prothrombin time

B. Elevated bilirubin

C. Decreased sodium and potassium

D. Impaired synthesis of vitamin K

Unit Ten

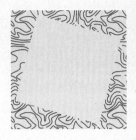

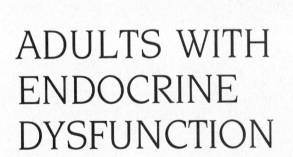

ADULTS WITH ENDOCRINE DYSFUNCTION

Chapter Twenty-nine

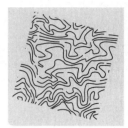

KNOWLEDGE BASIC TO THE NURSING CARE
of Adults with
Endocrine Dysfunction

Learning Objectives

1.0 Review the Function of the Endocrine System.

1.1 Identify the Major Endocrine Glands on a Diagram.
1.2 Identify Specific Hormones Secreted by each Specific Gland.
1.3 Match Specific Hormones with Their Primary Hormonal Functions.

2.0 Demonstrate an Understanding of the Specific Manifestations of Endocrine Dysfunctions.

2.1 Identify Assessment Data that is Characteristic of Endocrine Dysfunction.
2.2 Demonstrate Application of the Nursing Process when Caring for a Patient with an Endocrine Dysfunction.

Learning Activities

Identify

1. On the diagram, identify the major endocrine glands.

   A. Pituitary
   B. Thyroid
   C. Parathyroid
   D. Adrenals

   E. Pancreatic islets
   F. Kidneys
   G. Ovaries
   H. Testes

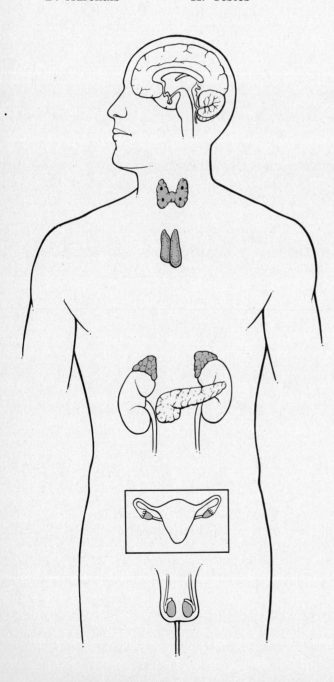

Fill In

2. Hormones can affect a _____ or can have a general effect on the entire body.

3. One way that the concentration of hormones in the blood is maintained is by _____ .

4. The pituitary gland is also known as _____ .

5. Secretion of insulin in the pancreas occurs in the _____ .

Next to each endocrine, fill in the principal hormone it secretes.

6. Thymus gland:

7. Pineal gland:

8. Hypothalamus:

9. Pituitary gland:

10. Thyroid:

11. Adrenal glands:

12. Pancreatic islets:

27. _____ Secondary glandular dysfunction is usually permanent.

Matching

Match each of the hormones with its primary function.

A. Insulin   F. Thyroxine
B. Glucagon   G. Calcitonin
C. Estrogen   H. Adrenalin
D. Testosterone   I. Aldosterone
E. Somatotropin   J. Antidiuretic hormone

13. _____ Promotes sodium and water retention, potassium excretion.

14. _____ Regulates energy production and growth and development.

15. _____ Stimulates closure of the epiphyseal plates at puberty.

16. _____ Stimulates the stress response.

17. _____ Regulates osmolality of extracellular fluids.

18. _____ Regulates metabolism of fat, protein, and carbohydrates.

19. _____ Increases the rate that calcium is deposited in the bones.

20. _____ Necessary for the maturation of the reproductive system.

21. _____ Stimulates the growth of cells, bones, and muscles.

22. _____ Raises blood glucose levels by promoting hepatic glycogenolysis.

True or False

23. _____ A cell will not respond to a hormone unless it has receptor sites for that hormone.

24. _____ The functions of the adrenal cortex are nonessential.

25. _____ Dysfunction of one endocrine gland often affects the function of another.

26. _____ Hypersecretion from an endocrine gland is often the result of a tumor.

Questions

28. The nurse would monitor for signs of glucose intolerance when a patient has:

    A. Acromegaly

    B. Cushing's disease

    C. Pheochromocytoma

    D. Graves' disease

29. An individual with abnormal production of _____ is at risk for developing osteoporosis.

    A. Adrenalin

    B. Aldosterone

    C. Calcitonin

    D. Cortisol

30. A deficiency in the production of this hormone will lead to symptoms of diabetes insipidus.

    A. Insulin

    B. Glucagon

    C. Estrogen

    D. Antidiuretic hormone

31. A deficiency in the production of this hormone will lead to symptoms of diabetes mellitus.

    A. Glucagon

    B. Insulin

    C. Prolactin

    D. Epinephrine

32. When a patient has an alteration in serum calcium and phosphorus levels, the nurse would suspect an alteration in function of this gland.

    A. Thyroid

    B. Parathyroid

    C. Pancreas

    D. Adrenal

33. When an individual is subjected to a very stressful experience, he or she would have increased amounts of _____ secreted.

A. Epinephrine

B. Insulin

C. Estrogen

D. Thyroxine

34. One of the most noticeable age-related changes in the endocrine system is:

A. Decrease in the ability to respond to stress

B. Increase in the number of endocrine disorders

C. Change in glucose production

D. Erratic production of hormones

CLINICAL SITUATION

Situation ■ 1

A patient is admitted with a suspected endocrine abnormality. Symptoms include: alteration in blood sugar, weakness, and irritability.

1. Diagnostic testing to determine the cause of the problem will mainly include:

A. X-ray

B. Laboratory studies

C. Ultrasound

D. MRI

2. Based on the initial symptoms, the nurse would suspect an alteration in the function of which gland?

A. Adrenal

B. Thyroid

C. Pancreas

D. Parathyroid

3. If this condition is a primary endocrine gland dysfunction, this implies:

A. The gland is secreting too much or too little hormone because of a defect in the gland itself

B. The gland is secreting abnormal amounts of hormone in response to changes in the pituitary gland

C. There is idiopathic hyperplasia of the affected gland

D. The primary gland is causing the dysfunction of the secondary gland

4. While collecting the medical history from the patient, it would be important to:

A. Determine if patient knows the reason for admission

B. Have someone familiar with the patient present

C. Determine if symptoms developed gradually or rapidly

D. Determine if patient has characteristic symptoms

E. All of the above

5. Emotional support and teaching are probably the most important nursing functions to help the individual, because:

A. The disease is usually life-threatening

B. It is almost impossible to comply with the many restrictions the patient will have

C. The individual will need to make adjustments in lifestyle and take lifelong medications

D. The disease will require a change of profession and much less activity

Chapter Thirty

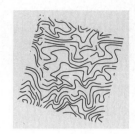

NURSING CARE
of Adults with Diabetes Mellitus

Learning Objectives

1.0 Demonstrate an Understanding of the Pathophysiology of Diabetes Mellitus.

1.1 Demonstrate an Understanding of the Hormonal Regulation of Blood Glucose Levels.
1.2 Identify Clinical Manifestations of the Patient with Diabetes Mellitus.
1.3 Identify Characteristics of Type I and Type II Diabetes.
1.4 Identify How the Diagnosis of Diabetes Mellitus Is Made.

2.0 Demonstrate an Understanding of the Medical Management of Diabetes Mellitus.

2.1 Identify Medications Used in the Treatment of Diabetes Mellitus.
2.2 Identify Ways to Manage the Diabetic Patient During Illness.

3.0 Demonstrate an Understanding of the Complications That Can Occur in the Patient with Diabetes.

3.1 Identify Symptoms of Short- and Long-Term Complications of Diabetes Mellitus.
3.2 Demonstrate Application of the Nursing Process When Caring for the Patient with Diabetes Mellitus.
3.3 Write a Nursing Care Plan for the Patient with Diabetes Mellitus.

Learning Activities

Questions

1. The effects of insulin on carbohydrate metabolism are to _____ glucose metabolism, _____ blood glucose concentration, and _____ glycogen stores.

   A. Increase; increase; increase

   B. Decrease; decrease; increase

   C. Increase; decrease; increase

   D. Increase; decrease; decrease

2. Insulin promotes fatty acid synthesis by converting _____ into fatty acids.

   A. Fats

   B. Glucose

   C. Carbohydrates

   D. Amino acids

3. The process of converting glycogen back into glucose, called glycogenolysis, is done by the _____.

   A. Liver

   B. Pancreas

   C. Pituitary gland

   D. Islets of Langerhans

4. All of the following EXCEPT _____ are counterregulatory hormones and will oppose the action of insulin.

   A. Glucagon

   B. Cortisol

   C. Growth hormone

   D. Antidiuretic hormone

5. When a patient with hyperglycemia is admitted, the nurse would assess carefully for signs of:

   A. Dehydration, electrolyte depletion

   B. Fluid retention, high potassium levels

   C. Cardiac arrhythmias

   D. Infection, pain

6. If the fasting blood glucose level is over _____ mg/dl on more than one occasion, the diagnosis of diabetes can be made.

   A. 80

   B. 100

   C. 140

   D. 180

7. When the patient with diabetes has insufficient insulin to metabolize carbohydrates, there will be a/an:

   A. Decrease in breakdown of fats

   B. Increase in the production of ketones

   C. Decrease in breakdown of ketones

   D. Development of respiratory alkalosis

8. The major characteristic of Type II diabetes is:

   A. Impaired receptor sites

   B. Excess of insulin

   C. Lack of insulin

   D. Insulin resistance

9. The main difference between Type I and Type II diabetes is that the Type I diabetic:

   A. Must follow a diabetic diet

   B. Must take daily insulin

   C. Has more complications

   D. Has a history of obesity

10. The diagnosis of diabetes is based on:

    A. Glucose tolerance test; hormone testing

    B. Presence of symptoms, fasting glucose levels

    C. Symptoms of polyuria, polydipsia, polyphagia

    D. Family history, current complaint

11. An appropriate diet for a diabetic should include _____ carbohydrate, _____ fat, and _____ protein.

    A. 30%; 30%; 40%

B. 40%; 20%; 40%

C. 60%; 15%; 25%

D. 55%; 25%; 20%

12. It is important for the nurse to instruct the patient with diabetes about the value of exercise since exercise:

   A. Acts as a hypoglycemic

   B. Can help to normalize blood sugar

   C. Can eliminate the need for insulin

   D. Helps prevent infections

13. When an elderly patient with Type II diabetes develops influenza, he or she is at risk for developing:

   A. Hypoglycemia

   B. Diabetic ketoacidosis

   C. Hyperglycemic hyperosmolar nonketotic syndrome

   D. Systemic infection

14. It would be important for the nurse to instruct diabetic patients that if they become ill, they should:

   A. Monitor blood sugar levels every 4 to 6 hours

   B. Stop taking their insulin until symptoms subside

   C. Come to the hospital immediately

   D. Follow any diet that makes them feel better

15. When a diabetic patient is admitted for surgery, the methods of administering insulin would be:

   A. Give the normal dose of insulin

   B. Give 1/3 to 1/2 the usual dose of long-acting insulin

   C. Make the patient NPO and withhold insulin

   D. Give regular insulin every 2 hours

16. When a patient has diabetic neuropathy, it is very important for the nurse to monitor for:

   A. Neurologic changes

   B. Changes in the skin on the lower extremities

   C. Signs of nausea, vomiting, diarrhea

   D. Signs of infection

17. The rationale for the measurement of hemoglobin A_{1c} is:

   A. Be sure the patient is taking insulin

   B. To see if the patient is following the diet

   C. To see blood glucose levels over the previous 3 months

   D. So that the patient doesn't have to do the daily blood glucose testing

18. Emergency treatment for the patient admitted with diabetic ketoacidosis would include:

   A. Rapid administration of D_5W and insulin

   B. Replacement of fluid, electrolytes, and dextrose

   C. Administration of 0.45% saline and insulin per pump

   D. Use of 0.9% saline, sodium bicarbonate, and potassium

19. What is the reason that the patient should be instructed to bring insulin to room temperature before injecting it?

   A. It will hurt if the insulin is cold

   B. Cold temperatures can affect the rate of absorption

   C. To prevent hypoglycemia

   D. It is harder to draw up when it is cold

20. If a diabetic patient exhibits symptoms of shaking, sweating, weakness, hunger, and drowsiness, the nurse should:

   A. Administer 4 oz fruit juice or regular soda

   B. Administer 8 oz of juice with two lumps of sugar

   C. Administer 1 amp of 50% dextrose

   D. Administer regular insulin as ordered

21. When a patient is to be discharged with an insulin pump, he or she needs to be instructed on possible complications. The most common complication is:

   A. Hypoglycemia

   B. Ketoacidosis

   C. Infection at site

   D. Pump failure

22. Which of the following patients would be the best candidate for a pancreas transplant?

    A. Insulin-dependent male, 20 years old

    B. Patient who is poorly controlled with insulin and has frequent episodes of hypoglycemia/hyperglycemia

    C. Patient who is unable to learn how to administer insulin or follow diet

    D. Elderly female, age 70, who can no longer take oral hypoglycemics

23. The nurse would monitor the patient with a pancreas transplant for early signs of rejection, which would include:

    A. Hypoglycemia

    B. Hyperglycemia

    C. Fever, weakness

    D. Nausea, vomiting

24. If a patient with diabetes has a hyperglycemic reaction, typical symptoms would include:

    A. Diaphoresis, hunger, confusion

    B. Blurred vision, thirst, nausea, vomiting

    C. Cool, clammy skin, dizziness, drowsiness

    D. Any of the above

25. For the patient with diabetic nephropathy, an important nursing measure is:

    A. Administration of antihypertensives

    B. Providing dietary instruction

    C. Contacting a support group

    D. Administration of insulin

26. The _____ is characterized by periods of hypoglycemia followed by rebound hyperglycemia.

    A. Dawn phenomenon

    B. Degenerative effect

    C. Somogyi phenomenon

    D. Ketosis effect

27. The main treatment for diabetic retinopathy is:

    A. Medication

    B. Corrective lens

    C. Laser treatment

    D. Surgical correction

28. When a patient with peripheral neuropathy develops muscle weakness and sensory loss, the primary nursing goal would be to:

    A. Prevent pain

    B. Prevent injury

    C. Treat symptoms

    D. Educate patient

29. When a diabetic patient has symptoms that include hyperglycemia, proteinuria, hypertension, and edema, this suggests:

    A. Diabetic nephropathy

    B. Diabetic retinopathy

    C. Diabetic neuropathy

    D. Diabetic ketosis

30. If the nurse administers 35 units of Humulin NPH insulin at 7:30 am, it would be important for the patient to receive a snack at:

    A. 11 am

    B. 1 pm

    C. 4 pm

    D. 8 pm

31. To help determine if a patient with symptoms of hyperglycemia has diabetic ketoacidosis of hyperglycemic, hyperosmolar, nonketotic syndrome (HHNKS), which laboratory finding would the nurse check?

    A. Blood sugar

    B. Potassium

    C. White blood count

    D. Ketones

True or False

32. _____ Opened bottles of insulin may be stored at room temperature.

33. _____ Patients with Type II diabetes mellitus may initially have none of the classic symptoms.

34. _____ The sulfonylureas should be considered oral insulin.

35. _____ Hypoglycemic reactions cannot occur when the patient takes sulfonylureas.

36. _____ The diabetic patient must assume responsibility for management of his or her condition.

37. _____ The diabetic diet is the cornerstone of treatment for the diabetic patient.

38. _____ It is very important to exercise if the blood glucose level is higher than 250 mg/dl.

39. _____ Humulin insulin comes from cadaver pancreases.

40. _____ Diabetic patients should stop taking their insulin if they become ill.

Questions

41. Write a care plan for the patient with diabetes mellitus.

    Nursing   Diagnosis: Altered   health   maintenance related to insufficient knowledge of diabetic self-management

    Patient Outcome:

    Nursing Interventions:

CLINICAL SITUATIONS

Situation ■ 1

A young adult is admitted to the hospital with a severe respiratory infection. Lab results show a blood glucose level of 450 mg/dl. Further testing establishes that the patient has diabetes Type I. The patient denies any prior history or symptoms of the disease.

1. Why would this patient develop diabetes at this time?

    A. The acute infection precipitated the event

    B. The patient used up all his or her insulin

    C. The patient is in the high-risk age group

    D. The patient must have parents with the disease

2. The treatment of choice for this patient will include: (Check all that apply.)

    A. Diet

    B. Insulin

    C. Exercise

    D. Oral hypoglycemics

    E. Pancreatic transplant

3. The nurse would instruct the patient to watch for signs of hypoglycemia when he is taking insulin. Causes of this condition include all EXCEPT:

    A. Too much insulin

    B. Too much food

    C. Too much activity

    D. Ingestion of alcohol

4. Because of the long-term complications that often occur with the Type I diabetic, the nurse would instruct the patient to:

    A. Have a yearly eye exam

    B. Join a health club

    C. Check his feet daily

    D. Have a yearly exam by a cardiologist

Situation ■ 2

A 50-year-old male was found to have a blood glucose level of 288 mg/dl during a spot check at a local health fair. He is very surprised by this.

1. Which of the characteristic findings might the nurse expect to find in the patient's medical history? (Check all that apply.)

    A. Obesity

    B. Inactivity

    C. Family history

    D. Recent infection

2. What is the most likely diagnosis for this patient?

    A. Type I diabetes

    B. Type II diabetes

    C. Gestational diabetes

    D. Impaired glucose tolerance

3. The treatment of choice for this patient will probably involve:

    A. Insulin and diet

    B. Exercise and diet

C. Oral hypoglycemics and diet

D. Insulin and antibiotics

4. This individual is most at risk for developing which of the following complications?

A. Diabetic retinopathy

B. Diabetic foot ulcer

C. Hypoglycemia

D. Diabetic ketoacidosis

Situation ■ 3

A 75-year-old female is admitted to the hospital from a nursing home. She has a history of Type II diabetes, arthritis, and stroke. Currently she is dehydrated and having diarrhea. Laboratory findings show a blood sugar level of 880 mg/dl and an osmolality of 400 mOsm/kg.

1. Based on the above information, the nurse would suspect that this individual has:

A. Hyperglycemia

B. Diabetic ketoacidosis

C. HHNKS

D. Sepsis

2. Appropriate treatment would involve:

A. Fluid replacement, correction of electrolyte deficiency

B. Giving NPH insulin and 0.9% saline for dehydration

C. Insulin drip, 10% dextrose in saline

D. Electrolyte replacement; sodium bicarbonate

3. On the second day, the nurse finds her talking incoherently. She is shaky, diaphoretic, tachycardiac, and very anxious. These symptoms suggest:

A. Hyperglycemia

B. Hypoglycemia

C. Dehydration

D. Stroke

4. An appropriate nursing intervention at this time would be:

A. Stop the insulin infusion and check the blood glucose

B. Call the physician

C. Draw blood gases

D. Increase the IV fluids and give the patient simple sugar

Chapter Thirty-one

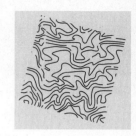

NURSING CARE
of Adults with Pituitary Disorders

Learning Objectives

1.0 Demonstrate an Understanding of the Pathophysiology of Pituitary Disorders.

1.1 Demonstrate an Understanding of the Role of Hormonal Regulation in Pituitary Disorders.
1.2 Identify the Clinical Manifestations of the Patient with a Pituitary Disorder.

2.0 Demonstrate an Understanding of the Disorders of the Anterior Pituitary.

2.1 Identify the Clinical Manifestations of Neoplasms of the Anterior Pituitary.
2.2 Identify the Clinical Manifestations of Hypersecretion Disorders of the Anterior Pituitary.
2.3 Identify Medications Used in the Treatment of Anterior Pituitary Disorders.
2.4 Identify the Nonmedical Management of the Patient with a Pituitary Disorder.
2.5 Demonstrate an Understanding of the Nursing Interventions Used in Caring for the Patient with an Anterior Pituitary Disorder.
2.6 Write a Nursing Care Plan for the Patient with an Anterior Pituitary Disorder.

3.0 Demonstrate an Understanding of the Disorders of the Posterior Pituitary.

3.1 Identify the Clinical Manifestations of Diabetes Insipidus.
3.2 Identify the Management Technique for the Patient with Diabetes Insipidus.
3.3 Demonstrate an Understanding of the Nursing Interventions Used in Caring for the Patient with Diabetes Insipidus.

Learning Activities

Questions

1. Pituitary hormones which directly affect the secretory functions of other endocrine glands are referred to as _____ hormones.

   A. Secretory

   B. Direct

   C. Tropic

   D. Target

2. The most common manifestation of a pituitary tumor is:

   A. Frequent headaches

   B. Visual disturbances

   C. Dizziness

   D. Vomiting

3. When a patient has had surgical removal of a pituitary neoplasm, the nurse would monitor carefully for the earliest sign of increasing intracranial pressure, which is:

   A. Lethargy

   B. Narrowing pulse pressure

   C. Tachycardia

   D. Agitation

4. Following surgery for a pituitary adenoma, the nurse would monitor for signs of the most common complication, which is:

   A. Fluid retention

   B. Diabetes insipidus

   C. Seizures

   D. Panhypopituitarism

5. A woman who has a prolactinoma will often seek medical attention because of:

   A. Headache

   B. Double vision

   C. Amenorrhea

   D. All of the above

6. The medical treatment of prolactinoma involves administration of:

   A. Antibiotics

   B. Corticosteroids

   C. Immunosuppressants

   D. Dopamine antagonist

7. When an individual has excess secretion of somatotropin, symptoms would include:

   A. Coarsening of features

   B. Kyphosis

   C. Muscle weakness

   D. Overgrowth of soft tissue

   E. Any of the above

8. Individuals with excess secretion of somatotropin are at high risk for development of:

   A. Renal failure

   B. Cardiac disease

   C. Diabetes mellitus

   D. Infections

9. The most accurate way to test for an excess of growth hormone is by:

   A. CT scan

   B. Laboratory testing

   C. MRI

   D. Radioimmunoassay

10. The treatment of choice for the individual with severe symptoms of acromegaly would be:

    A. External irradiation

    B. Treatment with parlodel

    C. Transsphenoidal microsurgery

    D. Chemotherapy

11. Clinical manifestations that the individual with deficiency of pituitary hormones would exhibit include:

    A. Weakness, cold intolerance, change in sex characteristics

    B. Heat intolerance, confusion, memory loss

    C. Change in body features, weight gain

    D. Agitation, weight loss, inappropriate behavior

12. Discharge instructions for the patient with a deficiency in pituitary hormone would include:

    A. Information on lifelong hormone replacement

    B. Information on proposed surgery

    C. Information on diabetes insipidus

    D. Information on diet therapy

13. Regulation of secretion of ADH is controlled by receptors in the hypothalamus which respond to changes in fluid _____ .

    A. Electrolytes

    B. Osmolality

    C. Vasopressin

    D. Levels

14. In the patient with diabetes insipidus, the nurse would monitor carefully for signs of:

    A. Hypoglycemia

    B. Dehydration and sodium depletion

    C. Hyperglycemia

    D. Vascular overload

15. Short-term medical treatment of diabetes insipidus would include administration of:

    A. Vasopressin

    B. Desmopressin acetate

    C. Lypressin

    D. Parlodel

16. A patient who develops the syndrome of inappropriate antidiuretic hormone would be treated by:

    A. Insulin, saline, electrolytes

    B. Antibiotics, analgesics

    C. Fluid replacement, potassium

    D. Fluid restriction, diuretics

True or False

17. _____ The posterior lobe of the pituitary gland is neural in origin.

18. _____ The anterior lobe of the pituitary gland is glandular in structure.

19. _____ Secretion of all anterior pituitary hormones is monitored by the hypothalamus.

20. _____ Pituitary adenomas are usually malignant.

21. _____ Following treatment for acromegaly, the symptoms will be reversed.

22. _____ Diabetes insipidus is caused by a deficiency in antidiuretic hormone.

23. _____ The incidence of pituitary disorders is higher in the elderly.

Questions

24. Write a nursing care plan for the patient who has had surgical removal of a pituitary adenoma.

    Nursing Diagnosis: Altered tissue perfusion: cerebral related to increased intracranial pressure secondary to surgical trauma

    Patient Outcome:

    Nursing Interventions:

CLINICAL SITUATION

Situation ■ 1

Mr. Mayhem has just returned to the unit following surgery for removal of a pituitary adenoma. The following questions relate to his care.

1. When a patient has had a hypophysectomy, which position should the patient be placed in?

    A. Prone

    B. Supine

C. High Fowler's

D. Elevated 30 degrees

2. Which of the following nursing interventions would be CONTRAINDICATED for this patient?

A. Avoid activities that cause exertion

B. Cough and deep breathe 10 times each hour

C. Medicate promptly if nauseated

D. Report urine output of > 100 ml to physician

3. Assessment for signs of nuchal rigidity or headaches should be performed because:

A. The patient may be septic

B. The patient may have meningitis

C. This is a sign of decreased ICP

D. These signs may precede a seizure

4. Discharge instructions for this patient would include:

A. Take antibiotics for 2 weeks

B. Rinse frequently with mouthwash

C. Use foam toothette and dental floss daily

D. Continue to do cough and deep breathing exercises four times a day

Chapter Thirty-two

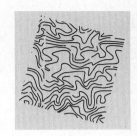

NURSING CARE
of Adults with
Adrenal Disorders

Learning Objectives

1.0 Demonstrate an Understanding of the Pathophysiology of Adrenal Disorders.

1.1 Demonstrate an Understanding of the Role of Hormonal Regulation in Adrenal Disorders.
1.2 Match the Specific Corticosteroids with Their Characteristics.

2.0 Demonstrate an Understanding of the Diagnosis and Treatment of Adrenocortical Insufficiency.

2.1 Identify the Etiology of Adrenocortical Insufficiency.
2.2 Identify the Clinical Manifestations of the Patient with Addison's disease.
2.3 Identify Medications Used in the Treatment of Adrenocortical Insufficiency.
2.4 Identify Nursing Interventions Used with Patients with Addison's Disorders.
2.5 Write a Nursing Care Plan for the Patient in Addison's crisis.

3.0 Demonstrate an Understanding of the Diagnosis and Treatment of the Patient with Adrenocortical Excess.

3.1 Identify the Etiology of Adrenocortical Excess.
3.2 Identify the Clinical Manifestations of the Patient with Cushing's Syndrome.
3.3 Identify the Treatment Protocols for the Patient with Cushing's Syndrome.
3.4 Identify the Nursing Interventions Appropriate for the Patient with Cushing's Syndrome.
3.5 Write a Nursing Care Plan for the Patient with Cushing's Syndrome.

4.0 Demonstrate an Understanding of the Treatment of the Patient with Dysfunction of the Adrenal Medulla.

4.1 Identify the Clinical Manifestations of the Patient with Pheochromocytoma.
4.2 Identify the Treatment Protocols for the Patient with Pheochromocytoma.
4.3 Identify the Nursing Interventions Appropriate for the Patient with Pheochromocytoma.

Learning Activities

Matching

A. Mineralocorticoids
B. Glucocorticoids
C. Androgen

1. _____ Promote sodium retention and potassium excretion

2. _____ Influence development of secondary sex characteristics

3. _____ Stimulate gluconeogenesis by the liver

4. _____ Aldosterone is an example of these

5. _____ Secretion is controlled by adrenocorticotropic hormone (ACTH) secretion

6. _____ Cortisol is the primary example of these

True or False

7. _____ Secondary adrenocortical insufficiency is caused by decreased secretion of ACTH.

8. _____ Individuals who develop Cushing's syndrome from taking steroids should stop the drug.

9. _____ Any illness can precipitate an Addison's crisis.

10. _____ Adrenal carcinoma is a common cause of increased aldosterone secretion.

11. _____ Treatment for Cushing's syndrome might involve administration of adrenal suppressant drugs.

12. _____ Epinephrine secretion has a major effect on the cardiovascular system.

Questions

13. The primary etiology of Addison's disease is thought to be:

A. Tumor of the gland

B. Autoimmune process

C. Secondary to pituitary failure

D. Histoplasmosis organism

14. What is one of the reasons that Addison's disease is difficult to diagnose?

A. Symptoms develop early and progress very slowly

B. Changes do not occur until 90% of the tissue is gone

C. The pituitary gland takes over its function

D. It is usually seen in the elderly

15. The result of aldosterone deficiency in the individual with Addison's disease will be:

A. Increased sodium and potassium retention

B. Retention of sodium, chloride, and water

C. Excretion of sodium; increased potassium retention

D. Excretion of sodium, water, potassium, and chloride

16. If the symptoms of Addison's disease were to continue without intervention, the end result would be:

A. Septic shock

B. Inability to fight infection

C. Renal failure

D. Circulatory collapse and hypovolemic shock

17. Often the individual with Addison's disease seeks medical attention because of:

A. Headache, change in elimination patterns

B. Severe weakness, fatigue, and debilitation

C. Weight gain, fluid retention, edema

D. Generalized discomfort, chest pain

18. Discharge instructions for the individual with Addison's disease would include how to prevent precipitating a crisis by avoiding:

A. Stress

B. Dehydration

C. Illness

D. All of the above

19. In making a diagnosis of primary Addison's disease, the nurse would expect to see which laboratory results?

A. Low levels of cortisol

B. Elevated levels of ACTH

C. Low levels of ACTH and cortisol

D. Low levels of androgens, low sodium, and potassium

20. The medical management for the adult with Addison's disease would include administration of:

A. Mineralocorticoids

B. Hydrocortisone, Florinef

C. ACTH

D. Cortisone, androgen

21. A primary nursing intervention for the individual with adrenocortical insufficiency would be:

A. Prevention of infection

B. Teaching administration of insulin

C. Teaching self-management

D. Teaching the patient to decrease medication during stress

22. The most appropriate diet for the patient with Addison's disease would be:

A. Low sodium, high carbohydrate

B. High sodium, low potassium, high fluid intake

C. Low protein, high carbohydrate, high fat

D. Low fat, low sodium

23. When caring for the patient in Addison's crisis, the most important nursing goal would be aimed at:

A. Preventing infection

B. Preventing a rise in intracranial pressure

C. Lowering blood pressure

D. Reestablishing fluid and electrolyte balance

24. The primary cause of Cushing's syndrome is:

A. Hyperplasia of the adrenal cortices

B. Oversecretion by the hypothalamus

C. Tumor of the adrenal cortex

D. High doses of steroids

25. Assessment of the patient with Cushing's syndrome involves observation for typical symptoms such as:

A. Thin skin with increased pigmentation

B. Truncal obesity, thin extremities, moon face

C. Weight gain, obesity, edema

D. Loss of hair, ecchymotic areas

26. To confirm a medical diagnosis of Cushing's disease, the nurse would expect which laboratory findings?

A. Decrease in cortisol and hydrocorticosteroid levels

B. High cortisol level, hypoglycemia, hypernatremia

C. High plasma cortisol and urinary ketosteroid levels

D. Elevation of plasma ACTH level

27. The nurse should monitor the patient with Cushing's syndrome for signs of activity intolerance. Symptoms might include:

A. Bradycardia, dizziness

B. Nausea, vomiting, anorexia

C. Hypertension, headache, tachypnea

D. Tachycardia, dyspnea, fatigue

28. Unregulated hypersecretion of aldosterone will result in:

A. Decreased fluid volume, hypotension

B. Increased sodium retention and excess potassium excretion

C. Hypotension, retention of potassium and sodium

D. Excessive secretion of sodium, potassium, fluids

29. The treatment of choice for the patient with primary aldosteronism would be:

A. Steroid-blocking agents

B. Antihypertensives, antibiotics

C. Unilateral adrenalectomy

D. Diet control, steroids

30. When a patient with primary aldosteronism exhibits a positive Chvostek's sign, the nurse would monitor for signs of:

A. Tetany

B. Respiratory distress

C. Cardiac irregularities

D. Hyporeflexia

31. The symptoms associated with pheochromocytoma are due to:

A. Overstimulation of the sympathetic nervous system

B. Decreased production of catecholamines

C. Overproduction of corticosteroids

D. Oversecretion of pituitary and adrenal hormones

32. The most common clinical feature of pheochromocytoma is:

A. Nausea, vomiting

B. Hypertension

C. Hypotension, tachycardia

D. Headaches, bradycardia

33. Treatment for the patient with pheochromocytoma would involve:

A. Administration of steroids

B. Laser treatment

C. Surgical excision and corticosteroid therapy

D. Hormonal blocking agents

34. When a patient has had an adrenalectomy, it would be important for the nurse to monitor postoperatively for complications such as:

A. Hyperreflexia

B. Pulmonary edema

C. Hypertensive crises

D. Hypovolemic shock

35. Write a nursing care plan for the patient in Addison's crisis.

Nursing Diagnosis: Fluid volume deficit related to extracellular sodium and water loss secondary to vomiting, diarrhea, and adrenocorticoid insufficiency

Patient Outcome:

Nursing Interventions:

36. Write a nursing care plan for the patient with Cushing's syndrome.

Nursing Diagnosis: High risk for infection related to impaired immune response and tissue repair

Patient Outcome:

Nursing Interventions:

37. Write a nursing care plan for the patient with a pheochromocytoma.

Nursing Diagnosis: Anxiety related to overstimulation of the nervous system

Patient Outcome:

Nursing Interventions:

CLINICAL SITUATION

Situation ■ 1

A patient is admitted to the hospital with a diagnosis of possible Addison's crisis.

1. During the initial assessment, the nurse would observe for symptoms of the disease, which include:

A. Respiratory distress, edema

B. Hyporeflexia, hypertension, bradycardia

C. Hypotension, hypoglycemia, hyponatremia

D. Hyporeflexia, hypotension

2. Treatment should be initiated quickly and the nurse would anticipate administration of:

A. Fluids and steroids

B. Insulin and dextrose

C. Ventilatory support

D. Surgical intervention

3. It would be important for the nurse to observe for complications such as:

A. Infection, septic shock

B. Hypovolemic shock, dysrhythmias

C. Fluid overload, pulmonary edema

D. Thrombophlebitis, pulmonary emboli

4. Which statement by the patient would signify an event that may have precipitated this crisis? (Check all that apply.)

A. I started a new diet

B. I recently lost my job

C. I am taking a new medication

D. I have a new baby

5. One of the ways that an individual with Addison's disease can prevent a crisis from occurring would be:

A. Reduce the level of activity

B. Follow dietary restrictions

C. Stop medications during the illness

D. Increase medication during stressful times or illness

Chapter Thirty-three

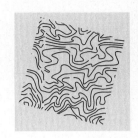

NURSING CARE
of Adults with
Thyroid Disorders

Learning Objectives

1.0 Demonstrate an Understanding of the Pathophysiology of Thyroid Disorders.

1.1 Demonstrate an Understanding of the Role of Hormonal Regulation in Thyroid Disorders.
1.2 Identify Clinical Manifestations of the Patient with a Thyroid Disorder.
1.3 Identify Symptoms of Thyroid Hypersecretion.
1.4 Identify Symptoms of Thyroid Hyposecretion.

2.0 Demonstrate an Understanding of the Diagnosis and Management of Thyroid Disorders.

2.1 Identify Tests Used to Diagnose Thyroid Disorders.
2.2 Identify Medications Used in the Treatment of Thyroid Disorders.
2.3 Identify Treatment Modalities Used with the Functional Thyroid Disorders.
2.4 Demonstrate an Understanding of the Nursing Interventions Used with Patients with Thyroid Disorders.
2.5 Write a Nursing Care Plan for the Patient with a Thyroid Disorder.

Learning Activities

Fill In

1. Adequate daily intake of _____ and _____ is necessary for the synthesis of thyroid hormones.

2. The production and secretion of thyroxine is controlled by secretion of _____.

3. List two of the primary functions of T_3 and T_4.

   1.

   2.

4. The thyroid also secretes _____, which lowers serum calcium.

5. The most common form of chronic thyroiditis is known as _____.

Questions

6. One of the earliest clinical manifestations seen with chronic thyroiditis is:

   A. Pain

   B. Goiter

   C. Redness

   D. Hoarseness

7. Lab results for the patient with chronic lymphocytic thyroiditis would show:

   A. High levels of thyroid hormones

   B. Low levels of TSH

   C. High titers of antithyroid antibodies

   D. High levels of calcitonin

True or False

8. _____ Thyroid function is usually abnormal with acute thyroiditis.

9. _____ Radioactive iodine uptake is subnormal with subacute thyroiditis.

10. _____ Treatment for hypothyroidism usually lasts 6 to 9 months.

11. _____ Primary hypothyroidism is due to a deficiency of TSH.

12. _____ Many patients who have hypothyroidism remain undiagnosed for years.

13. _____ Hyperthyroidism may be precipitated by stress.

14. _____ Over 50% of the patients with hyperthyroidism can achieve remission with medication.

Matching

Match each of the following diagnostic tests with its description.

A. Radioactive Iodine Uptake

B. Thyroid scan

15. _____ Produces an image of iodine concentration in the thyroid gland.

16. _____ Measures the rate that iodine is taken up by the thyroid.

Questions

17. A patient with tertiary hypothyroidism will have a low level of:

   A. TSH

   B. T_4

   C. T_3

   D. All the above

18. Early symptoms of hypothyroidism would include:

   A. Mental deterioration

   B. Puffy appearance to tissue

C. Dull, sparse hair, loss of hair

D. Fatigue, lethargy, increased somnolence

19. Chronic headaches in a patient with hypothyroidism are significant because they may indicate:

A. Decreased metabolism

B. Cerebral hypoxia

C. Brain damage

D. Paresthesia

20. A patient is admitted with myxedema coma. The nursing diagnosis which would have priority would be:

A. High risk for infection

B. Altered health maintenance

C. Impaired skin integrity

D. Altered tissue perfusion

21. For a patient with primary hypothyroidism, the nurse would expect laboratory results to show high levels of:

A. TRH

B. TSH

C. T_3

D. Radioactive iodine uptake

22. Medical treatment of primary hypothyroidism includes:

A. Surgery

B. Radiation therapy

C. Thyroid replacement

D. Iodine replacement

23. Which of the following medications would be contraindicated for a patient receiving thyroid replacement therapy?

A. Estrogen

B. Antibiotics

C. Aspirin

D. Feosol

24. A patient who will be taking thyroid replacement therapy should be taught to monitor for side effects, which would include:

A. Palpitations, tachycardia

B. Chest pain, headache

C. Nausea, diarrhea, anorexia

D. Menstrual irregularities

E. Any of the above

25. Elderly patients starting thyroid replacement therapy should increase the dose gradually in order to:

A. Avoid cardiovascular side effects

B. Avoid a rapid slowdown of metabolic rate

C. Avoid nausea and vomiting

D. Prevent psychotic reactions

26. Increased secretion of thyroid will cause:

A. Hypermetabolic states

B. Increased oxygen consumption

C. Sympathetic nervous system stimulation

D. All of the above

27. When a patient with Graves' disease develops exophthalmos, this is due to:

A. Increased volume of the orbital contents

B. Inflammation of the extraocular muscles

C. Pretibial edema

D. Unknown etiology

28. When assessing a patient with Graves' disease, the nurse would monitor for clinical manifestations such as: (Check all that apply.)

A. Nervousness

B. Insomnia

C. Tachycardia

D. Impaired coordination

E. Fatigue

F. Warm, moist skin

29. Dietary recommendations for the patient with hyperthyroidism would include:

A. Low-residue, high-calorie, high-fat diet

B. Low-calorie, low-fat, no-simple-sugar diet

C. High-calorie, high-protein, high-carbohydrate diet

D. Low-protein, low-potassium, low-sodium diet

30. A patient who is taking antithyroid drugs should not stop them abruptly because it may precipitate:

    A. Respiratory distress

    B. Hypothyroidism

    C. Exophthalmos

    D. Thyroid crisis

31. The drug of choice to treat hyperthyroidism is:

    A. Levothyroxine

    B. Methimazole

    C. Prednisone

    D. Propylthiouracil

32. Teaching the patient who is to have radioactive iodine therapy would include providing information about:

    A. Thyroid replacement therapy

    B. Type of anesthesia

    C. Precautions to follow

    D. Postoperative care

33. Following a subtotal thyroidectomy, the nurse would monitor the patient for complications such as:

    A. Infection

    B. Hemorrhage

    C. Tetany

    D. Vocal cord paralysis

    E. B & C

    F. B,C,D

34. Write a nursing care plan for a patient with hypothyroidism.

    Nursing Diagnosis: Altered health maintenance related to insufficient knowledge of self-management

    Patient Outcome:

    Nursing Interventions:

35. Write a nursing care plan for a patient with hyperthyroidism.

    Nursing Diagnosis: Altered tissue perfusion: systemic related to dehydration, hyperthermia, and decreased cardiac output

    Patient Outcome:

    Nursing Interventions:

CLINICAL SITUATIONS

Situation ■ 1

An elderly patient has been diagnosed as having primary thyroid dysfunction as a result of thyroiditis.

1. During the initial interview, the nurse would assess for clinical manifestations of the disease such as: (Check all that apply.)

    A. Low blood pressure, low heart rate

    B. Impaired wound healing

    C. Pale, cool skin

    D. Anorexia and diarrhea

    E. Heat intolerance

    F. Slowed speech, forgetfulness

2. This disorder can be very serious in the elderly because it can lead to myxedema coma. _____ can precipitate coma.

    A. Exposure to temperature extremes

    B. Use of CNS depressants

    C. Use of caffeine, alcohol

    D. Immobility

3. Which medication would be the drug of choice to treat this patient?

    A. Dessicated thyroid

    B. Cytomel

    C. Levothyroxine

    D. Iodine

4. To avoid an overdose of her medication, the nurse would instruct the patient to monitor:

    A. Pulse

B. Weight

C. Urine output

D. Diet

Situation ■ 2

Mrs. Bates is admitted for thyroid surgery for Graves' disease after other methods of treatment were unsuccessful.

1. Prior to surgery, the patient states she has been taking:

   A. Synthroid

   B. Cytomel

   C. Ampicillin

   D. Propylthiouracil

2. A subtotal thyroidectomy is performed. Six hours after surgery, the patient complains of numbness of the toes and the nurse notices muscle twitching. This suggests:

   A. Hyperthyroidism

   B. Hypothyroidism

   C. Tetany

   D. Cerebral hypoxia

3. After receiving appropriate medical orders, the nurse would administer:

   A. Potassium

   B. Calcium

   C. Dilantin

   D. Morphine

4. Mrs. Bates is having difficulty breathing and is becoming anxious. An appropriate nursing intervention is

   A. To assess the patient's vital signs.

   B. To release the dressing and check for bleeding.

   C. To obtain a tracheostomy set.

   D. All of the above.

5. Mrs. Bates is stabilized and the rest of the hospitalization is uneventful. Check statements that the nurse would include in the discharge teaching.

   A. Need to continue antithyroid medications

   B. Need to monitor blood level of thyroid hormone

   C. Possible need to take hypothyroid medication

   D. Side effects of therapy

Chapter Thirty-four

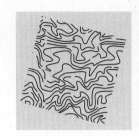

NURSING CARE
of Adults with
Parathyroid Disorders

Learning Objectives

1.0 Demonstrate an Understanding of the Pathophysiology of Parathyroid Disorders.

1.1 Demonstrate an Understanding of the Role of Hormonal Regulation in Parathyroid Disorders.
1.2 Identify Clinical Manifestations of the Patient with a Parathyroid Disorder.
1.3 Identify Symptoms of Parathyroid Hypersecretion.
1.4 Identify Symptoms of Parathyroid Hyposecretion.

2.0 Demonstrate an Understanding of the Management of Parathyroid Disorders.

2.1 Identify Medications Used in the Treatment of Parathyroid Disorders.
2.2 Identify the Nonmedical Management of the Patient with a Parathyroid Disorder.
2.3 Demonstrate an Understanding of the Nursing Interventions Used with Patients with Parathyroid Disorders.
2.4 Write a Nursing Care Plan for the Patient with a Parathyroid Disorder.

Learning Activities

Fill In

1. The primary function of the parathyroid gland is to _____ .

2. Serum calcium levels will _____ as parathyroid hormone is secreted.

Questions

3. Explain how parathyroid hormone raises serum calcium levels in the body by acting on:

   Bones:

   Kidneys:

   Intestines:

4. The most common cause of hypoparathyroidism is:

   A. Trauma

   B. Irradiation of neck

   C. Accidental removal

   D. Any of the above

5. Early manifestations of acute hypocalcemia would include:

   A. Difficulty breathing, stridor

   B. Cardiac arrhythmias, hypertension

   C. Irritability, muscle cramps, photophobia

   D. Change in level of consciousness

6. The nurse is assessing a patient for signs of low serum calcium by tapping the facial nerve. This is known as:

   A. Chvostek's sign

   B. Trousseau's sign

   C. Homans' sign

7. Dietary recommendations for a patient with chronic hypoparathyroidism would include:

   A. High calcium, high phosphorus, low sodium

   B. High calcium, low phosphorus, vitamin D supplement

   C. High calcium, high potassium, high sodium

8. A patient is admitted with signs of hypoparathyroidism. Which information in the history is a possible cause of the current condition?

   A. History of diabetes

   B. History of chronic renal failure

   C. History of steroid use

   D. History of hypertension

9. A condition that could precipitate secondary hyperparathyroidism in a patient is:

   A. Diabetes

   B. Hypothyroidism

   C. Acromegaly

   D. Congestive heart failure

10. The majority of patients with hyperparathyroidism are known to develop:

    A. Renal calculi

    B. Vitamin D deficiency

    C. Anemia

    D. Osteoporosis

11. The medical management of the patient with primary hyperparathyroidism includes:

    A. Vitamin C and D supplements, phosphate salts

    B. Diuretics, antihypertensives

    C. Limiting fluids, increasing calcium, decreasing phosphate

    D. Increasing fluids, decreasing calcium, increasing phosphate

12. Which of the following medications might be

administered to help promote phosphorus excretion?

A. Calcium

B. Amphojel

C. Feosol

D. Lasix

13. The nurse would recommend that a patient with high calcium levels include _____ in their diet.

A. Dairy products

B. Red meats

C. Cranberry or tomato juice

D. Complex carbohydrates

True or False

14. _____ Acute hypocalcemic tetany is a medical emergency.

15. _____ Adequate intake of vitamin D is necessary for calcium absorption.

16. _____ Calcium supplements should be taken between meals to help with absorption.

17. _____ Following parathyroidectomy, patient will be given calcium supplements.

Questions

18. Write a nursing care plan for the patient with hypoparathyroidism.

Nursing Diagnosis: High risk for injury: suffocation, trauma related to increased neuromuscular irritability and tetany

Patient Outcome:

Nursing Interventions:

CLINICAL SITUATION

Situation ■ 1

A patient with renal failure is admitted for therapy. Laboratory results show a high level of potassium, magnesium, phosphate, BUN and creatinine.

1. Based on the laboratory results, the nurse would monitor the patient for signs of:

A. Hypocalcemia

B. Hypercalcemia

2. Medications which the nurse administers to the patient that will help this condition include:

A. Maalox

B. Epogen

C. Milk of Magnesia

D. Multivitamins

3. The patient begins to complain of a tingling sensation in her hands and feet. While the nurse is waiting to hear from the physician, the patient begins breathing rapidly. An appropriate action would be:

A. Administer oxygen

B. Elevate the bed

C. Initiate rebreathing in a paper bag

D. Administer a sedative

4. The patient continues to exhibit neuromuscular irritability. The nurse prepares to administer:

A. Potassium

B. Calcium gluconate

C. Dilantin

D. Morphine sulfate

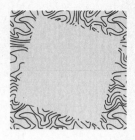

Unit Eleven

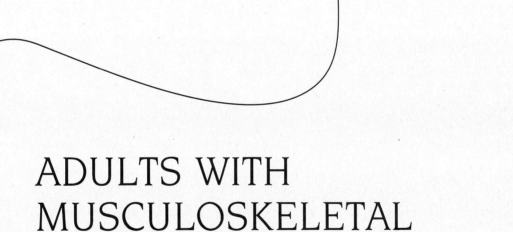

ADULTS WITH MUSCULOSKELETAL DYSFUNCTION

Chapter Thirty-five

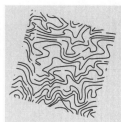

KNOWLEDGE BASIC TO THE NURSING CARE
of Adults with Musculoskeletal Dysfunction

Learning Objectives

1.0 *Review the Anatomy and Physiology of the Musculoskeletal System.*

1.1 List the Parts of the Musculoskeletal System.
1.2 List the Functions of the Musculoskeletal System.
1.3 Explain the Stages of Bone Repair.
1.4 List Factors that Affect How Damaged Bone Heals.

2.0 *Demonstrate an Understanding of Assessment Data Related to the Musculoskeletal System.*

2.1 Identify Symptoms of Musculoskeletal Dysfunction.
2.2 Identify the Clinical Manifestation of Musculoskeletal Dysfunction.
2.3 Match the Diagnostic Tests Used to Identify Musculoskeletal Dysfunction with Their Descriptions.

3.0 *Demonstrate an Understanding of Interventions used to Treat Adults with Musculoskeletal Dysfunction.*

3.1 Identify Types of Nonsurgical Treatment of Musculoskeletal Dysfunctions.
3.2 Demonstrate an Understanding of the Use of Casts in Treating Musculoskeletal Dysfunction.
3.3 Demonstrate an Understanding of the Principles of Traction.
3.4 Identify Surgical Interventions used to Treat Musculoskeletal Dysfunction.
3.5 Plan the Nursing Care for an Adult with a Dysfunction of the Musculoskeletal System.

Learning Activities

Questions

1. List the parts of the musculoskeletal system.

   1.

   2.

   3.

   4.

   5.

2. List the functions of the musculoskeletal system.

   1.

   2.

3. List and briefly explain the five stages of bone healing.

   1.

   2.

   3.

   4.

   5.

4. List six of the factors that can affect how damaged bone heals.

   1.

   2.

   3.

   4.

   5.

   6.

Fill In

5. The process of bone formation is called _____ .

6. Axial skeletal growth is completed by the end of _____ .

7. Throughout life the _____ deposits newly formed bone, while the _____ resorb or thin the bone.

8. Bones are enclosed in a tough fibrous tissue called _____ .

9. The diaphysis of a long bone is made up of _____ , whereas the epiphysis is made up of _____ bone.

10. Skeletal muscle contracts in response to impulses from the _____ .

11. To produce _____ , muscles contract over bones.

12. The primary energy source for muscle activity is the breakdown of _____ .

Matching

Match the following musculoskeletal tissues with their descriptions.

A. Ligaments   C. Cartilage
B. Tendons

13. _____ Strong, nonelastic fibrous connective tissue cords.

14. _____ Smooth, resilient supporting tissue composed of collagen.

15. _____ Fibrous connective tissue bands which bind bones to other bones.

16. _____ Provides a cushion that absorbs shock and reduces stress on joint surfaces.

Match the following diagnostic tests with their descriptions.

A. Arthrogram   D. MRI
B. Bone scan   E. Electromyography
C. CT scan   F. Thermography

17. _____ Uses magnetic force to provide pictures of internal structures.

18. _____ X-ray of a joint after a radiopaque dye or air has been injected into the joint.

19. _____ Determines the electrical activity of skeletal muscle and its ability to respond to stimulus.

20. _____ Combines x-rays with computer technology to produce pictures of internal structures.

21. _____ Uses an infrared camera to determine the amount of heat radiating from soft tissue.

22. _____ X-ray of skeletal bone using a gamma camera scanner after an injection of a radioactive substance.

True or False

23. _____ Muscles can atrophy in a short time from lack of use.

24. _____ Without mobility, bone destruction occurs at a greater rate than bone production.

25. _____ The MRI can be easily used with all patients.

26. _____ Heat is applied to sore joints to promote circulation.

27. _____ Casts made of plaster of Paris are ready for weight-bearing in 6 hours.

28. _____ Internal fixation devices are usually made of polyethylene.

29. _____ Once a joint has been replaced, it will last a lifetime.

30. _____ Extended use of traction is usually a treatment of choice for the elderly.

Questions

31. Which of the following assessment findings would indicate a possible musculoskeletal disorder?

A. Pain

B. Change in gait

C. Change in elimination

D. Diminished pulses

32. Following a musculoskeletal injury the most appropriate intervention is:

A. Application of cold

B. Application of heat

C. Splinting the extremity

D. Transport to emergency room

33. When caring for the patient in a full body cast, one of the most important nursing responsibilities is to:

A. Assess for infection

B. Assess for restricted chest expansion

C. Assess for fluid imbalance

D. Assess for ineffective coping

34. To prevent problems with tissue perfusion when a patient has a full leg cast, the nurse should

A. Maintain bedrest

B. Assess for pulses every shift

C. Keep legs in a nondependent position when not out of bed

D. Keep legs below heart level to increase circulation

35. All of the following are complications of immobility EXCEPT:

A. Alteration in elimination

B. Discoloration of the skin

C. Alteration in nutrition

D. Symptoms of infection

36. If the patient in a spica cast develops abdominal distention and vomiting, this may be due to:

A. Pressure on the mesenteric artery

B. Pressure on the aorta

C. Pressure on the diaphragm

D. Pressure on the spine

37. When a patient is in traction, the counter traction is usually generated by:

A. Weights

B. Pulleys

C. Height of bed

D. Patient's weight

38. Which of the following conditions would not require the use of traction?

    A. Reduction of compound fracture

    B. Fracture of the pelvis

    C. Nondisplaced fracture of radius

    D. Displaced fracture of femur

39. The amount of weight that is used with the application of skin traction is:

    A. 2–4 pounds

    B. 5–7 pounds

    C. 7–12 pounds

    D. 10–15 pounds

40. The amount of weight that is used with the application of skeletal traction is:

    A. 5–7 pounds

    B. 10–15 pounds

    C. 15–25 pounds

    D. 20–30 pounds

41. The reason that skeletal traction is effective in reducing and maintaining alignment of fracture fragments is because:

    A. It can be used intermittently

    B. It controls rotation as well as longitudinal pull

    C. It can maintain a position of hyperextension

    D. There is a low rate of infection

42. Skin traction is contraindicated when:

    A. There is a fracture of the upper extremities

    B. Impaired circulation is present

    C. The patient is over the age of 65

    D. Other injuries are present

43. The reason that the halo apparatus is connected to the body jacket when a patient has Crutchfield tongs is:

    A. To permit ambulation

    B. To prevent infection

    C. To prevent rotation of the spine

    D. To keep the patient immobilized

44. The purpose of an external fixation device is to:

    A. Compress bone fragments and maintain alignment

    B. Promote external rotation and alignment

    C. Prevent infection

    D. Promote rapid healing of injuries

45. All of the following would be indications for external fixation therapy EXCEPT:

    A. Open fracture with nerve damage

    B. Leg lengthening

    C. Open contaminated fracture

    D. Closed fracture with swelling

46. When caring for the patient with traction, which of the following observations by the nurse would be important to report at once?

    A. Low-grade fever

    B. Pain and drainage at pin site

    C. Generalized discomfort

    D. Loss of appetite

47. One of the problems associated with the use of internal fixation devices is:

    A. Tissue reaction to a foreign substance

    B. Infection can occur on surface of device

    C. Infection can occur long after surgery

    D. All of the above

48. The purpose of total joint replacement is:

    A. To prevent problems related to immobility

    B. To relieve pain and provide improved joint function

    C. To remove a severely infected joint

    D. To stop further joint degeneration

49. The reason that a patient experiences phantom sensation following a limb amputation is:

    A. The inability to distinguish pain site

    B. Nerve endings in the pathway are still being stimulated

    C. The intensity of the pain at the site of the amputation

    D. Severe stress increases the pain perception

50. When considering whether or not a patient is a candidate for an external prosthesis, which of the following factors should be considered?

    A. General health of individual

    B. Weight and strength of individual

    C. Lifestyle and activity of individual

    D. Potential for rehabilitation

    E. All of the above

51. Write a nursing care plan for the adult experiencing immobility problems.

    Nursing Diagnosis: Knowledge deficit: nature of immobility problems and prevention of complications

    Patient Outcome:

    Nursing Interventions:

52. Write a nursing care plan for the patient with an external fixation device.

    Nursing Diagnosis: Knowledge deficit: nature of care for the external fixation device, pin site care, and mobility management

    Patient Outcome:

    Nursing Interventions:

CLINICAL SITUATIONS

Situation ■ 1

Jeremy is injured when he is hit by a car. Medics identify a fracture of the leg and possibly the arm. He is assessed, an IV is started and pain medication is given. He is immobilized and transported to the hospital.

1. The most important measure taken by the medics to ensure further injury did not occur was:

    A. Correct identification of injury

    B. Immobilization of injuries

    C. Adequate pain medication

    D. Transport to proper emergency room

2. Jeremy is diagnosed as having fractures of the femur, tibia, and clavicle. He is placed in traction. All of the following principles of traction are true EXCEPT:

    A. Sufficient countertraction must be maintained.

    B. Weights must hang free.

    C. Avoid friction on ropes or weights.

    D. Remove weight only when linens are changed.

3. His injuries are healed sufficiently to allow for a cast to be placed. Following the application of a plaster cast, the nurse should:

    A. Dry the cast with a hair dryer

    B. Ambulate within 2 hours

    C. Assess for adequate circulation

    D. Assess for respiratory distress

4. Jeremy is discharged and returns in 6 weeks for cast removal. Following cast removal, it will be important for the nurse to:

    A. Inspect the limb for atrophy, weakness, and loss of range of motion

    B. Teach Jeremy how to use a walker

    C. Teach Jeremy proper use of pain medication

    D. Inspect for signs of infection

Situation ■ 2

Mr. Nolan is admitted for a below-the-knee amputation because of severe peripheral vascular disease. He refuses to talk about the proposed surgery.

1. The most appropriate nursing diagnosis for this patient is:

    A. Alteration in tissue perfusion

    B. Impaired skin integrity

    C. Dysfunctional grieving

    D. Anxiety

2. Following the surgery, Mr. Nolan complains of severe pain in the amputated extremity. The appropriate nursing action is:

    A. Medicate as needed

    B. Reinforce the absence of the extremity

C. Notify the physician

D. Explain that pain is only psychological

3. The proper position for the residual limb immediately following surgery is:

A. Elevated on pillow

B. Dependent position

C. Position of comfort

D. In abduction

4. In preparation for discharge, it would be important for the nurse to instruct Mr. Nolan in:

A. Proper wrapping of the limb

B. Proper skin care

C. Proper nutrition

D. All of the above

Chapter Thirty-Six

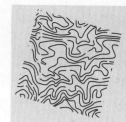

NURSING CARE
of Adults with Musculoskeletal Disorders

Learning Objectives

1.0 Demonstrate an Understanding of the Infections and Inflammations of the Musculoskeletal System.

1.1 Define Several of the Infections and Inflammatory Disorders of the Musculoskeletal System.
1.2 Identify Characteristics of Infections and Inflammations of the Musculoskeletal System.
1.3 Identify Types of Medical Management for Infections and Inflammations of the Musculoskeletal System.
1.4 Identify Nursing Interventions Used with Patients with Infectious Musculoskeletal Disorders.
1.5 Write a Nursing Care Plan for a Patient with an Inflammatory Musculoskeletal Disorder.

2.0 Demonstrate an Understanding of the Structural Disorders of the Musculoskeletal System.

2.1 Identify Characteristics of Specific Structural Disorders of the Musculoskeletal System.
2.2 Identify the Medical Management of Structural Disorders of the Musculoskeletal System.
2.3 Identify Nursing Interventions Used with Patients with Structural Disorders of the Musculoskeletal System.

3.0 Demonstrate an Understanding of Traumatic Injuries to the Musculoskeletal System.

3.1 Identify Signs and Symptoms of Musculoskeletal Injuries.
3.2 Identify Types of Medical Management for Musculoskeletal Injuries.
3.3 Identify Types of Surgical Treatment of Musculoskeletal Injuries.
3.4 Identify Nursing Interventions Used with Patients with Musculoskeletal Injuries.
3.5 Write a Nursing Care Plan for the Patient with a Traumatic Injury.

279

4.0 Demonstrate an Understanding of the Neoplasms that Affect the Musculoskeletal System.

4.1 Define Several of the Musculoskeletal Neoplasms.
4.2 Identify Medical and Surgical Treatments of Musculoskeletal Neoplasms.
4.3 Identify Nursing Interventions Used with Patients with Musculoskeletal Neoplasms.

Learning Activities

Define

1. Osteomyelitis:

2. Arthritis:

3. Osteoarthritis:

4. Ankylosing spondylitis:

5. Gout:

6. Lyme disease:

7. Osteomalacia:

8. Osteoporosis:

True or False

9. _____ The cause of rheumatoid arthritis is unknown.

10. _____ Osteomyelitis can only be contracted by direct contamination of the bone.

11. _____ Fractures are more common in the geriatric patient.

12. _____ Arthritis is a leading cause of immobility.

13. _____ Osteoarthritis is the most serious form of arthritis.

14. _____ Presence of the rheumatoid factor is considered to be diagnostic for rheumatoid arthritis.

15. _____ A patient can have both rheumatoid and osteoarthritis.

16. _____ Hip fractures with complications are a leading cause of mortality in the elderly.

Questions

17. _____ is one of the organisms most frequently associated with osteomyelitis.

   A. *Escherichia coli*

   B. *Staphylococcus aureus*

   C. *Streptococcus viridans*

   D. *Pseudomonas*

18. Treatment of osteomyelitis would involve:

   A. Analgesics

   B. Debridement of necrotic tissue

   C. Antibiotics

   D. All of the above

19. A complication of acute osteomyelitis that the nurse would monitor for is:

   A. Meningitis

   B. Pulmonary emboli

   C. Pneumonia

   D. Compartment syndrome

20. A review of the x-ray of the patient with chronic osteomyelitis would reveal:

   A. Mild inflammation

B. Synovitis

C. Areas of sequestrum

D. Ankylosis

21. Individuals with chronic osteomyelitis are at risk for developing:

A. Malnutrition

B. Muscle contractions

C. Septicemia

D. Cardiac arrhythmias

22. All of the following risk factors have been associated with the development of osteoporosis EXCEPT:

A. High level of stress

B. Low intake of calcium

C. Caucasian over the age of 50

D. Immobility

23. The type of diagnostic test that is done to help in determining if a patient has osteoporosis is:

A. CT scan

B. Nuclear scanning

C. Bone densitometry

D. Chest x-ray

24. Osteomalacia is caused by a lack of:

A. Calcium

B. Vitamin A

C. Intrinsic factor

D. Vitamin D

25. From the foods below, which one would have the highest calcium content?

A. 1 cup low-fat yogurt

B. 1 oz swiss cheese

C. 1 cup cottage cheese

D. 1 cup spinach

26. The early joint changes that are evident in the patient with rheumatoid arthritis are caused by:

A. Joint calcification

B. Kyphosis

C. Ankylosis

D. Synovitis

27. When a patient has osteoporosis, the nurse would implement interventions to prevent:

A. Altered nutrition

B. Cardiac arrhythmias

C. Pathologic fractures

D. Pain

28. When a patient is in the second stage of Lyme disease, the nurse would monitor for:

A. Cardiac manifestations

B. Musculoskeletal involvement

C. Macular lesions

D. Joint destruction

29. Because of the type of pain experienced by the patient with rheumatoid arthritis, an appropriate nursing intervention would involve:

A. Having patient exercise upon arising

B. Having patient take analgesics before rising

C. Using cold compresses on affected joints daily

D. Staying in bed for prolonged periods of time

30. The area that is most often affected when a patient has gout is:

A. Ankle

B. Large toe

C. Fingers

D. Spine

31. This type of arthritis is characterized as being a chronic systemic disease with inflammation of the joints and extra-articular manifestations.

A. Rheumatoid arthritis

B. Osteoarthritis

C. Osteogenic sarcoma

D. Osteochondrosis

32. When a patient with ankylosing spondylitis has developed rigid kyphosis, an important nursing intervention would be:

A. Teach breathing exercises

B. Use application of heat

C. Administer NSAIDs

D. Maintain bedrest in supine position

33. Diagnostic testing for the patient with gout would most likely reveal:

A. High BUN and creatinine

B. High uric acid

C. High white count

D. Low hemoglobin and hematocrit

34. Diagnostic testing for the patient with Paget's disease would most likely reveal an elevated:

A. White count

B. Uric acid

C. Erythrocyte sedimentation rate

D. Serum alkaline phosphatase

35. Medical management of the patient with gout involves administration of medications to inhibit bone resorption, such as:

A. Calcitonin

B. Vitamin D

C. Allopurinol

D. Indocin

36. The drug of choice for the patient during an acute episode of gout is:

A. Allopurinol

B. Colchicine

C. Probenecid

D. Aspirin

37. A patient is to be instructed to follow a diet low in purine. Which food should be avoided?

A. Bread

B. Ice cream

C. Sardines

D. Green vegetables

38. While examining a patient, the nurse hears crepitus when moving the knees. The patient also has nodules on the fingers. These symptoms suggest:

A. Rheumatoid arthritis

B. Osteomyelitis

C. Osteoarthritis

D. Gouty arthritis

39. The type of surgery that might provide some relief of pain for the patient with osteoarthritis is:

A. Synovectomy

B. Arthrodesis

C. Incision and drainage

D. Joint replacement

40. A secretary who works on a computer for long hours is complaining of pain, numbness, and tingling in the thumb and middle finger. These symptoms suggest:

A. Paget's disease

B. Carpal tunnel syndrome

C. Dupuytren's contracture

D. Volkmann's Syndrome

Matching (medications)

A. NSAIDs

B. Uricosurics

C. Oral calcium

D. Antipagetics

41. _____ Produce an anti-inflammatory, analgesic, and antipyretic effect.

42. _____ Inhibit bone resorption and reduce bone vascularity.

43. _____ Effective in controlling serum uric acid levels.

44. _____ Used primarily to treat osteoarthritis and rheumatoid arthritis.

45. _____ Individuals on these medications should also be on a low-purine diet.

46. _____ Supplements are indicated for prevention of osteomalacia and osteoporosis.

47. _____ Older adults should be closely monitored for liver impairment when on these medications.

Questions

48. Nursing care of the patient who has had a total hip replacement should include:

A. Preventing injury

B. Preventing infection

C. Maintaining skin integrity

D. All of the above

49. Discharge planning for the patient who has had arthroscopic surgery for a tear of the cruciate ligament of the knee should include which of the following?

A. Explanation of cast care

B. Explanation of full-leg immobilizer

C. Explanation of use of walker

D. Any of the above

50. Fractures may be caused by which of the following?

A. Direct blow to the bone

B. Demineralization of the bone

C. Sudden, strong muscle contraction

D. Any of the above

51. Which of the following types of fracture can be considered to be a life-threatening injury?

A. Closed fracture

B. Comminuted fracture

C. Compound fracture

D. Greenstick fracture

52. The immediate care of the patient with a fracture would include:

A. Splinting the injured part in correct alignment

B. Padding or protecting the injured area

C. Administering an analgesic

D. All of the above

53. When a patient with a fractured pelvis becomes restless, agitated, and confused, the nurse should assess for:

A. Hypovolemic shock

B. Sepsis

C. Compartment syndrome

D. Pulmonary embolus

54. An early sign of compartment syndrome that the nurse would monitor for is:

A. Loss of the distal pulse

B. Paresthesia

C. Severe pain in area not relieved by narcotics

D. Falling blood pressure and rise in pulse

55. Medical management for the patient with compartment syndrome would include:

A. Application of traction

B. Incision and drainage

C. Debridement

D. Fasciotomy

56. When a patient has had an internal fixation for a fractured leg, it is important to monitor for:

A. Infection

B. Problems related to immobility

C. Correct traction set up

D. Nutritional deficits

57. A potentially fatal complication of long bone fractures and multiple trauma is:

A. Fat embolism

B. Cardiac arrhythmias

C. Cerebral vascular accident

D. Pulmonary edema

58. A complication of severe trauma that can occur from a lack of circulation to the tissue is:

A. Compartment syndrome

B. Septicemia

C. Avascular necrosis

D. Sympathetic dystrophy

Define

Define the following neoplasms.

59. Osteochondroma:

60. Hemangioma:

61. Osteosarcoma:

62. Fibrosarcoma:

63. Multiple myeloma:

Questions

64. The treatment of choice for osteosarcoma is:

    A. Removal of segment of bone

    B. Chemotherapy

    C. Radiation therapy

    D. Amputation

65. The nurse should suspect _____ in a patient who has Bence Jones protein in the urine.

    A. Osteogenic sarcoma

    B. Multiple myeloma

    C. Leukemia

    D. Osteoporosis

66. The most common malignant bone tumor is:

    A. Osteosarcoma

    B. Multiple myeloma

    C. Fibrosarcoma

    D. Hemangioma

67. Write a nursing care plan for the patient with rheumatoid arthritis.

    Nursing Diagnosis: Impaired physical mobility related to disease process and pain

    Patient Outcome:

Nursing Interventions:

68. Write a nursing care plan for the patient with a compound fracture of the tibia.

    Nursing Diagnosis: Altered tissue perfusion; peripheral related to trauma.

    Patient Outcome:

    Nursing Interventions:

CLINICAL SITUATIONS

Situation ■ 1

Mr. Wasserman, age 75, has been diagnosed as having chronic rheumatoid arthritis. He has been treated for many years by his family physician. He has been slowly losing mobility.

1. Laboratory values that would be increased with this condition include:

    A. RBC

    B. ESR

    C. WBC

    D. BUN

2. The office nurses finds deformities in his hands which interfere with ADLs. This is called:

    A. Subluxation

    B. Ankylosis

    C. Synovitis

    D. Sjögren's syndrome

3. The goals in the medical management of this condition would be aimed at:

    A. Curing the condition

    B. Preventing a recurrence

    C. Relieving pain and maintaining mobility

    D. Referral to a nursing home in the future

4. A medication that is tried with Mr. Wasserman in the hopes of inducing a remission is:

    A. Parenteral gold salts

B. NSAIDs

C. Enteric aspirin

D. Steroids

Situation ■ 2

Keith was playing football with some college friends when he fell and injured his shoulder. Clinical manifestations include marked joint deformity, loss of joint function, and ecchymosis.

1. These symptoms suggest:

   A. Subluxation

   B. Dislocation

   C. Fracture

   D. Ankylosis

2. The usual medical management of this condition would involve:

   A. Surgical intervention

   B. Closed reduction

   C. Application of a cast

   D. Application of a sling

3. Following the procedure, it is important for the nurse to assess:

   A. Neurovascular status

   B. Cardiac status

   C. Mobility status

   D. Cerebrovascular status

4. Part of the discharge instructions should include:

   A. Explanation of the need to limit activity

   B. Explanation of antibiotic therapy

   C. Demonstration of exercise regimen

   D. Explanation of cast care

Situation ■ 3

Mrs. Meyers, age 78, fell in the bathroom at the local nursing home. She is admitted to the hospital with a suspected hip fracture.

1. The x-ray studies reveal an intertrochanteric fracture. Typical symptoms associated with this type of injury include:

   A. Involved limb is of normal length and position, with pain radiating to groin

   B. Involved limb appears shortened and externally rotated

   C. Involved limb is internally rotated and deformed

   D. Involved limb appears normal, but extreme pain is felt upon movement

2. Mrs. Meyers has the fracture treated by open reduction and internal fixation under a general anesthesia. Postoperative complications might include: (Check all that apply.)

   A. Paralytic ileus

   B. Disorientation

   C. Cardiac arrhythmias

   D. Fluid and electrolyte imbalance

   E. Thromboembolism

3. Following the surgery, the most important nursing observation includes looking for:

   A. Impaired skin integrity

   B. Signs of confusion

   C. Signs of compromised circulation

   D. Problems with the traction

4. On the second postoperative day, Mrs. Meyers complains of headache and lethargy. She appears confused. Other symptoms include tachycardia, tachypnea, and dyspnea. The nurse suspects:

   A. Pneumonia

   B. Fat embolism

   C. Pneumothorax

   D. Atelectasis

5. Arterial blood gases are: pH 7.2; PaO_2 50%; $PaCO_2$ 60%; HCO_3 22. The nurse would anticipate:

   A. Administering oxygen per nasal cannula

   B. Administering oxygen per mask, suctioning frequently

   C. Having patient cough and deep breathe every 4 hours

   D. Mechanically ventilating with positive end-expiratory pressure

Unit Twelve

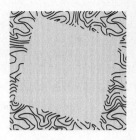

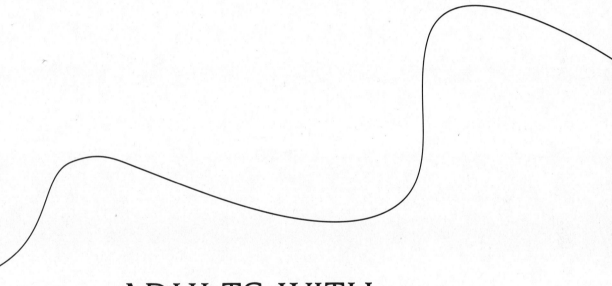

ADULTS WITH NEUROLOGIC DYSFUNCTION

Chapter Thirty-seven

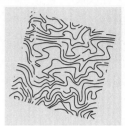

KNOWLEDGE BASIC TO THE NURSING CARE
of Adults with
Neurologic Dysfunction

Learning Objectives

1.0 Review the Anatomy and Physiology of the Nervous System.

1.1 Label the Parts of the Nervous System.
1.2 Demonstrate an Understanding of Nerve Impulse Transmission.
1.3 List the Functions of the Nervous System.
1.4 Identify Causes of Altered Levels of Consciousness.
1.5 Identify Reasons for Increases in Intracranial Pressure.

2.0 Demonstrate an Understanding of the Assessment Data Related to the Neurologic System.

2.1 Demonstrate an Understanding of the Way to Assess the Nervous System.
2.2 Interpret Assessment Data Related to the Neurologic System.
2.3 Identify Clinical Manifestations of Neurologic Dysfunctions.
2.4 Identify Dysfunctions of Language and Speech.
2.5 Identify Several Types of Diagnostic Tests.
2.6 Plan the Nursing Care for a Patient Undergoing Diagnostic Testing.

3.0 Demonstrate an Understanding of the Interventions Used to Manage Neurologic Dysfunctions.

3.1 Identify Medical and Surgical Management Techniques for the Patient with a Neurologic Dysfunction.
3.2 Identify Ways to Treat Increases in Intracranial Pressure.
3.3 Plan the Nursing Care of the Patient Having a Craniotomy.
3.4 Write a Nursing Care Plan for the Patient Having Spinal Surgery.
3.5 Plan the Nursing Care for a Patient with an Altered Level of Consciousness.
3.6 Write a Nursing Care Plan for the Patient with a Visual Field Disturbance.

Learning Activities

Identify

1. On the figure below, label the following parts of the central nervous system.

    A. Cerebrum   E. Diencephalon
    B. Brain stem   F. Pons
    C. Cerebellum   G. Medulla
    D. Midbrain   H. Spinal cord

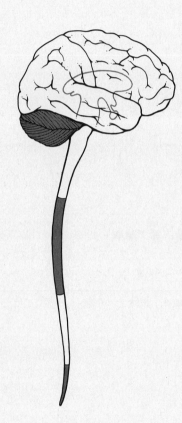

Fill In

2. The central nervous system is composed of the _____ and the _____.

3. The peripheral nervous system is composed of:
    1.
    2.
    3.

4. _____ conduct impulses to the cell body, and _____ conduct impulses away from the cell body.

5. The membranes that cover the brain and spinal cord and provide support and protection are the _____.

6. Cerebrospinal fluid is formed primarily in the _____.

7. The purpose of cerebrospinal fluid is _____
_____

8. Cerebrospinal fluid is reabsorbed constantly into the _____.

9. In the spinal cord, _____ pathways carry sensory impulses to the brain, and _____ pathways carry motor impulses from the brain.

10. Superficial receptors of pain, temperature, and light touch are located throughout the skin in regions known as _____.

Questions

11. Intracranial pressure is:

12. Normal intracranial pressure is:

13. Decreased level of consciousness is caused by:

Matching

Match the following diagnostic tests with their descriptions.

A. MRI
B. CT scan
C. PET scan
D. Evoked potential studies
E. EMG
F. Doppler studies
G. Angiography
H. Lumbar puncture
I. EEG
J. Myelogram

14. _____ Uses a powerful magnet and radio frequency to scan the head and body, then a computer creates pictures.

15. _____ Noninvasive procedure to evaluate carotid arterial blood flow.

16. _____ Uses an x-ray scanner, computer, and display mechanism to print images of the brain.

17. _____ Imaging technique that uses radioactive tracers to produce images which measure physiologic and biochemical activities of the brain.

18. _____ Invasive procedure to allow visualization of the intracranial vasculature.

19. _____ Performed to determine CSF pressure.

20. _____ Measures the electrical impulses of the brain.

21. _____ Measures the brain waves to determine cerebral response to peripheral sensory stimulation.

22. _____ Records electrical impulses of the peripheral nerves.

23. _____ Introduces contrast medium into the subarachnoid space, which can diagnose herniated disk.

Questions

24. In the event of neuron trauma or injury, which of the nerves have the ability to recover?

    A. Cranial nerves

    B. Spinal nerves

    C. Peripheral nerves

    D. None

25. During the depolarization process of nerve impulse transmission, the following will occur:

    A. Cell membrane becomes permeable to sodium

    B. Neuron has a negative membrane potential

    C. Influx of potassium occurs

    D. Chloride and potassium ions move into the cells

26. During neuromuscular transmission of the nerve impulse, what process occurs?

    A. Neurotransmitters cause repolarization at the neuron junction

    B. Acetylcholine binds with acetylcholinesterase at the myoneuron junction, causing release of calcium and contraction of the muscle

    C. Acetylcholine is released and travels across the synaptic cleft to bind with receptor sites

    D. Acetylcholinesterase is released, which stimulates the release of calcium to stimulate contraction

27. The protective membrane which adheres to the brain and spinal cord is the:

    A. Dura mater

    B. Arachnoid

    C. Pia mater

28. The part of the cerebral hemisphere which is thought to be the seat of abstract thought, judgment, and emotion is the:

    A. Frontal lobe

    B. Temporal lobe

    C. Parietal lobe

    D. Occipital lobe

29. The area in the cerebral hemisphere which is responsible for speech is known as:

    A. Wernicke's area

    B. Broca's area

    C. Rolando's area

    D. Lateral fissure

30. In most individuals, the right hemisphere of the cerebrum is responsible for:

    A. Understanding speech and expression of speech

    B. Sensation of touch, position, and pressure

C. Perception of spatial orientation and perspective

D. Conscious awareness of pain

31. The respiratory centers of the brain are located here:

A. Midbrain

B. Pons

C. Medulla oblongata

D. Cerebellum

Matching

A. Autonomic nervous system
B. Sympathetic system
C. Parasympathetic system

32. _____ Associated with fight or flight response.

33. _____ Composed of the sympathetic and parasympathetic systems.

34. _____ Associated with a conservation of energy.

35. _____ The neurotransmitter acetylcholine is associated with this system.

36. _____ The neurotransmitter noradrenalin is associated with this system.

Questions

37. An activity which can result in an increase in intracranial pressure is:

A. Coughing

B. Performing the Valsalva maneuver

C. Flexing the head

D. All of the above

38. The reason that pupil checks are important when a change in ICP is suspected is because:

A. High pressure clouds the vision

B. Pupil changes can be caused by pressure on the ocular nerve

C. Hemorrhages will cause visual impairment

D. Pupil dilation is the first sign of increase in ICP

39. The nurse is aware that the most sensitive indicator of increased intracranial pressure in a patient is:

A. Increase in blood pressure

B. Decrease in level of consciousness

C. Agitation and hostility

D. Rise in temperature

40. Displacement of intracranial components from one compartment to another is called:

A. Deceleration

B. Herniation

C. Decortication

D. Tamponade

41. Brain stem compression which will result in a change in vital signs is called:

A. Cushing's response

B. Decerebrate response

C. Hypothalamic response

D. Glasgow response

42. A patient with an altered level of consciousness exhibits a downward drifting of an extended hand. This may indicate:

A. A developing hemiparesis

B. Increasing intracranial pressure

C. Overdose of medication

D. Alteration in electrolytes

43. A patient exhibits the following posturing: rigid spine, flexed and abducted arms, and extended legs. This is called:

A. Decerebrate posturing

B. Hyperreflexia posturing

C. Decorticate posturing

D. Persistent vegetative state

44. The nurse is assessing a patient with an altered level of consciousness. The assessment reveals eye opening to painful stimuli, abnormal extension of extremities, and no verbal respone. The Glasgow coma scale total for this patient would be:

A. 5

B. 7

C. 9

D. 12

45. An impairment of consciousness occurs when there is a disruption in this circuit system:

A. Cerebellar area

B. Reticular activating system

C. Myoneural junction

D. Bundle of His

46. An altered level of consciousness can be the result of:

A. Metabolic disorders

B. Infectious processes

C. Psychiatric disorders

D. All of the above

47. Medical management of increased intracranial pressure will include medications such as:

A. Osmotic diuretics

B. Corticosteroids

C. Anticonvulsants

D. Any or all of the above

48. When a patient is receiving mannitol, the nurse would monitor:

A. Serum osmolarity

B. Hemoglobin and hematocrit

C. Serum electrolytes

D. Arterial blood gases

49. When a patient has an increase in ICP, the nurse would place him or her in a _____ position.

A. Trendelenburg

B. Reverse Trendelenburg

C. Semi-Fowler's

D. Supine

50. When a patient has receptive aphasia, the nurse is aware that this is the result of injury to:

A. Broca's area

B. Wernicke's area

C. cerebrum

D. lateral fissure

51. Assessment data of a patient reveals involuntary twisting movements of the body and trunk. This condition is called:

A. Dystonia

B. Bradykinesia

C. Hemiparesis

D. Torticollis

52. Following a stroke, a patient keeps walking into the wall on the right side. This type of visual field disturbance is known as:

A. Nystagmus

B. Diplopia

C. Tinnitus

D. Hemianopia

53. Write a nursing care plan for the patient who has an intracranial bleed.

Nursing Diagnosis: Alteration in tissue perfusion

Patient Outcome:

Nursing Interventions:

54. Write a nursing care plan for the unconscious patient.

Nursing Diagnosis: Impaired physical mobility: related to inability to participate in movement.

Patient Outcome:

Nursing Interventions:

Matching

A. Aphasia   C. Alexia
B. Agraphia

55. _____ Dysfunction of spoken language

56. _____ Impairment of language function

57. _____ Impairment of reading ability

Questions

58. Write a nursing care plan for a patient who has expressive aphasia as a result of a stroke.

    Nursing Diagnosis:

    Patient Outcome:

    Nursing Interventions:

59. Write a nursing care plan for the patient with a visual field deficit.

    Nursing Diagnosis: High risk for injury.

    Patient Outcome:

    Nursing Interventions:

Matching

Which test would give information on the status of the following?

A. Sensory system   C. Motor function
B. Speech and language   D. Abstract thinking

60. _____ Proprioception
61. _____ Arm drift
62. _____ Reflex testing
63. _____ Ask patient to explain a proverb
64. _____ Ask patient to identify objects
65. _____ Check resistance to movement

Questions

66. The nurse is aware that if a lumbar puncture is performed on a patient who has an increase in intracranial pressure the following complication may occur:

    A. Herniation syndrome

    B. Hydrocephalic syndrome

    C. Intracranial hemorrhage

    D. Sepsis

67. Nursing care following angiography would involve:

    A. Monitoring neurologic signs for 24 hours

    B. Immobilization of puncture site for 8 hours

    C. Assessment of distal pulses

    D. All of the above

68. A patient who has returned from a cerebral angiogram is complaining of inability to understand questions. The nurse is aware that this may indicate:

    A. Increase in intracranial pressure

    B. Cerebral vascular accident

    C. Hemorrhage

    D. Renal shutdown

69. When a patient is scheduled for a myelogram, which medication should be discontinued several days prior to the procedure?

    A. Calcium channel blockers

    B. Diuretics

    C. MAO inhibitors

    D. Analgesics

70. Which of the following nursing interventions would be implemented for the patient after a myelogram?

    A. Limit fluids

    B. Elevate bed to 45 degrees for 6 hours

    C. Keep bed flat for 24 hours

    D. Check peripheral pulses every hour for 6 hours

71. Which of the following symptoms, when present, indicates a possible allergic reaction to the contrast medium given during a myelogram?

    A. Vomiting

    B. Raised rash

    C. Pain in flank area

    D. Anorexia

72. Plan the nursing care for the patient who has had spinal surgery.

    Nursing Diagnosis: Pain

Patient Outcome:

Nursing Interventions:

CLINICAL SITUATIONS

Situation ■ 1

The nurse is caring for a 25-year-old male who was the victim of a motorcycle accident. He was not wearing a helmet. Severe head injury is suspected.

1. Assessment of this patient shows him to be restless, with inappropriate verbal response. BP is 140/50; pulse is 50. The most likely reason for these signs and symptoms is:

   A. Hypovolemic shock

   B. Hemorrhage

   C. Increased intracranial pressure

   D. Post-traumatic stress syndrome

2. Medical management of this patient would include administration of osmotic diuretics such as:

   A. Lasix

   B. Mannitol

   C. Dyazide

   D. Aldomet

3. The physician orders Decadron to be administered intravenously every 6 hours. Which of the following symptoms, if present, would indicate a side effect of this therapy?

   A. Rapid heart rate

   B. Hyperglycemia

   C. Vomiting and nausea

   D. Blurred vision

4. Nursing care of the patient who has a head injury would include:

   A. Increasing fluid intake

   B. Keeping the patient in a prone position

C. Maintaining the head of the bed at a 30-degree angle

D. Monitoring neurologic status every 4 hours

Situation ■ 2

Ms. York is admitted with a possible brain tumor. She is 66 years old and has a history of diabetes and heart disease with a pacemaker inserted 10 years ago. She is scheduled for diagnostic testing and possible surgery.

1. Ms. York is scheduled for a complete workup. Which of the following tests would not be appropriate for this patient?

   A. Cerebral angiogram

   B. CT scan

   C. MRI

   D. EEG

2. The diagnosis of a cerebral neoplasm is confirmed and Ms. York is scheduled for a craniotomy. The physician is likely to order which of the following medications prior to surgery?

   A. Dilantin

   B. Ancef

   C. Lasix

   D. Potassium

3. Following the surgery, one of the most important nursing goals would be:

   A. Preventing alteration in fluid and electrolytes

   B. Maintaining adequate cardiac output

   C. Maintaining adequate breathing patterns

   D. Preventing increased intracranial pressure

4. Which of the following symptoms, when present, would indicate a serious complication of the surgery?

   A. Nausea and vomiting

   B. Change in level of consciousness

   C. Rise in temperature

   D. Decrease in urine output

Chapter Thirty-eight

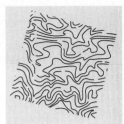

NURSING CARE
of Adults with
Nervous System Disorders

Learning Objectives

1.0 Demonstrate an Understanding of the Infections and Inflammations that Affect the Nervous System.

1.1 Identify Characteristics of the Infections and Inflammations of the Nervous System.
1.2 Assess Clinical Manifestations of Several of the Abnormalities of the Nervous System.
1.3 Define Several of the Infectious and Inflammatory Disorders of the Nervous System.
1.4 Write a Nursing Care Plan for an Individual with Multiple Sclerosis.
1.5 Write a Nursing Care Plan that Addresses the Nutritional Needs of the Patient with Encephalitis.

2.0 Demonstrate an Understanding of the Degenerative Disorders that can Affect the Nervous System.

2.1 Identify Characteristic Symptoms of Degenerative Disorders of the Nervous System.
2.2 Pick Appropriate Nursing Interventions Used in Caring for the Patient with a Degenerative Disorder.
2.3 Identify the Pathology of Several of the Degenerative Disorders.
2.4 Plan the Nursing Care for the Patient with a Degenerative Disorder.

3.0 Demonstrate an Understanding of the Functional Disorders of the Nervous System.

3.1 Identify Symptoms of Functional Disorders.
3.2 Plan the Nursing Care for the Patient with a Functional Disorder.
3.3 Write a Nursing Care Plan for the Patient with a Seizure Disorder.

4.0 Demonstrate an Understanding of the Structural Disorders of the Nervous System.

4.1 Identify Characteristics of Structural Disorders.
4.2 Review Appropriate Medical Interventions for the Patient with a Structural Disorder.
4.3 Write a Nursing Care Plan for the Patient with a Cerebrovascular Accident.

5.0 Demonstrate an Understanding of Traumatic Injuries of the Nervous System.

5.1 Identify Symptoms of Head Injuries.
5.2 Identify the Symptoms of Spinal Shock.
5.3 Write a Nursing Care Plan for the Patient with a Spinal Injury.

6.0 Demonstrate an Understanding of the Neoplasms which Affect the Nervous System

6.1 Assess the Characteristics of Neoplasms of the Nervous System.
6.2 Write a Nursing Care Plan for the Patient with a Brain Tumor.

Learning Activities

Define

1. Encephalitis:

2. Guillain-Barré syndrome:

3. Amyotrophic lateral sclerosis:

4. Multiple sclerosis:

5. Neurogenic bladder:

6. Muscular dystrophy:

7. Alzheimer's disease:

8. Status epilepticus:

Questions

9. In a patient with suspected meningococcal meningitis, the nurse would assess for:

   A. Petechial rash or ecchymosis

   B. Nausea and vomiting

   C. Change in consciousness

   D. Pupil changes

10. The nurse is assessing a patient who is admitted with a neurologic disorder. The nurse performs an assessment and finds that when the patient flexes the head toward the chest, it results in flexion of the thighs and legs. This is known as:

    A. Nuchal rigidity

    B. Kernig's sign

    C. Brudzinski's sign

    D. Cortical irritation

11. In order to make a definitive diagnosis of meningitis, the nurse would expect the physician to order a/an:

    A. CT scan

    B. MRI scan

    C. Angiography

    D. Lumbar puncture

12. The focus of the medical management of the patient with bacterial meningitis is _____ .

    A. Corticosteroids

    B. Antiviral agents

    C. Antibiotic agents

    D. Chemotherapeutic agents

13. The nurse's responsibility in preventing transmission of herpes simplex virus type 2 would be:

    A. Testing of all college-aged students

    B. Determining presence of virus in pregnant women

    C. Treating all sexually active men

    D. Random screening in drug clinics

14. Nursing care of the patient who has viral encephalitis would include:

    A. Administration of antibiotics

    B. Administration of antiviral agents

C. Providing nutritional support

D. Providing emotional support

15. Plan the nursing care for the patient with encephalitis who is unable to eat.

Nursing Diagnosis:

Patient Outcome:

Nursing Interventions:

16. When a patient with herpes simplex encephalitis develops neurologic symptoms such as hemiparesis or behavioral changes, the nurse would monitor closely for:

A. Signs of increased intracranial pressure

B. Loss of bladder and bowel control

C. Respiratory distress

D. Cardiac arrhythmias

17. Medical management of the patient with herpes simplex encephalitis will include:

A. Antibiotics

B. Fluid restrictions

C. Antiviral agents

D. Analgesics

18. An individual who has a severe mastoiditis is at risk for developing:

A. Hearing loss

B. Brain abscess

C. Encephalitis

D. Septic shock

19. When assessing a patient who has Guillain-Barré syndrome, the nurse notices asymmetric facial expressions. This may indicate:

A. There is cranial nerve involvement

B. There is permanent paralysis

C. There is an increase in intracranial pressure

D. There has been brain damage

20. Because the patient with Guillain-Barré syndrome often develops flaccid paralysis, the nursing management is primarily directed toward:

A. Preventing dehydration

B. Promoting independence

C. Preventing development of contractures

D. Maintaining bowel and bladder control

21. The most common motor neuron disease in adults is:

A. Multiple sclerosis (MS)

B. Amyotrophic lateral sclerosis (ALS)

C. Muscular dystrophy

D. Myasthenia gravis

22. The nurse is assessing a patient with a nervous system disorder. All of the following symptoms would indicate ALS EXCEPT:

A. Difficulty swallowing

B. Decreased sensation

C. Hyperreflexia

D. Slurred speech

23. In caring for a patient with a diagnosis of ALS, the nurse should be chiefly concerned with?

A. Maintaining highest functioning level of the patient

B. Maintaining adequate nutritional intake

C. Returning the patient to prior activity level

D. Preventing atrophy of muscles

24. The nurse should have which equipment available when feeding the patient with ALS?

A. Cardiac monitor

B. Oxygen

C. Suction machine

D. Oral airway

25. A patient has been diagnosed with multiple sclerosis. This means:

A. There is decreased impulse transmission at the myoneuron junction

B. The motor neurons in the cerebral cortex are beginning to degenerate

C. There is deactivation of anticholinesterase

D. There is demyelination and scarring along the central nervous system

26. In the patient with multiple sclerosis, the nurse would anticipate which of the following alterations to be present?

    A. Sensory alterations

    B. Motor alterations

    C. Visual alteration

    D. Emotional lability

    E. Any or all of the above

27. Which statement best describes the clinical course of multiple sclerosis?

    A. The disease will often go into total remission after aggressive treatment

    B. The disease is chronic and has a steady downhill course

    C. The disease is characterized by exacerbation and remissions which are unpredictable

    D. The disease is curable if recognized and diagnosed early

28. A patient with multiple sclerosis has severe spasticity of the lower extremities. The nurse would anticipate that _____ would be used.

    A. Lioresal

    B. Tylenol

    C. Decadron

    D. Gantrisin

29. Write a nursing care plan for the patient with MS who has a neurogenic bladder.

    Nursing Diagnosis:

    Patient Outcome:

    Nursing Interventions:

30. Which description would be most appropriate in explaining the pathophysiology of myasthenia gravis?

    A. It is a hereditary autoimmune disease of the motor neurons.

    B. It is a progressive degeneration of the myelin sheath of the spinal cord.

    C. It is a disease which affects the acetylcholine released at the neuromuscular junction.

    D. It is an acute disease which has effective treatment regimens.

31. The nurse is assisting the physician in making a diagnosis of myasthenia. What is an appropriate nursing action?

    A. Have Tensilon ready for administration

    B. Explain to the patient that this test may cure the disease

    C. Keep the patient on NPO status

    D. Have the patient sign a consent form

32. The nurse is educating a patient on when to take his Mestinon after discharge. What information should the nurse obtain from the patient?

    A. What time he goes to bed

    B. What time he eats meals

    C. How often he urinates daily

    D. What types of activity he can do

33. If a patient with myasthenia gravis has a severe infection, the nurse realizes that he or she is at risk for developing:

    A. Cholinergic crisis

    B. Myasthenic crisis

    C. Septic shock

    D. Respiratory arrest

34. A hereditary neurologic condition which is characterized by progressive degeneration and weakness of the voluntary muscles is known as:

    A. Multiple sclerosis

    B. Lou Gehrig's disease

    C. Muscular dystrophy

    D. Alzheimer's disease

35. Parkinson's disease is a neurologic condition which is characterized by degenerative changes in the:

    A. Cerebral cortex

    B. Medulla oblongata

    C. Basal ganglia

    D. Longitudinal fissures

36. When the nurse is assessing a patient with Par-

kinson's disease, findings would most likely include:

A. Tremors, weakness, muscle atrophy

B. Shuffling gait, spastic leg movement

C. Blurred vision, weakness, fatigue

D. Tremors, muscle rigidity, bradykinesia

37. In evaluating a patient for Parkinson's disease, the nurse would expect to see a decreased urine level of:

A. Homovanillic acid

B. Uric acid

C. Catecholamines

D. Acetylcholine

38. The medical treatment for the individual with Parkinson's disease would include the use of anticholinergic drugs such as:

A. Levodopa

B. Sinemet

C. Cogentin

D. Decadron

39. The nurse is assisting a patient with Parkinson's disease to plan meals. Which foods would the nurse instruct the patient to limit?

A. Chicken and turkey

B. Cereal and whole grains

C. Milk and eggs

D. Green vegetables

40. Write a nursing care plan for the individual with Parkinson's disease; focus on problems with mobility.

Nursing Diagnosis:

Patient Outcome:

Nursing Interventions:

41. An appropriate nursing intervention for the patient with Alzheimer's disease would be:

A. Increase verbal and environmental cues

B. Restrain the individual so he or she cannot harm him or herself

C. Speak loudly and slowly

D. Involve the patient in new activities

42. A patient is admitted with a possible herniated disc. Which information given by the patient might indicate the cause of the current condition?

A. I like to jog in the morning

B. I am 20 pounds overweight

C. I smoke 2 packs of cigarettes a day

D. I helped my neighbor move his furniture yesterday

43. A test which is used to diagnose a herniated disc because it can provide clear images of the spinal cord anatomy is the:

A. Spinal x-ray

B. Lumbar puncture

C. Magnetic resonance imaging

D. Ultrasound

44. The most comfortable position for the patient with a herniation of a lumbar disk is:

A. Prone without a pillow

B. Semi-Fowler's

C. Side-lying with knees flexed

D. Supine

45. The nurse is assessing a patient who is admitted with seizures. During examination, the patient has a 2-minute period of lack of awareness of the environment. This was most likely a:

A. Simple partial seizure

B. Complex partial seizure

C. Petit mal seizure

D. Tonic-clonic seizure

46. If a patient develops status epilepticus, the physician might order:

A. Dilantin

B. Phenobarbital

C. Valium

D. Any or all of above

47. One of the most important nursing interventions for the patient with a seizure disorder is:

A. Provide a safe environment

B. Maintain effective gas exchange

C. Provide appropriate knowledge of condition

D. Instruct the patient in self-care activities

48. The rationale for treating migraine headaches with medications such as Inderal and Catapres is to:

A. Promote analgesia and sedation

B. Promote vasodilatation

C. Reduce stress and anxiety

D. Inhibit vasodilatation

49. When a patient is admitted with a diagnosis of communicating hydrocephalus, which information in the past medical history is most relevant?

A. History of myocardial infarction

B. History of meningitis

C. History of seizures

D. History of adrenal insufficiency

50. Mr. Pasterman, 64 years old, is admitted with a diagnosis of normal pressure hydrocephalus. Which assessment data is related to this problem?

A. Gait disturbance, impaired memory

B. Mood swings, depression, aphasia

C. Headache, dizziness, sensory deficit

D. Hemiplegia, agnosia

51. Mr. Pasterman has a ventricular shunt inserted to correct the problem. Following the surgery, the nurse would consider which of the following a serious complication?

A. Patient complains of tenderness at insertion site

B. Patient has urinary incontinence

C. Patient is anxious

D. Patient is lethargic and hard to arouse

52. The nurse is aware that a cerebrovascular accident (CVA) is often the result of:

A. Sudden increase in cardiac output

B. Interruption of blood flow to the brain

C. Sudden change in electrolyte balance

D. Seizure disorder

53. In differentiating between a TIA and a CVA, the nurse is aware that a TIA:

A. Has sudden onset and short duration

B. Has slow insidious onset and lasts up to 48 hours

C. Is progressive in nature

D. Is often undetected but will always lead to a stroke

54. A patient who is admitted with a left-sided cerebrovascular accident will most likely have:

A. Aphasia

B. Ataxia

C. Dyslexia

D. Quadriplegia

55. Which position would be most appropriate for the nurse to use for positioning the patient with a right CVA who is nonresponsive?

A. Prone position

B. Right side with knees flexed

C. Left side with the head of the bed at 30 degrees

D. Trendelenburg's position

56. A patient has a CVA with left-sided paralysis. The nurse positions the bed table on the left side. The rationale for this is:

A. To encourage self-care

B. To keep the environment uncluttered

C. To prevent unilateral neglect

D. To prevent falls from the bed

57. Write a nursing care plan for the patient who has been admitted with a CVA and is hemiplegic and aphasic.

Nursing Diagnosis: Impaired physical mobility related to hemiplegia

Patient Outcome:

Nursing Interventions:

Nursing Diagnosis: Impaired verbal communication

Patient Outcome:

Nursing Interventions:

True or False

58. _____ The mortality rate associated with subarachnoid hemorrhages is > 30%.

59. _____ Cerebral aneurysms are often asymptomatic until they rupture.

60. _____ Individuals with arteriovenous malformations may have headaches and seizures.

61. _____ The presenting symptom associated with a subarachnoid hemorrhage is severe dizziness.

62. _____ Individuals with a subarachnoid hemorrhage are immediately started on heparin.

Questions

63. Which of the following clinical manifestations is present in a large percentage of the individuals who have brain tumors?

    A. Frontal headache
    B. Projectile vomiting
    C. Papilledema
    D. Seizures

64. Which of the following diagnostic tests is often contraindicated when an individual is being evaluated for a possible brain tumor?

    A. CT scan
    B. Lumbar puncture
    C. Angiography
    D. MRI scan

65. The nurse is assessing a patient who has a possible skull fracture as a result of an accident. A finding of ecchymosis over the mastoid bone is indicative of:

    A. Linear skull fracture
    B. Scalp laceration
    C. Basilar skull fracture
    D. Leakage of cerebrospinal fluid

66. The nurse is aware that the drug of choice for reducing cerebral edema is:

    A. Mannitol
    B. Dexamethasone
    C. Heparin
    D. Cephalozolin

67. When caring for the patient with a skull fracture, the nurse would explain to the patient that the following activity would be contraindicated:

    A. Blowing the nose
    B. Ambulating in the unit
    C. Sitting in a chair
    D. Urinating while standing

68. A traumatic accident that causes the brain to strike the internal surfaces of the skull, resulting in bruising of brain tissues, is a:

    A. Contusion
    B. Concussion
    C. Hematoma
    D. Herniation

69. A patient is admitted with a head injury. During the initial assessment, he was unconscious 1 hour. Now he is awake, but 3 hours later he begins to lose consciousness. This suggests:

    A. Cerebrovascular accident
    B. Transient ischemia
    C. Epidural hematoma
    D. Subdural hematoma

70. A patient who is admitted with an epidural hematoma is deteriorating rapidly. An appropriate nursing measure would be:

    A. Transfer the patient to intensive care
    B. Prepare the patient for surgery
    C. Notify the code team
    D. Monitor vital signs closely

71. The nurse is assessing a patient with a spinal cord injury. Symptoms which would indicate spinal shock would include:

    A. Flaccid paralysis of skeletal musculature below the level of the lesion

    B. Spastic paralysis of skeletal musculature below the level of injury

    C. Rigidity of the lower extremities with flaccidity of upper extremities

    D. Total lack of sensation and motor activity

72. A patient who has a spinal injury is to be fitted with a halo device. The nurse realizes that one advantage of this device is:

    A. Reduction in time healing

    B. Improvement in mobility

    C. Decrease in complications

    D. Prevention of spinal shock

73. Write a nursing care plan for the patient who has sustained a head injury.

    Nursing Diagnosis: Altered thought processes related to acute head injury

    Patient Outcome:

    Nursing Interventions:

74. Write a nursing care plan for the patient with a spinal cord injury.

    Nursing Diagnosis: High risk for injury related to unstable vertebral column

    Patient Outcome:

    Nursing Interventions:

1. The nurse's first priority should be:

    A. Remove everyone from the area

    B. Move her to the floor

    C. Insert a padded tongue blade between her teeth

    D. Ask a bystander what precipitated the seizure

2. Immediately following the seizure, the student is incontinent of urine and difficult to arouse. Based on this information, the nurse should:

    A. Call the paramedics

    B. Do a thorough neurologic check every 5 minutes

    C. Shake her frequently so she doesn't fall asleep

    D. Place her on her side and let her sleep

3. After a thorough workup, it is determined that Kathy is suffering from epilepsy. She is started on Dilantin. Which information would the nurse emphasize?

    A. Less medication will be needed as she gets older

    B. Medication should never be stopped suddenly

    C. Medication should be discontinued if side effects occur

    D. Medication will probably not totally control seizures

4. Kathy is to be married next year. She wonders if she should have children. Which of the following statements would the nurse make?

    A. When you decide to get pregnant, ask your physician to change your medication.

    B. Your children won't have any increased risk of having seizures.

    C. It is often impossible to become pregnant when a woman has a seizure disorder.

    D. Unless you stop having seizures, you shouldn't consider having children.

CLINICAL SITUATIONS

Situation ■ 1

Kathy, a college-aged student, is waiting in the health clinic when she suddenly begins to experience a generalized tonic-clonic seizure.

Situation ■ 2

Mr. Smith, 75 years old, is admitted with a diagnosis of left hemispheric cerebrovascular accident. He is lethargic and nonverbal at present.

1. During the acute phase, the nurse is aware that a priority is:

   A. Maintaining mobility

   B. Maintaining fluid and electrolyte balance

   C. Maintaining patent airway

   D. Preventing skin breakdown

2. Based on the type of CVA which has occurred, the nurse will anticipate that Mr. Smith will have:

   A. Language and speech impairment, motor plegia

   B. Left-sided neglect, self-care deficit

   C. Normal speech but plegia on right side

   D. Normal return of function in 6–8 months

3. It is determined that Mr. Smith has had his stroke as a result of a cerebral embolus. Based on this information, the nurse would expect what type of treatment?

   A. Heparin therapy

   B. Aspirin therapy

   C. Diuretic therapy

   D. Antibiotic therapy

4. It is now 1 week later; Mr. Smith is more alert. He is placed on Coumadin, Minipress, and Digoxin. The nurse is reviewing Mr. Smith's lab findings. Which lab result demonstrates a therapeutic response to treatment?

   A. PT of 10.0

   B. PT of 16.3

   C. PTT of 60.0

   D. PTT of 35.3

5. Mr. Smith has been incontinent of both urine and feces since his stroke. Which nursing measure would be most appropriate in helping Mr. Smith regain bladder control?

   A. Change the bed pads frequently

   B. Get an order for a Foley catheter

   C. Apply an external urinary catheter

   D. Keep the urinal within easy reach

6. Mr. Smith has expressive aphasia. Which technique should the nurse use to facilitate communication with him?

   A. Speak loudly and slowly

   B. Face the patient and speak normally

   C. Use pantomime and gestures frequently

   D. Write down everything and show to him

Situation ■ 3

Steven, 18 years old, was involved in a climbing accident. He fell from a ledge, and a spinal cord injury is suspected.

1. A nurse is in the area and is the first one to find him. Steven is lying on his back and says he can't move his legs. An appropriate action on the part of the nurse would be:

   A. Turn him on his side

   B. Send for help and keep him still

   C. Have him bend his knees to relieve the pain

   D. Carry Steven to the road and summon help

2. In the emergency room, Steven is alert but anxious. His heart rate and respirations are increasing, while his BP is falling. These findings suggest:

   A. Autonomic dysreflexia

   B. Hypovolemic shock

   C. Spinal shock

   D. Cardiogenic shock

3. Once his condition stabilizes, he is moved to the rehabilitation unit. The nurse notices that he is uncooperative and hostile. This behavior indicates:

   A. Normal grief reaction

   B. Normal anxiety reaction

   C. Sign of depression

   D. Reaction to being in intensive care

Situation ■ 4

A patient is admitted with a diagnosis of bacterial meningitis. The admitting symptoms include headache, fever, and petechial rash.

1. The nurse is examining the patient. Which of the following signs, if present, indicate meningeal irritation?

A. Severe headache

B. Seizure activity

C. Positive Homans' sign

D. Positive Kernig's sign

2. Medical treatment is initiated immediately. The nurse would anticipate administration of medications such as:

A. Analgesics

B. Anti-inflammatory drugs

C. Antibiotics

D. Antipyretics

3. The nurse realizes it is important to observe the patient for any signs of increased intracranial pressure. A sign of increased ICP would be:

A. Difficulty breathing

B. Irregularity of heart rate

C. Rapid pulse

D. Seizure activity

4. Which would be the best method for the nurse to administer Dilantin 100 mg IV to the patient?

A. Dilute with 100 ml dextrose and administer over 30 minutes

B. Dilute with 10 ml dextrose and give within 5 minutes to get the maximum therapeutic effect

C. Dilute in 100 ml of normal saline and administer over 30–60 minutes

D. Administer cautiously from syringe within 20 minutes and flush with any IV solution

Unit Thirteen

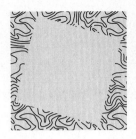

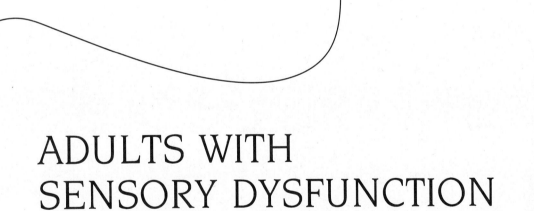

ADULTS WITH SENSORY DYSFUNCTION

Chapter Thirty-nine

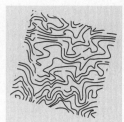

KNOWLEDGE BASIC TO THE NURSING CARE of Adults with Dysfunction of the Eye

Learning Objectives

1.0 Review the Anatomy and Physiology of the Eye.

1.1 Identify the Structures of the Eye.
1.2 Explain the Process of Vision.
1.3 Match the Parts of the Eye with Their Functions.

2.0 Demonstrate an Understanding of the Assessment Data Related to Dysfunction of the Eye.

2.1 Review the Assessment Data Specific to the Eye.
2.2 Identify Clinical Manifestations of Eye Dysfunction.
2.3 Match the Diagnostic Procedures Used to Identify Visual Dysfunctions with Their Correct Definitions.

3.0 Demonstrate an Understanding of the Interventions Used to Treat Eye Dysfunctions.

3.1 Identify Several Medications Used to Treat Eye Dysfunctions.
3.2 Identify Surgical Interventions Used to Treat Eye Dysfunctions.
3.3 Demonstrate an Application of the Nursing Process When Caring for a Patient with a Dysfunction of the Eye.
3.4 Demonstrate an Understanding of the Postoperative Care of the Patient Who Has Undergone Eye Surgery.

Learning Activities

Identify

1. On the diagram below, label the structures of the eye.

A. Cornea
B. Ciliary body
C. Vitreous humor

D. Sclera
E. Retina
F. Lens

G. Iris
H. Optic disk
I. Choroid

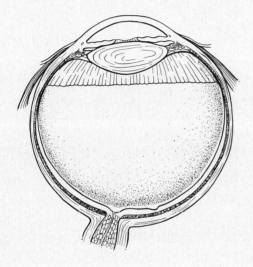

Fill In

2. Tears are produced by the _____ gland.

3. The _____ is responsible for regulating the amount of light entering the eye.

4. The _____ is a vascular membrane that nourishes the retina.

5. The inner coat of the eye, which forms the visual image, is known as the _____ .

6. The fluid responsible for maintaining the intraocular pressure is known as _____ .

7. The _____ refracts or bends light rays so that they converge on the retina.

Questions

8. Explain how the visual image is produced in the retina.

9. When you see the pupillary finding recorded as PERRLA in the patient record, this means:

10. The muscles that control the movement of the eye are under the control of which cranial nerves?

   1.

   2.

   3.

Matching

Match the parts of the eye with their functions.

A. Iris
B. Choroid
C. Retina

D. Cones
E. Rods

11. _____ Posterior portion of the middle coat; absorbs light rays to prevent reflection.

12. _____ Responsible for color vision and visual acuity.

13. _____ Regulates the amount of light entering the eye.

14. _____ Covers the choroid; forms visual images.

15. _____ Gives support to the posterior cavity.

16. _____ Allow for vision in dim light.

Matching

Match the eye dysfunctions with their descriptions.

A. Floaters
B. Photophobia
C. Scotoma
D. Diplopia
E. Photopsia
F. Nystagmus

17. _____ Involuntary twitching eye movements.

18. _____ Appearance of flashing light in the visual field.

19. _____ Seeing one object as two.

20. _____ Unusual intolerance to light.

21. _____ Fixed defects or "spots" in the visual field.

22. _____ Moving spots in the visual field.

Questions

23. During the admission process, a patient tells the nurse that he has blurred vision. Which information in his history may be related?

A. History of hypertension
B. History of ulcer
C. History of angina
D. History of leg cramps

24. Which of the following is a primary symptom of nonocular conditions such as meningitis and migraine headaches?

A. Floaters
B. Photophobia
C. Scotoma
D. Blurred vision

25. The most common cause of blurred vision is:

A. Drug overdose
B. Congenital defect
C. Refractory error
D. Ocular muscle weakness

26. The sudden appearance of flashing lights in the visual field can be a symptom of _____ .

A. Retinal detachment
B. Diabetes mellitus
C. Hypertension
D. Glaucoma

27. Sudden loss of vision is associated with which of the following?

A. Retinal detachment
B. Cataracts
C. Glaucoma
D. Diabetic retinopathy

28. Visual acuity is usually tested by use of a:

A. Ophthalmoscope
B. Penlight
C. Snellen's chart
D. Otoscope

29. Legal blindness is defined as:

A. Corrected vision of < 20/100
B. Corrected vision of < 20/200
C. Uncorrected vision of < 20/100
D. Uncorrected vision of < 20/300

30. Consensual response when testing the pupillary reaction to light is:

A. Constriction of the pupil in response to light.
B. Constriction of the pupil of the opposite eye.
C. Dilation of the pupil when light is removed.
D. Inward movement of the eye in response to light.

31. If a patient is unable to see any letters during a visual exam, the nurse should:

A. Notify the physician
B. Check the ability to count fingers
C. Have the patient put on his or her glasses
D. Use the ophthalmoscope

32. To test for _____ , the nurse would hold a finger 6 inches from the patient's nose and have the patient look behind him or her and then back at the finger.

    A. Direct response

    B. Consensual response

    C. Extraocular movement

    D. Accommodation

33. Which of the following pharmacologic agents would be used for treatment of a foreign body in the eye?

    A. Anesthetic

    B. Anti-infective

    C. Anti-inflammatory

    D. Autonomic drug

34. After eye surgery, which of the following activities would be permitted during the postoperative period?

    A. Smoking

    B. Lying on the unaffected side

    C. Lying on the stomach

    D. Frequent coughing to expand the lung

Matching (Diagnostic Testing)

Match the following diagnostic procedures with their descriptions.

A. Tonometry   C. Gonioscopy
B. Fluorescein staining   D. Ultrasonography

35. _____ Measurement of intraocular pressure.

36. _____ Used in the diagnosis of glaucoma.

37. _____ Used to detect corneal abrasions.

38. _____ Uses sound waves to detect tumors.

Fill In

39. In the eye, drugs which cause sympathetic stimulation are called _____ . They cause the pupil to _____ .

40. Drugs that cause parasympathetic stimulation are called _____ . They cause the pupil to _____ .

41. Carbonic anhydrase inhibitors _____ intraocular pressure by causing a decrease in the amount of _____ .

42. Mannitol is an example of a drug which moves fluid rapidly by _____ .

Questions

43. The drug of choice to suppress hyperemia, photophobia, and pain is _____ .

    A. Analgesic

    B. Antipyretic

    C. Corticosteroid

    D. Antibiotic

44. When a sympatholytic drug is to be used in treating an eye condition, it should be used cautiously for a patient with _____ .

    A. Diabetes

    B. Cardiac disease

    C. Hepatic disease

    D. Skin disease

45. If a patient has angle closure glaucoma, the preferred medical treatment would be:

    A. Carbonic anhydrase inhibitors

    B. Sympathomimetic drugs

    C. Parasympatholytic drugs

    D. Sympatholytic drugs

True or False

46. _____ Eye surgery is generally done using local anesthesia.

47. _____ Miotic agents are given before surgery to dilate the pupil.

48. _____ Postoperatively, the operated eye is usually covered with an eye patch.

49. _____ Drainage following surgery is a cause for concern.

50. _____ Severe eye pain can indicate a complication such as hemorrhage.

51. _____ Laser therapy is a noninvasive procedure done on an outpatient basis.

52. _____ Peripheral vision generally narrows with aging.

Define

53. Vitrectomy:

54. Iridectomy:

55. Scleral buckling:

56. Keratoplasty:

57. Enucleation:

Questions

58. Describe three optical aids which are available to assist with vision.

    1.

    2.

    3.

59. Write a nursing care plan for the patient having eye surgery.

    Nursing diagnosis: Knowledge deficit: related to preoperative experience and the expected effect on vision

    Patient Outcome:

Nursing Interventions:

CLINICAL SITUATIONS

Situation ■ 1

Ms. Minor has had eye surgery to correct a visual deficit. The following questions relate to the postoperative period.

1. Why would the nurse encourage her to refrain from smoking following the surgery?

    A. Smoking will lower her blood pressure

    B. Smoking will irritate her vision

    C. Smoking will cause increased ocular pressure

    D. Smoking will increase her heart rate

2. Which of the following symptoms in the immediate postoperative period warrants immediate attention?

    A. Patient complains of nausea

    B. Patient complains of constipation

    C. Patient complains of headache

    D. Patient complains of thirst

3. The nurse tells Ms. Minor that she should lie on her back and have the bed elevated slightly. What is the reason for this instruction?

    A. To prevent hemorrhage

    B. To prevent an infection

    C. To avoid pressure on the eye

    D. To provide for effective coughing

Situation ■ 2

A patient is to have a corneal transplant because of degeneration.

1. Preoperatively, the nurse would administer:

    A. Antibiotic eye drops, pilocarpine hydrochloride

    B. Antibiotics and analgesics

    C. Mydriatics and analgesics

    D. Osmotic diuretics

2. Which of the following information is true about the procedure?

   A. It is done under general anesthesia

   B. Patients stay in the hospital for 3–5 days

   C. Local anesthesia is used; the stay is overnight

   D. A living donor is used

3. Postoperative teaching by the nurse would include: (Check all that apply.)

   A. Instruction on fluid restrictions

   B. Information on use of eyepatch and shield

   C. Information on antibiotics

   D. Information on activity limits

   E. Information on how to instill eyedrops

Chapter Forty

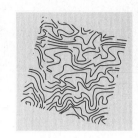

NURSING CARE
of Adults with
Eye Disorders

Learning Objectives

1.0 Demonstrate an Understanding of the Infections and Inflammations that Affect the Eye.

1.1 Identify the Clinical Manifestations of Several of the Infections and Inflammations of the Eye.
1.2 Identify the Etiology and Pathophysiology of Several Infections and Inflammations of the Eye.
1.3 Define Several of the Infections of the Eye.
1.4 Plan the Nursing Care for the Patient with an Infection or Inflammation of the Eye.
1.5 Pick the Appropriate Medical Interventions for the Patient with an Infection or Inflammation.
1.6 Write a Nursing Care Plan for the Patient with an Inflammation of the Eye.

2.0 Demonstrate an Understanding of the Structural Disorders of the Eye.

2.1 Identify the Clinical Manifestations of Several Structural Disorders.
2.2 Identify the Etiology and Pathophysiology of Several Structural Disorders.
2.3 Plan the Nursing Care for the Patient with a Structural Disorder.
2.4 Pick Appropriate Medical and Surgical Interventions for the Patient with a Structural Disorder.
2.5 Write a Nursing Care Plan for the Patient with a Structural Disorder of the Eye.

3.0 Demonstrate an Understanding of the Degenerative Disorders of the Eye.

3.1 Identify the Clinical Manifestations of Several Degenerative Disorders.
3.2 Pick Appropriate Nursing Interventions for the Patient with a Degenerative Disorder.

4.0 Demonstrate an Understanding of Traumatic Disorders of the Eye.

4.1 Identify the Correct Assessment of the Patient with Eye Trauma.
4.2 Identify Appropriate Interventions for the Patient with Eye Trauma.

Learning Activities

Define

1. Blepharitis:

2. Chalazion:

3. Conjunctivitis:

4. Dacryocystitis:

5. Keratitis:

6. Endophthalmitis:

Questions

7. If left untreated, staphylococcal blepharitis can cause:

    A. Permanent loss of vision

    B. Eyelashes to fall out

    C. Scar tissue to form on the cornea

    D. Systemic infection

8. Left untreated, chalazia can cause:

    A. Blindness

    B. Scarring of eye

    C. Astigmatism

    D. All of the above

9. When a patient has blepharitis or hordeola, the nurse would provide information about:

    A. Cold compresses

    B. Antiviral medications

    C. Application of warm compresses

    D. Proposed surgery

10. Symptoms such as itching, burning, photophobia, and the sensation of a foreign body in the eye suggest:

    A. Blepharitis

    B. Hordeola

    C. Chalazia

    D. Conjunctivitis

11. Which of the following eye disorders would by considered the most serious?

    A. Keratitis

    B. Blepharitis

    C. Endophthalmitis

    D. Conjunctivitis

12. Which information would the nurse obtain from a patient who has recurrent conjunctivitis?

    A. History of hypertension

    B. Use of antibiotics

    C. Exposure to irritants

    D. Recent loss of vision

13. The number one cause of corneal ulceration is:

    A. Herpes simplex virus

    B. *Streptococcus viridans*

    C. *Escherichia coli*

    D. *Staphylococcus*

14. All of the following symptoms may be present with bacterial keratitis EXCEPT:

    A. Reduced visual acuity

    B. Photophobia

C. Mucopurulent discharge

D. Ocular pain

E. Scratchy feeling in eye

15. One of the main treatment objectives with keratitis is:

A. Controlling pain

B. Protecting the cornea

C. Administering corticosteriods

D. All of the above

16. In caring for a patient with endophthalmitis, the nurse would do all the following EXCEPT:

A. Keep the room well lit

B. Provide distraction with music

C. Monitor intraocular pressure as ordered

D. Administer pain medications

Matching

Match the following structural disorders with their symptoms.

A. Epiphora   D. Hypermetropia
B. Photophobia   E. Myopia
C. Hypopyon

17. _____ Excessive tearing

18. _____ Purulent material in the anterior chamber

19. _____ Farsightedness

20. _____ Sensitivity to light

21. _____ Nearsightedness

Questions

22. A patient with symptoms such as visual fatigue, discomfort, or headache may have a:

A. Corneal abrasion

B. Refractory error

C. Traumatic injury

D. Sensitivity to light

23. One of the problems with using rigid contact lenses is that they:

A. Are easily damaged

B. Can harbor microorganisms

C. Are easily broken

D. Cause dry eyes or corneal warping

24. Write a nursing care plan for the patient with a corneal ulcer.

Nursing Diagnosis: Sensory perceptual alteration, vision: related to corneal transparency

Patient Outcome:

Nursing Interventions:

25. A structural eye disorder that can occur with aging is:

A. Primary glaucoma

B. Entropion

C. Astigmatism

D. All of the above

26. Which of the following eye medications should be used with caution in the elderly with cardiac disease?

A. Diamox

B. Pilocar

C. Tearisol

D. Timoptic

27. Evidence exists that cataracts can be seen in most patients over age 70.

A. True

B. False

28. The chief clinical manifestation of a cataract is:

A. Gradual painless blurring of distance vision

B. Sudden loss of peripheral vision

C. Pain and mucoid discharge from the eye

D. Excessive tearing of eyes

29. The preferred method of treating patients with significant visual loss is:

A. Surgical excision and intraocular lens implant

B. Laser surgery and contact lenses

C. Cataract spectacles

D. Radiation therapy and lens implants

30. Write a nursing care plan for the patient undergoing cataract surgery.

Nursing Diagnosis: High risk for injury

Patient Outcome:

Nursing Interventions:

31. Which statement best describes the pathophysiology of glaucoma?

A. Intraocular pressure decreases gradually

B. Vitreous humor is overproduced

C. Aqueous humor is produced faster than it can be drained

D. Obstructive processes in the eye canal occur

32. A patient is complaining of sudden onset of severe unilateral ocular pain, nausea, vomiting, and seeing haloes around the eye. These symptoms suggest:

A. Primary-open angle glaucoma

B. Angle-closure glaucoma

C. Secondary glaucoma

D. Unilateral cataract

33. Oral hyperosmotics may be used to reduce intraocular pressure (IOP) in a patient. Side effects that the nurse would observe for include:

A. Cardiac arrhythmias

B. Ataxia, paresthesia

C. Bradycardia, hypotension

D. Headaches, confusion, disorientation

34. When pharmacologic treatment for primary open-angle glaucoma is ineffective, the physician may suggest:

A. Adding a second medication

B. Argon laser trabeculoplasty

C. Intraocular surgery

D. Intraocular shunting

35. One of the earliest changes that occurs in individuals with diabetes is thickening in the blood vessel's basement membrane. This results in:

A. Blood cell abnormalities

B. Micro-aneurysms

C. Macular edema

D. Increased ocular pressure

36. The nurse would explain to a patient with diabetic retinopathy that the best way to control the problem is:

A. Keep blood glucose and blood pressure well controlled

B. Take osmotic diuretics as ordered

C. Undergo laser surgery

D. Undergo intraocular procedures

37. When a patient suddenly complains of seeing flashes of bright light or spots before the eye, this suggests:

A. Diabetic retinopathy

B. Macular degeneration

C. Retinal detachment

D. Conjunctivitis

38. Following a scleral buckling procedure, the nurse would administer antibiotics and steroid eye drops such as:

A. Timoptic

B. Atropine

C. Pred-G

D. Diamox

39. When educating the patient about macular degeneration, the nurse would explain:

A. Treatment with miotic drugs can control symptoms

B. Laser surgery may be used if medication is ineffective

C. Total blindness is inevitable

D. Vision loss is permanent but total loss is rare

40. To help the patient with macular degeneration cope with sensory-perceptual alteration, the nurse would:

A. Assist the patient in maximizing existing vision

B. Explain how to instill eye drops

C. Explain the use of an eye patch

D. Explain proposed surgical procedures

41. When a traumatic injury has been sustained, the first diagnostic procedure should be:

A. Ophthalmoscopy

B. Fluorescein exam

C. Visual acuity

D. Ultrasonography

42. Emergency treatment of chemical burns of the eye would involve:

A. Flushing the eye with a large amount of water

B. Patching the eye immediately

C. Transporting the patient to emergency room

D. Instilling antibiotic eye drops

43. The usual treatment for the patient with choroidal melanoma is: (Check all that apply.)

A. Analgesics and antibiotics

B. Laser surgery

C. Radioactive plaque therapy

D. Enucleation

CLINICAL SITUATIONS

Situation ■ 1

Jane Naeman has returned to the unit following cataract surgery this morning. The following questions relate to the surgery and follow-up care.

1. Which statement best describes the type of pain control that Jane will need? (Check all that apply.)

A. Narcotics will be used for the first 24 hours

B. Pain is usual and Tylenol is usually effective

C. Pain may persist for 3–5 days

D. Pain unrelieved by Tylenol should be reported to the physician

2. Which intervention would be included under the nursing diagnosis: High risk for impaired home maintenance? (Check all that apply.)

A. Use eye drops every 2 hours

B. Don't bend at the waist or lift more than 20 pounds

C. Wear an eyeshield as ordered

D. Resume normal activity

3. Signs and symptoms of complications which Jane should report immediately include:

A. Spots in vision

B. Flashes of light

C. Change in vision

D. All of the above

Situation ■ 2

A patient was diagnosed with primary open-angle glaucoma 2 years ago. The following questions refer to this condition.

1. Which statement best describes the initial symptoms experienced by most patients with this condition?

A. Onset is acute; severe eye pain is the primary symptom

B. Onset is slow, with vision suddenly changing

C. Patients are often symptomatic with complaints of foggy vision

D. Symptoms include headache, nausea, and photophobia

2. Which of the following manifestations of this condition are evident during the eye exam?

A. Retinal vessels are tortuous

B. Sclera is red; cornea looks steamy

C. Lens is gray and bulging

D. Optic disk is pale or gray

3. Because of the many side effects of the medications which reduce IOP, which condition in this patient would contraindicate use of Timpotic?

A. Ulcerative colitis

B. Diabetes

C. Migraine headache

D. Renal disease

4. Because medications have not been effective in controlling IOP, the patient is scheduled for laser surgery. Which statement best describes what the patient can expect?

   A. Following the procedure, medication is no longer necessary

   B. IOP is lowered in 80% of patients, but effectiveness may be lost over time

   C. If laser surgery is ineffective, the patient is immediately taken for intraocular surgery

   D. Effects are immediate, and often full vision is restored

5. Following the laser surgery, the nurse would:

   A. Monitor vital signs every 4 hours

   B. Keep patient flat in bed for 8 hours

   C. Monitor IOP on arrival and after administering Iopidine

   D. Keep both eyes patched and room dim

Chapter Forty-one

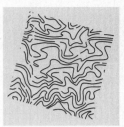

KNOWLEDGE BASIC TO THE NURSING CARE
of Adults with Dysfunction of the Ear

Learning Objectives

1.0 Review the Anatomy and Physiology of the Ear.

1.1 Locate the Parts of the External Ear.
1.2 Locate the Parts of the Internal Ear.
1.3 Explain the Process of Hearing.

2.0 Demonstrate an Understanding of the Assessment Data Related to the Ear.

2.1 Review the Assessment of Hearing Status.
2.2 Identify Clinical Manifestations of Adults with Dysfunction of the Ear.
2.3 Identify Specific Types of Hearing Loss.
2.4 Define Specific Symptoms of Hearing Disorders.
2.5 Match Diagnostic Procedures used to Evaluate Ear Disorders with their Definitions.

3.0 Demonstrate an Understanding of the Interventions used to Treat Adults with Dysfunction of the Ear.

3.1 Identify Surgical Procedures used to Treat Dysfunction of the Ear.
3.2 Identify Types of Medical Treatment used for the Patient with Dysfunction of the Ear.
3.3 Identify the Needs of the Patient Having Ear Surgery.
3.4 Write a Nursing Care Plan for the Patient Having Ear Surgery.

Learning Activities

Identify

1. On the diagram below, identify the structures of the ear.

   A. Malleus
   B. External ear
   C. Stapes

   D. Incus
   E. Tympanic membrane
   F. Eustachian tube

   G. Semicircular canals
   H. Cochlea
   I. Cochlear nerve

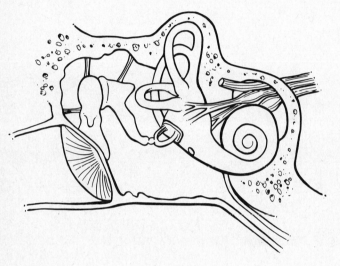

Define

2. Otalgia:

3. Tinnitus:

4. Otorrhea:

5. Vertigo:

6. Presbycusis:

Fill In

7. The _____ is a bony, tubelike structure that contains the organ of hearing.

8. The term used to express a unit of frequency is _____ .

9. Intensity of sound is measured in _____ .

10. In assessing the auditory canal, an _____ is used to detect obstructions.

Questions

11. Explain in detail how the process of hearing occurs.

12. When obtaining a patient history from an individual with an ear disorder, the nurse would obtain information in regard to:

    1.

    2.

    3.

4.

5.

Matching

Match the types of hearing loss with their descriptions.

A. Sensorineural hearing loss
B. Conductive hearing loss
C. Functional hearing loss

13. _____ Any condition that interferes with transmission of sound waves from the external or middle ear to the sensorineural apparatus of the inner ear.

14. _____ Psychogenic problem with no organic cause.

15. _____ Results from a problem within the internal ear.

Questions

16. The major clinical manifestation of ear disorders is:

    A. Pain in the ear

    B. Dizziness

    C. Drainage from ear

    D. Loss of hearing

17. Which information in the medical history can be a cause of an ear disorder in adulthood? (Check all that apply.)

    A. History of measles

    B. History of allergies

    C. Chronic use of aspirin

    D. Listening to loud music

18. Repeated upper respiratory infections can predispose an individual to a _____ hearing loss.

    A. Conductive

    B. Sensorineural

    C. Mixed

    D. Functional

19. Repeated exposure to loud noise may result in a _____ hearing loss.

    A. Conductive

    B. Sensorineural

    C. Mixed

    D. Functional

20. When a patient with an ear disorder suffers from vertigo, the nurse would instruct the patient to:

    A. Avoid sudden changes in position

    B. Use warm compresses on the ear

    C. Take analgesics as ordered

    D. Take a prescribed course of antibiotics

21. One of the medications that may be prescribed for the individual with mild vertigo is:

    A. Prednisone

    B. Dramamine

    C. Valium

    D. Tylenol

22. The nurse would closely monitor the patient taking _____ for signs of ear toxicity.

    A. Gentamicin

    B. Streptomycin

    C. Furosemide

    D. All of the above

Matching

Match the following diagnostic procedures with their descriptions.

A. Rinne test   D. Pneumatoscopy
B. Caloric test   E. Tuning fork test
C. Audiometry   F. Weber's test

23. _____ Tests the ability of the eardrum to adjust to changes in air pressure in the middle ear.

24. _____ Tests hearing ability between air and bone conduction.

25. _____ Used to categorize types and severity of hearing loss.

26. _____ Measures the acuity of the sense of hearing for frequencies of sound waves.

27. _____ Tests the function of the vestibular system.

28. _____ Tests hearing by bone conduction.

Questions

29. The organ of hearing is the _____ .

    A. Stapes

    B. Malleus

    C. Cochlea

    D. Ochlear nerve

30. Progressive hearing loss that occurs as an apparent part of the aging process is known as:

    A. Mixed hearing loss

    B. Labyrinthitis

    C. Presbycusis

    D. Malleatitis

31. When a patient has a sensation of dizziness or vertigo, it may be due to:

    A. Pressure behind the tympanic membrane

    B. Movement of fluid in the semicircular canals

    C. Decrease in the fluid in the cochlea

    D. Interference in conduction of sound waves

32. The function of the _____ is to amplify the force of sound.

    A. Stapes

    B. Auditory meatus

    C. Ossicles

    D. Cochlea

33. To visualize the auditory canal in an adult, the auricle should be pulled:

    A. Downward and backward

    B. Upward and forward

    C. Upward and backward

    D. Downward and forward

34. When the Rinne test is positive, this indicates:

    A. Air conduction is longer than bone conduction

    B. Bone conduction is longer than air conduction

    C. Air conduction and bone conduction are equal

35. A patient who has been complaining of ataxia and dizziness would probably be given which test?

    A. Weber test

    B. Past-pointing test

    C. Caloric test

    D. Rinne test

36. A patient with a sensorineural hearing loss, when given the Weber test, will hear better in the _____ ear.

    A. Affected

    B. Unaffected

    C. Neither

37. A patient with a sensorineural hearing loss would score _____ during the speech discrimination test.

    A. Low

    B. Normal

    C. High

38. For an individual with suspected middle ear pathology, the best diagnostic test would be:

    A. Weber test

    B. Caloric test

    C. Vestibular test

    D. Impedance audiometry

39. When the patient with a hearing disorder also has tinnitus, which test would be appropriate?

    A. Impedance audiometry

    B. Vestibular test

    C. Audiometric test

    D. Rinne test

40. The normal response of the patient to a caloric test should be:

A. Jerking movement of the eye toward or away from water instillation

B. Ringing in the ear when water is instilled

C. Sensation of dizziness and headache with water instillation

D. No abnormal response should be noted if the test is normal

41. For which of the following conditions would a myringotomy be an appropriate intervention?

A. Rupture of eardrum

B. Otorrhea

C. Presbycusis

D. Eustachian tube blockage

42. Following a mastoidectomy, the nurse would position the patient:

A. Supine

B. Low Fowler's position

C. Trendelenburg's position

D. Position of comfort

True or False

43. _____ Many ear disorders can be treated with drug therapy.

44. _____ Ear surgery may be done if drug therapy is ineffective.

45. _____ The major complication of ear surgery is hemorrhage.

46. _____ A tympanoplasty may be done to improve hearing.

47. _____ Cochlear implants are a solution for the profoundly deaf.

48. _____ After a cochlear implant, normal hearing is restored.

Questions

49. Write a nursing care plan for the patient who has had a tympanoplasty.

Nursing Diagnosis: Sensory perceptual alteration related to vertigo secondary to surgical manipulation

Patient Outcome:

Nursing Intervention:

CLINICAL SITUATIONS

Situation ■ 1

Susan Parker has been admitted with a ruptured eardrum and is scheduled for a myringoplasty (type 1).

1. Responsibilities of the nurse during the preoperative assessment include gathering information about:

A. Allergies

B. Medications

C. Special Diets

D. A and C

E. A, B, C

2. Susan asks if she will have her hair shaved off. The surgeon plans to use an endaural approach. The appropriate response would be:

A. No, that isn't necessary.

B. Yes, we will shave a small area behind the ear.

C. Yes, we shave 6 inches around the ear for asepsis.

3. A correct explanation of the surgical procedure is:

A. A skin graft will be sutured in place and covered with gelfoam.

B. A bone graft will be sutured in place and then packing will be inserted.

C. The membrane will be sutured shut and then bedrest maintained for 4 days.

4. It is apparent that Susan has a good understanding of her discharge instructions when she states:

A. I will follow my special diet.

B. I am glad that I don't have any physical restriction.

C. I know I should avoid blowing my nose.

D. I will lie flat in bed after the procedure.

Situation ■ 2

Lee Jordan, 20 years old, is admitted for a tympanoplasty. He has had severe otitis media for several years. Current medical treatment has been ineffective.

1. On assessment, findings consistent with otitis media would be:

   A. Retracted membrane, gray in color

   B. Bulging of the membrane, whitish in color

   C. Absence of the membrane, pus in the canal

2. Nursing care of the patient scheduled for surgery involves explaining the procedure. A correct explanation of this surgery would be:

   A. A local anesthesia is used, and an incision is made into the eardrum.

   B. A general anesthesia is used, and an incision is made into the eardrum, followed by a graft.

   C. A short-acting general anesthesia is used, and a single incision will be made in the eardrum.

3. Discharge planning should include information about complications such as:

   A. Primary infection

   B. Secondary infection

   C. Hearing loss

   D. Hemorrhage

4. Discharge instruction would involve giving Lee information on which of the following? (Check all that apply.)

   A. Wipe away any excess drainage

   B. Change the dressing frequently

   C. Shower as desired

   D. Avoid lifting or straining

   E. Take antihistamines as prescribed

   F. Report fever or increased pain

Chapter Forty-two

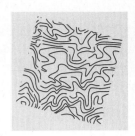

NURSING CARE
of Adults with
Ear Disorders

Learning Objectives

1.0 Demonstrate an Understanding of the Infections and Inflammations of the Ear.

1.1 Define Several Inflammatory Processes of the Ear.
1.2 Identify the Clinical Manifestations of Several Inflammatory Processes of the Ear.
1.3 Identify the Medical Treatment of Ear Disorders.
1.4 Describe the Nursing Interventions for a Patient with an Ear Disorder.
1.5 Write a Nursing Care Plan for the Patient with an Infection of the Ear.

2.0 Demonstrate an Understanding of Structural Disorders of the Ear.

2.1 Identify Clinical Manifestations of Structural Disorders.
2.2 Identify the Medical Treatment of Structural Disorders.
2.3 Review the Surgical Treatment of Structural Disorders.
2.4 Plan the Nursing Care for a Patient with a Structural Disorder.

Learning Activities

Define

1. External otitis:

2. Otomycosis:

3. Furuncle:

4. Otitis media:

5. Mastoiditis:

6. Labyrinthitis:

7. Meniere's disease:

Questions

8. List three symptoms specific to Meniere's Disease.
   1.
   2.
   3.

Matching

Based on your understanding of the clinical manifestations of the various disorders, match the findings with the disorder.

A. External otitis   C. Acute otitis media
B. Serous otitis media D. Mastoiditis

9. _____ Eardrum is red and bulging with fluid

10. _____ Eardrum is dull, thickened, swollen

11. _____ Eardrum is retracted

12. _____ Red, swollen external ear canal

Questions

13. Which ear condition often results from swimming in contaminated water?
    A. External otitis
    B. Otomycosis
    C. Otitis media
    D. Mastoiditis

14. Medical management of external otitis involves:
    A. Intravenous antibiotics
    B. Oral antibiotics and warm compresses
    C. Topical antibiotics and steroids
    D. Analgesics and betadine soaks

15. Symptoms of acute otitis media include:
    A. Severe earache and total hearing loss
    B. Earache and mild hearing loss, fever, nausea
    C. Purulent drainage, vertigo, hypertension
    D. Ear pain, severe headache, sore throat

16. Symptoms of serous otitis media include:
    A. Earache, fever, nausea
    B. Earache, fever, tinnitus

C. Purulent drainage, pain, tinnitus

D. Tinnitus, conductive hearing loss

17. In viral labyrinthitis, the hearing loss is usually:

A. Sudden and profound and permanent

B. Sudden and profound but temporary

C. Gradual and permanent

D. Gradual but temporary

18. _____ may be administered intravenously to control dizziness in the patient with labyrinthitis.

A. Valium

B. Vistaril

C. Demoral

D. Haldol

19. Which information in the health history might explain why a patient has a perforation of the tympanic membrane?

A. History of ear infection

B. History of ear trauma

C. History of recent diving competition

20. The most common cause of progressive hearing loss is:

A. Otitis media

B. Labyrinthitis

C. Mastoiditis

D. Otosclerosis

21. Medical treatment for Meniere's disease would include:

A. Antibiotics and steroids

B. Analgesics and sedatives

C. Sedatives and antivert

D. All of the above

22. During an acute attack of Meniere's disease the patient would be advised to:

A. Stay in bed

B. Follow a low-sodium diet

C. Restrict fluids

D. All of the above

23. The most appropriate nursing diagnosis for a patient with Meniere's disease is:

A. Pain related to inner ear disorder

B. Altered health maintenance

C. High risk for infection

D. Impaired verbal communication

24. The reason that the patient with Meniere's disease should avoid use of nicotine or caffeine is:

A. They cause vasodilation, which causes too much fluid in the inner ear

B. They cause the patient to be overstimulated

C. They cause vasoconstriction, which can decrease circulation to the inner ear

D. None of the above

True or False

25. _____ Otitis media is usually caused by a bacteria.

26. _____ Acute otitis media is frequently associated with an upper respiratory infection.

27. _____ Prednisone is the treatment of choice for acute otitis media.

28. _____ Sudden changes in atmospheric pressure can result in occlusion of the ear canal.

29. _____ Chronic otitis media often results in perforation of the eardrum.

30. _____ Cholesteatoma is the formation of an abscess.

31. _____ Brain infection is a major complication of mastoidectomy.

32. _____ Presbycusis is a progressive sensorineural hearing loss that is part of normal aging.

33. _____ A hearing aide is basically an amplifier.

Questions

34. Patient education for the individual with serous otitis media would include which information?

A. Blow the nose vigorously several times a day.

B. Take decongestants as indicated

C. Avoid exposure to allergens

D. All of the above

35. Discharge instructions for the patient following stapedectomy would include all of the following EXCEPT:

A. No showers for 6 weeks

B. Avoid forceful coughing

C. Avoid tub baths for 2 weeks

D. Avoid airplane travel as ordered

36. The reason that the patient must avoid bending or lifting after a stapedectomy is:

A. To prevent infection

B. To prevent displacement of prosthesis

C. To prevent rupture of eardrum

D. To help drain the ear

37. Write a nursing care plan for a patient with serous otitis media.

Nursing Diagnosis: Knowledge deficit related to prevention of recurrence of problem

Patient Outcome:

Nursing Interventions:

38. Write a nursing care plan for the patient who has a traumatic perforation of the eardrum.

Nursing Diagnosis:

Patient Outcome:

Nursing Interventions:

39. Write a nursing care plan for the patient with Meniere's disease.

Nursing Diagnosis: Ineffective individual coping related to the chronic nature of the disease

Patient Outcome:

Nursing Interventions:

40. Write a nursing care plan for an elderly individual with presbycusis.

Nursing Diagnosis: Impaired verbal communication related to hearing loss

Patient Outcome:

Nursing Interventions:

CLINICAL SITUATIONS

Situation ▪ 1

Ms. Williams has had four episodes of otitis media during the past 2 years. She is now scheduled for a tympanoplasty.

1. Prior to surgery, she explains that her medical treatment involved:

A. Antibiotic therapy for 2 weeks

B. Cleansing of the ear canal and topical antibiotics

C. Systemic sympathomimetic agents

2. As the primary nurse, how do you explain this surgery?

A. It is a surgical repair of the structure of the inner ear

B. It involves the insertion of a tube in the inner ear canal

C. It is the removal of cholesteatoma

3. Following the surgery, the patient complains of vertigo. What nursing diagnosis is appropriate at this time?

A. Alteration in comfort

B. Sensory-perceptual alteration

C. Alteration in self-concept

D. Potential for infection

4. Part of your nursing interventions include discharge instructions. These would include:

A. Clean the ear with a Q-tip daily.

B. Blow nose vigorously four times a day.

C. Avoid touching the ear; keep the dressing dry.

D. Avoid driving for 8 weeks.

Situation ■ 2

Mr. Parker is scheduled for a stapedectomy for progressive otosclerosis. He also states that he has had periods of dizziness. During the assessment, it is evident that he has a hearing loss.

1. Based on the diagnosis, the results of a Rinne test that confirm the diagnosis would be:

   A. Air conduction > bone conduction

   B. Bone conduction > air conduction

2. Mr. Parker is apprehensive about the proposed surgery. How would the nurse explain the procedure?

   A. The diseased bone is removed and tubes are inserted

   B. The stapes is removed and replaced with a prosthesis

   C. The stapes is scraped and a bone graft inserted

3. How does the nurse explain the operation?

   A. It is done under local anesthesia and takes about 20 minutes

   B. It is done under local anesthesia and takes about 2 hours

   C. It is done using general anesthesia and takes 1 hour

4. Which of the following statements is true about the postoperative course?

   A. Patient is up ad libitum and discharged in 48 hours

   B. Patient is on bedrest 48 hours, then discharged in 4 days

   C. Patient is on bedrest 4 days, then discharged in 1 week

5. Providing discharge instruction for Mr. Parker is part of the nursing care plan. What information should be emphasized?

   A. No swimming or showers for 6 weeks

   B. No heavy lifting or strenuous exercise

   C. Avoid coughing and nose blowing

   D. All of the above

Unit Fourteen

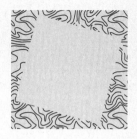

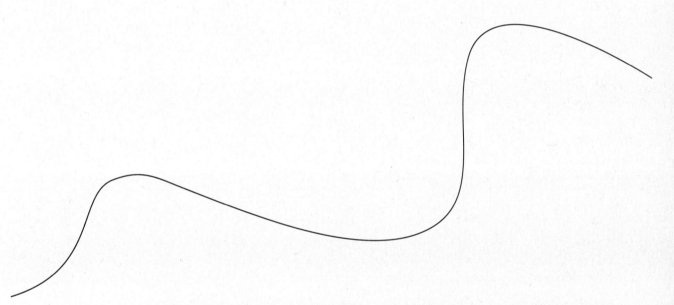

ADULTS WITH REPRODUCTIVE SYSTEM DYSFUNCTION

Chapter Forty-three

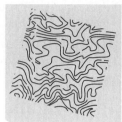

KNOWLEDGE BASIC TO THE NURSING CARE *of Women with Reproductive System Dysfunction*

Learning Objectives

1.0 *Review the Anatomy and Physiology of the Reproductive System.*

1.1 Identify the Parts of the Reproductive System.
1.2 Identify the Stages of Menstruation.
1.3 Demonstrate an Understanding of the Process of Menopause.
1.4 Identify Symptoms Associated with Menopause.
1.5 Write a Care Plan for the Menopausal Woman.

2.0 *Demonstrate an Understanding of the Assessment Data Related to the Female Reproductive System.*

2.1 Identify Symptoms of a Reproductive Dysfunction.
2.2 Identify Specific Reproductive Dysfunctions.
2.3 Identify Tests which are Used to Diagnose a Reproductive Dysfunction.
2.4 Identify Reasons for Laparoscopic Procedures.

3.0 *Demonstrate an Understanding of Interventions Used to Treat Women with Reproductive System Dysfunction.*

3.1 Identify Medical and Surgical Interventions Used to Treat Reproductive System Dysfunction.
3.2 Plan the Nursing Care for the Patient Having Laparoscopy.
3.3 Identify Complications Following Surgical Treatment of Reproductive Disorders.
3.4 Utilize the Nursing Process in Planning the Care for the Patient who has had a Hysterectomy.
3.5 List Interventions Related to the Psychological Needs of the Patient Having a Hysterectomy.

Learning Activities

Identify

1. Identify the correct parts of the woman's external genitalia.

   A. Mons pubis
   B. Clitoris
   C. Bartholin's glands
   D. Labia majora
   E. Vestibule
   F. Perineum
   G. Labia minora
   H. Hymen
   I. Urethral meatus

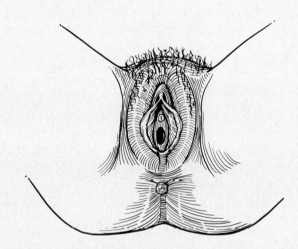

2. Identify the correct parts of the woman's internal genitalia.

   A. Vagina
   B. Fallopian tubes
   C. Fundus
   D. Cervix
   E. Ovaries
   F. Endometrium

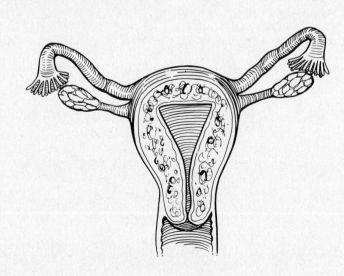

Fill In

3. The _____ is a muscular, tubelike organ which is lined with mucous membrane.

4. The _____ is a hollow, thick-walled, muscular organ shaped like an inverted pear.

5. The position of the uterus in the pelvic cavity is maintained by a series of _____.

6. The _____ transport ova from the ovaries to the uterus.

7. The _____ secrete the female sex hormones.

8. The purpose of the female sexual cycle is _____.

Questions

9. List three things which can affect the frequency of the menstrual cycle.

    1.

    2.

    3.

10. List four symptoms which have been associated with menopause.

    1.

    2.

    3.

    4.

Matching

Match the stages of menstruation with their descriptions.

A. Ischemic phase   C. Proliferative phase
B. Menstrual phase   D. Secretory phase

11. _____ Occurs from the end of menstruation until ovulation.

12. _____ Occurs during the 3 days prior to the next menses.

13. _____ The time of the menstrual flow.

14. _____ Occurs from ovulation until 3 days before the next menses.

True or False

15. _____ Menopause most often occurs between the ages of 35 and 55.

16. _____ Pregnancy can occur during menopause.

17. _____ Hot flashes are experienced by many women during menopause.

18. _____ Ovulation usually ends before the last menses.

19. _____ Research has found a potential link between estrogen therapy and cancer.

20. _____ Estrogen therapy is indicated when the patient has a history of breast cancer.

21. _____ Urinary symptoms are frequently manifestations of a gynecologic disorder.

22. _____ Pelvic examination assesses structural conditions of the reproductive organs.

23. _____ A Pap smear examines cells obtained from the uterus.

24. _____ A Pap smear is painful and requires local anesthesia.

Questions

25. What is the current recommended treatment for the individual who is having severe menopausal symptoms?

    A. Estrogen therapy 5 mg every day until symptoms subside

    B. Progesterone 20 mg every day and estrogen 2 mg twice a day for 6 months, then every day

    C. Estrogen therapy 0.625 mg every day for 25 days followed by progesterone therapy

26. Estrogen therapy is contraindicated with individuals who have had which of the following disorders?

    A. Breast cancer

    B. Endometrial cancer

C. Recurrent thrombophlebitis

D. All of the above

27. The nurse is helping a patient cope with the psychological effects of menopause. Evidence of success would be which of the following statements by the patient?

A. I realize that I can no longer get pregnant.

B. I realize that I can still work and be a wife.

C. I realize that the symptoms are all in my mind.

D. I realize that gaining weight is inevitable.

28. Abnormal uterine bleeding can be caused by:

A. Ectopic pregnancy

B. Threatened abortion

C. Intrauterine devices

D. Anticholinergic agents

E. All but D

F. All of the above

Matching

Match the following reproductive dysfunctions with their descriptions.

A. Dysmenorrhea   E. Polymenorrhagia
B. Metrorrhagia   F. Oligomenorrhea
C. Amenorrhea   G. Menorrhagia
D. Leukorrhea

29. _____ Absence of menstruation for 6 months.

30. _____ Frequent but regular episodes of bleeding.

31. _____ Bleeding which is excessive in amount and duration.

32. _____ Infrequent, irregular episodes of bleeding.

33. _____ Cyclic pain associated with menstruation.

34. _____ Vaginal discharge other than blood.

35. _____ Normal bleeding which is irregular.

Questions

36. Findings suggest that primary dysmenorrhea is due to excessive:

A. Vaginal discharge

B. Uterine contractility

C. Exercise during menstruation

D. Dietary habits

37. Recent research indicates which of the following as being responsible for the symptoms of primary dysmenorrhea?

A. High levels of prostaglandins

B. High levels of progesterone

C. High levels of estrogen

D. Low levels of estrogen

38. Which nursing intervention is likely to be effective in relieving symptoms associated with dysmenorrhea?

A. Administration of analgesics

B. Application of heat

C. Increase in exercise at start of menses

D. Bedrest with hot fluids

E. Any of the above

39. One reason that a physician may perform a colposcopy would be:

A. When the patient is having vaginal bleeding

B. When the cervix is normal but the Pap test is atypical

C. When the patient has symptoms and abdominal pain

D. All of the above

40. Why is a conization (cone biopsy) NOT performed on women who plan on bearing children?

A. There is a great risk of infection

B. It can cause prolapse of the uterus

C. It can lead to spontaneous abortion

D. It can cause incompetence of the cervix

41. The nurse is discharging a patient who has had a cone biopsy. All of the following would be emphasized EXCEPT:

A. Resume normal activity as soon as possible.

B. Avoid using tampons unless directed otherwise.

C. Don't remove vaginal packing until instructed to do so.

D. Do not douche until told to do so.

Matching

A. Ultrasonography
B. Hysteroscopy
C. Endometrial smear

42. _____ Allows direct visualization of the intrauterine cavity.

43. _____ Screening test for uterine cancer.

44. _____ Produces an image of the pelvic organs.

Questions

45. Which group of women would be at increased risk of developing postoperative depression following a hysterectomy?

A. Women in their early thirties

B. Women with less than two children

C. Women who are unmarried

D. All of the above

46. All of the following statements are true about laparoscopy EXCEPT:

A. It allows for visualization of the internal pelvic organs

B. It is done through an incision in the vaginal wall

C. It is used as a diagnostic procedure to evaluate abdominal pain

D. It can be used to determine the patency of the fallopian tubes

47. In a patient who is being considered for laparoscopy, which of the following information in the patient history would make the surgery contraindicated?

A. History of tubal ligation

B. History of diabetes

C. History of unstable angina

D. History of chronic cystitis

48. When assessing the patient 2 hours after having a laparoscopy, the nurse finds her complaining of shoulder pain and soreness in her chest. An appropriate nursing intervention would be:

A. Immediately notify the physician

B. Monitor vital signs and, if the heart rate is elevated, administer a narcotic

C. Record the findings and reassess in 1 hour

D. Reassure the patient that these are common symptoms and offer analgesics.

True or False

49. _____ Cryosurgery is a technique which uses exposure to cold to destroy tissue.

50. _____ Cryosurgery may be performed in a doctor's office without anesthesia.

51. _____ Following cryosurgery, bloody drainage occurs which lasts about 2 weeks.

52. _____ Electrocautery is done to burn away abnormal tissue.

53. _____ A tubal ligation may be done 24 hours after delivery.

54. _____ A vaginal approach for a tubal ligation is the preferred procedure.

55. _____ Sexual intercourse is restricted for 2 weeks following tubal ligation.

Questions

56. A patient had a dilation and curettage early in the morning. During the 4 pm assessment, she tells the nurse that she has changed her pad two times in the last hour. The nurse is aware that:

A. This amount of bleeding is normal during the first day.

B. This is excessive; pads should not require changing more than once every hour.

57. What intervention would be appropriate based on the above information?

A. Reassure her that everything is fine.

B. Call the physician immediately.

C. Check the amount of saturation on the pads.

58. The vaginal route is considered a preferred route for a hysterectomy when:

    A. There is a diagnosis of cancer

    B. The patient is young and in good health

    C. Vaginal repair is being done

    D. A salpingectomy is also performed

59. The nurse is aware that _____ is a frequent postoperative complication following abdominal hysterectomy.

    A. Cystitis

    B. Bladder fistula

    C. Evisceration

    D. Nerve damage

60. Which patient would have the highest risk for development of an incisional infection following an abdominal hysterectomy?

    A. 23 years old with cervical cancer

    B. 44 years old with uterine cancer, history of asthma

    C. 35 years old with benign tumors, history of cystitis

    D. 68 years old with ovarian cancer, history of diabetes

61. Following gynecologic surgery, patients have a high risk for development of _____.

    A. Thromboembolism

    B. Depression

    C. Sepsis

    D. Nutritional deficiency

62. List three nursing interventions to prevent this condition.

    1.

    2.

    3.

63. Write a care plan for the woman entering menopause.

    Nursing Diagnosis: Knowledge deficit: menopause and related self-care

    Patient Outcome:

    Nursing Interventions:

64. Write a nursing care plan for the patient who has had a total hysterectomy.

    Nursing Diagnosis: Anxiety related to the physical and psychosocial effects of impending surgery

    Patient Outcome:

    Nursing Interventions:

CLINICAL SITUATIONS

Situation ■ 1

A 19-year-old female is seen in the clinic with a complaint of severe menstrual pain. She has had menstrual pain since age 15, but never this severe.

1. During the history, she says, "My mother thinks I must have contracted VD because I have such severe pain." An appropriate response by the nurse would be:

    A. Painful menstruation does not have to be associated with any other problem.

    B. Painful menstruation is often related to secondary VD.

    C. Painful menstruation is usually caused by endometriosis.

    D. Painful menstruation is something women have to live with.

2. The nurse will discuss treatment options. This condition is often treated with:

    A. Analgesics, antibiotics, anticholinergics

    B. Antibiotics, sedatives, antispasmodics

    C. Analgesics, antispasmodics, heat, rest

    D. Relaxation therapy, narcotics

3. One medication which is ordered for this patient is Motrin (ibuprofen). Side effects which you will advise her to expect include:

    A. Rapid heart rate, palpitations

B. GI upset, headache

C. Constipation, urinary frequency

D. Irregular menstruation

4. The patient asks if it is advisable for her to use oral contraceptives to help with the dysmenorrhea. An appropriate reply would be:

A. No, that is not a recommended therapy.

B. Yes, that is probably a good idea.

C. Yes, if you also desire them as a contraceptive.

D. No, there are too many side effects.

Situation ■ 2

Anna Simmons, 28 years old, is admitted with chronic pelvic pain. She is scheduled for a laparoscopy in the morning.

1. The nurse is aware that the preoperative prep would include: (Check all that apply.)

A. NPO after midnight

B. Bowel cleaning with soapsuds enema

C. Shave abdomen from nipple line to knees

D. Instructing patient that general anesthesia will be used.

2. Anna has a diagnosis of possible endometriosis and blocked fallopian tubes. How is the patency of the tubes evaluated?

A. By intravenous injection of a dye

B. By injecting a dye via a cannula through the cervix

C. By abdominal ultrasound

D. By the use of the laparoscope

3. Following the procedure, the nurse is aware that the most serious complication of laparoscopy is:

A. Hemorrhage

B. Sepsis

C. Intestinal burns

D. Embolism

4. Anna has done well and is ready for discharge. It is apparent that she has a good understanding of her instructions when she states:

A. I must avoid sexual intercourse for 6 weeks

B. I should not experience any discomfort

C. I should avoid heavy lifting for a week

D. I may experience pain in my chest or shoulder

E. A, C, D

F. C, D

Situation ■ 3

Mrs. Devon is scheduled for a total abdominal hysterectomy (TAH) and bilateral salpingo-oophorectomy (BSO) for a malignancy. She has a history of breast cancer and diabetes.

1. Mrs. Devon asks if she will continue to menstruate after this procedure. The nurse would reply:

A. No, you will no longer menstruate.

B. Yes, you may have slightly irregular periods.

2. Mrs. Devon wonders why she is not having a vaginal approach like her friend had. How should the nurse respond?

A. Tell her that she needs to talk to her physician.

B. Tell her that everyone is different.

C. Tell her that this approach is preferred when the adnexae and uterus are to be removed.

3. Mrs. Devon is crying and says, "I know I no longer will feel like a woman. The doctor says he won't even prescribe estrogen for me. Why not?"

A. You explain that she needs to talk to the physician.

B. You ask her if she is upset about the surgery.

C. You explain that estrogen therapy may be contraindicated for individuals with her history.

D. You tell her that she is lucky to be alive.

4. On the second postoperative day, Mrs. Devon tells the nurse that she had to get up to urinate six times during the night. Her urine output is 300 ml. This suggests:

A. Mrs. Devon is in pain and should be medicated.

B. Mrs. Devon is probably bleeding, which is putting pressure on the bladder.

C. Mrs. Devon probably has urinary retention.

D. Mrs. Devon is very anxious and needs to talk.

5. During the assessment you find that Mrs. Devon has no bowel sounds. The physician orders an abdominal scan, which reveals a paralytic ileus. The reason that this complication occurs is:

    A. The patient has been immobilized.

    B. The patient has had nerve trauma from handling of the viscera.

    C. The patient has had too much anesthesia.

    D. The patient has not had any food or drink for 48 hours.

6. How can the nurse evaluate Mrs. Devon's psychological response to the surgery?

    A. Check vital signs every 4 hours, monitor the wound.

    B. Ask her if she has any questions.

    C. Monitor any changes in behavior.

Chapter Forty-four

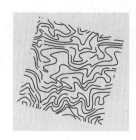

NURSING CARE
of Women with Disorders of the Reproductive System

Learning Objectives

1.0 Demonstrate an Understanding of the Inflammatory Processes within the Reproductive System.

1.1 Define Several of the Inflammatory Disorders.
1.2 Identify Assessment Data Relevant to Reproductive Disorders.
1.3 Identify the Causes, Signs, and Symptoms of Toxic Shock Syndrome.
1.4 Identify the Teaching Needs of the Patient with an Inflammatory Process.
1.5 Identify Appropriate Nursing Interventions for a Patient with an Infection.

2.0 Demonstrate an Understanding of Functional Disorders of the Reproductive System.

2.1 List Symptoms Related to Premenstrual Syndrome.
2.2 Write Nursing Interventions for the Patient with Premenstrual Syndrome.
2.3 Describe Current Treatment Options for the Patient with Endometriosis.
2.4 Describe the Emotional Problems of a Female with a Functional Abnormality.
2.5 Write a Nursing Care Plan for the Patient with Premenstrual Syndrome.

3.0 Demonstrate an Understanding of the Structural Disorders of the Female Reproductive System.

3.1 Define Several Structural Disorders.
3.2 Identify the Clinical Manifestations of a Structural Abnormality of the Reproductive System.
3.3 Identify Medical Interventions used for a Patient with a Weakened Pelvic Structure.
3.4 Plan the Nursing Care for a Patient Having Surgical Repair of a Structural Disorder.

4.0 Demonstrate an Understanding of the Types of Neoplasms that Affect the Reproductive System.

4.1 Identify Clinical Manifestations of Neoplasms.

4.2 Review Treatment Options for the Patient with a Neoplasm.

4.3 Identify the Psychological Needs of a Woman who has a Disorder of the Reproductive System.

4.4 Plan the Nursing Care for the Woman with a Radioactive Implant.

4.5 Plan the Nursing Care for the Woman with a Neoplasm of the Reproductive System.

Learning Activities

Define

1. Vaginitis:

2. Vulvitis:

3. Endometriosis:

4. Colpocele:

5. Urethrocele:

6. Rectocele:

7. Cystocele:

Questions

8. List two causes of vaginitis.

   1.

   2.

9. List three mechanical irritants which have been found to cause vaginitis.

   1.

   2.

   3.

10. List several interventions which would help control itching for the patient with vulvitis or vaginitis.

    1.

    2.

    3.

11. List four clinical manifestations of toxic shock syndrome.

    1.

    2.

    3.

    4.

12. List five symptoms related to premenstrual syndrome.

    1.

    2.

    3.

    4.

    5.

13. List two of the hormones used in the treatment of endometriosis.

    1.

    2.

Fill In

14. One of the primary causes of weakened pelvic support is damage due to _____ .

15. A genital fistula can be between the _____ or the _____ and the vagina.

Questions

16. Plan the nursing care for a 78-year-old woman with a draining fistula. List several nursing in-

terventions which will promote physical and psychological comfort.

Physical:

Psychological:

17. A classic clinical manifestation of vulvitis which the nurse would asses for is:

    A. Pruritus

    B. Vaginal discharge

    C. Dribbling of urine

    D. Perineal pain

18. When working with an individual who has vaginitis, an important nursing measure would be to:

    A. Provide pain medication

    B. Teach proper hygiene

    C. Explain treatment options

    D. Make sure antibiotics are taken

19. Organisms which have been found to cause vaginitis include:

    A. *Escherichia coli*

    B. *Trichomonas vaginalis*

    C. *Treponema pallidum*

    D. Herpes simplex

    E. Any of the above

20. There are many factors which predispose a woman to developing vaginitis. These would include all of the following EXCEPT:

    A. Malnutrition

    B. Stress

    C. Pregnancy

    D. Exercise

21. Culture results show that a patient has vaginitis caused by *E. coli*. The nurse knows that the patient understands how to prevent a recurrence of this problem when:

    A. She describes the proper way to wipe after a bowel movement

    B. She states that she should avoid tight clothing

    C. She states that she cannot have sexual relations

    D. She states that she is starting a new diet

22. The reason that atrophic vaginitis occurs in postmenopausal women is thought to be:

    A. The drop in estrogen levels

    B. The drop in progesterone levels

    C. The loss of vaginal mucosa

    D. The decrease in vaginal secretions

23. Which of the following clinical manifestations, when present, would indicate that a woman has atrophic vaginitis?

    A. Itching and yellow discharge

    B. Burning and brownish discharge

    C. Thin yellow discharge and burning

    D. Itching and foul-smelling discharge

24. Treatment for the patient with vaginitis might involve baths which contain:

    A. Antibiotics

    B. Tannic acid

    C. Baby oil

    D. Hydrogen peroxide

25. An effective therapy for a 65-year-old postmenopausal woman who has severe vaginitis might be:

    A. Estrogen creme

    B. Topical ointment

    C. Antibiotics

    D. Cessation of intercourse

26. Toxic shock syndrome is thought to be caused by:

    A. *Escherichia coli*

    B. *Candida albicans*

    C. *Staphylococcus aureus*

    D. Herpes simplex

27. Nursing care for the patient with toxic shock syndrome is designed to enable the woman to:

    A. Control the long-term side effects

    B. Return to psychosocial stability

C. Return to physiological stability

D. Effect a cure rapidly

28. The primary medical treatment for toxic shock would be:

    A. Life support

    B. Antibiotic therapy

    C. Intravenous therapy

    D. Nutritional support

29. A patient recovering from toxic shock syndrome exhibits the following symptoms: petechiae, hematoma on the legs, cool extremities with cyanotic nailbeds. These findings suggest:

    A. Acute renal failure

    B. Peripheral vascular collapse

    C. Disseminated intravascular coagulation

    D. Cardiogenic shock

30. The nurse is discharging a patient who has recovered from toxic shock syndrome. Which statement indicates she understands a contributory factor and ways to prevent a recurrence? The patient states:

    A. She will see the physician in 6 weeks

    B. She will change tampons every 4 hours

    C. She will stop using birth control pills

    D. She will only take baths

True or False

31. _____ Symptoms of PMS are very often the same for all women.

32. _____ PMS is thought to be caused by an estrogen-progesterone imbalance.

33. _____ Symptoms of PMS disappear when menstruation begins.

34. _____ During pregnancy, there is often an increase in symptoms related to PMS.

35. _____ Damage during childbirth is the main cause of weakened pelvic support.

36. _____ Uterine prolapse is visible on inspection.

37. _____ Repairs of pelvic relaxation can be done at any time.

38. _____ Pessaries should be recommended for patients with pelvic relaxation.

Questions

39. Write a nursing care plan for the woman with PMS.

    Nursing Diagnosis: High risk for ineffective coping

    Patient Outcome:

    Nursing Interventions:

40. The nurse is aware that women with PMS need specific information on lifestyle changes which have been shown to have some impact on the control of symptoms. Write an appropriate interventions under each area.

    Rest and activity:

    Diet:

    Fluids:

    Anxiety:

41. A patient has a diagnosis of endometriosis. She asks for an explanation of this disorder. The nurse explains:

    A. It is an inflammation of the endometrium.

    B. It is a condition in which tissue-like endometrium is found in other locations.

    C. It is a condition which causes severe abdominal pain and cessation of menstruation.

    D. It is a condition in which the lining of the endometrium is shed and passed as large clots.

42. During the assessment, the nurse finds that the symptom which caused this patient to seek medical help was:

    A. Fever

    B. Lengthy periods

    C. Dysmenorrhea

    D. Foul vaginal discharge

43. In the absence of significant clinical manifestations, the reason that women who have endometriosis often seek medical attention is:

A. Lack of interest in sexual activity

B. Frequent mood changes

C. Infertility

D. Changes in activity

44. One of the newest therapies to treat endometriosis is danazol. A disadvantage of this antigonadotropic drug is:

A. Serious side effects

B. Not approved by the FDA

C. Symptoms recur when discontinued

45. When a woman with endometriosis no longer desires children, surgery may be recommended to:

A. Relieve symptoms

B. Remove the scar tissue

C. Cure the disease

D. Prevent disease from becoming malignant

46. The nurse would teach the patient with endometriosis which of the following to help her cope with symptoms? (Check all that apply.)

A. Correct use of analgesics

B. Correct use of hormonal therapy

C. Correct application of heat

D. Correct application of cold packs

E. Pelvic exercises

F. Increased periods of rest

47. Identify the clinical manifestations of a weakened pelvis support. Check all the symptoms that may occur:

A. Lump protruding from the vagina

B. Foul-smelling vaginal discharge

C. Constipation

D. Pruritus

E. Changes in urination

F. Pain on intercourse

48. The primary reason that the patient with a cystocele seeks medical help is:

A. Constipation

B. Stress incontinence

C. Abdominal pain

D. Diarrhea and vomiting

49. The medical treatment for a patient with a weakened pelvic structure will most often involve:

A. Muscle relaxant medications

B. Antibiotic therapy

C. Surgical intervention

D. Aggressive exercise program

E. Insertion of a pessary

50. After posterior repair for a rectocele, a common problem is:

A. Infection

B. Constipation

C. Vaginal stenosis

D. Respiratory disorders

51. Following an anterior colporrhaphy, which symptom should be reported to the physician at once:

A. Inability to void

B. Refusal to get up

C. Nausea and vomiting

D. Constipation

52. For a patient with retrodisplacement of the uterus, which intervention might help alleviate the discomfort?

A. Warm sitz baths

B. Daily douching

C. Tylenol as ordered

D. Postural therapy

53. A patient is admitted with leakage of urine from the vagina. The nurse suspects:

A. Vaginitis

B. Vesicovaginal fistula

C. Urinary infection

D. Prolapse of uterus

54. An appropriate nursing diagnosis for this patient would be:

A. High risk for impaired skin integrity

B. Pain related to infectious process

C. Fluid volume excess

D. Impaired physical mobility

55. An important part of the instruction for this patient would involve:

A. Ways to control discomfort

B. Ways to maintain adequate nutrition

C. Ways to cope with constipation

D. Ways to decrease discharge

56. The first symptom of cervical cancer is often:

A. Abdominal pain

B. Excessive menstrual bleeding

C. Thin, watery discharge

D. Vaginal pain and foul discharge

57. How often should the PAP smear be done if a woman is not in a high risk group?

A. Every 6 months

B. Every 2 years

C. Every 3 years

D. Every 5 years

58. One of the main reasons that many women do not have routine gynecologic exams after menopause is:

A. They are no longer at risk

B. They have limited resources

C. Lack of knowledge

D. Lack of transportation

Matching

A. Polyp

B. Leiomyoma

C. Vulvar carcinoma

D. Dermoid cyst

59. _____ Benign smooth muscle tumor

60. _____ Benign ovarian neoplasm

61. _____ Tumor that has stalks

62. _____ Neoplasm in the vulvar epidermis

Questions

63. One of the primary symptoms of vulvar carcinoma is:

A. Pruritus

B. Thin, watery discharge

C. Painless bleeding

D. Protruding mass

64. All of the following would be ordered postoperatively for the patient who has had a radical vulvectomy EXCEPT:

A. Hemovac

B. Intravenous therapy

C. High residue diet

D. Foley catheter

65. The most common complication after a radical vulvectomy is:

A. Pulmonary embolus

B. Wound breakdown

C. Loss of sexual functioning

D. Stress incontinence

66. The nurse is aware that the patient who has had a radical vulvectomy is at risk for developing an infection. To prevent this, the nurse would:

A. Get the patient out of bed as soon as possible

B. Change the dressing frequently and clean the wound with a sterile solution

C. Provide a diet low in fiber and high in protein

D. Medicate as ordered every 4 hours

67. Plan the nursing care for the patient who has had a radical vulvectomy. Use the following diagnosis.

Nursing Diagnosis: High risk for impaired tissue integrity related to disruption of suture line

Patient Outcome:

Nursing Interventions:

68. The most common form of cancer of the female reproductive tract in young women is cancer of the:

    A. Vulva

    B. Cervix

    C. Uterus

    D. Ovaries

69. The classic symptom of cervical cancer is:

    A. Intermittent, painless bleeding

    B. Thick, foul-smelling discharge

    C. Heavy bleeding with clots

    D. Painful periods with heavy flow

70. Risk factors associated with cervical cancer include all of the following EXCEPT:

    A. Age of sexual activity

    B. Age of first pregnancy

    C. Number of pregnancies

    D. Ethnic background

    E. Nutritional status

    F. Socioeconomic status

71. The usual treatment for the woman who has a diagnosis of carcinoma in situ would be:

    A. Radiation therapy

    B. Chemotherapy

    C. Conization or hysterectomy

    D. Hysterectomy with bilateral salpingo-oophorectomy

72. A patient is admitted for insertion of an internal radiation device. A possible effect of this therapy is:

    A. Nausea

    B. Vomiting

    C. Malaise

    D. Cystitis

    E. Any of the above

73. When caring for the patient with a radiation implant, which nursing action is of primary importance?

    A. Maintain patient on strict bedrest

    B. Keep patient on NPO status

    C. Administer narcotics for pain control

    D. Maintain patency of NG tube and IV

74. Plan the nursing care for the patient with a radioactive implant using the following nursing diagnosis.

    Nursing Diagnosis: Knowledge deficit related to restrictions and safety precautions to be followed

    Patient Outcome:

    Nursing Interventions:

75. When reviewing a patient's chart, the nurse notices that the diagnosis is Stage III adenocarcinoma of the uterus. This means:

    A. The cancer is confined to the uterus and the cervix.

    B. The cancer extends outside the uterus but not outside the pelvis.

    C. The cancer involves the uterus and either the bladder or rectum.

    D. The cancer has spread beyond the uterus to the brain.

76. The recommended treatment for the patient with Stage III uterine cancer would include:

    A. Total abdominal hysterectomy with a bilateral salpingo-oophorectomy followed by adjunct therapy

    B. Radiation therapy followed by hormonal therapy

    C. Hysterectomy followed by chemotherapy

    D. Palliative therapy only

77. Plan the nursing care for a patient who has had a total hysterectomy. Use the following nursing diagnosis.

    Nursing Diagnosis: High risk for ineffective coping

    Patient Outcome:

    Nursing Interventions:

CLINICAL SITUATIONS

Situation ■ 1

Mrs. Winters has severe symptoms of PMS. She has severe mood swings and can't control her emotions. She has tried many methods of medical treatment without any success.

1. Nursing care for Mrs. Winter would include all of the following EXCEPT:

    A. Teaching her to accept a disease that has no known cure

    B. Teaching ways to implement changes in lifestyle

    C. Providing information on surgical alternatives

    D. Providing information on support groups

2. Mrs. Winters states that she feels fat and often gains 5 pounds prior to beginning menstruation. What advice would be appropriate?

    A. Reduce or eliminate alcoholic beverages

    B. Reduce intake of food high in sodium

    C. Eat food high in protein

    D. Reduce intake of water

3. The nurse is evaluating the teaching plan. Which statement by Mrs. Winters shows she has some misunderstandings?

    A. I will try to stop eating potato chips.

    B. I am going to try and walk daily.

    C. I hope the new medication will cure me.

    D. I will try to sleep 8 hours each night.

Situation ■ 2

Mrs. Collins is admitted because of weakened pelvic support. She has four children, is overweight, and spends all her time caring for her family. She says, "It feels like my insides are falling out."

1. Mrs. Collins is scheduled for an anterior and posterior surgical repair. She wonders if this surgery will interfere with her ability to have any more children. An appropriate response would be:

    A. Yes, you will be sterile after the surgery.

    B. Not always, but infertility may be a problem.

    C. No, in fact it will help any future deliveries.

    D. You need to discuss this with your doctor.

2. Which information from Mrs. Collins would be important to report to the physician?

    A. She has been using birth control pills

    B. She doesn't exercise regularly

    C. She received antibiotics preoperatively

    D. She has no known allergies

3. Postoperatively, nursing interventions should include all of the following EXCEPT:

    A. Clean perineal area with warm water every 4 hours

    B. Encourage the patient to cough and deep breathe

    C. Assess for adequate urinary output

    D. Monitor for positive Homans' sign

Situation ■ 3

Mrs. Patrick has ovarian cancer and is admitted for a total abdominal hysterectomy, with bilateral salpingo-oophorectomy. She is anxious and needs emotional support and teaching prior to her surgery. The surgery will be followed by radiation therapy.

1. Mrs. Patrick wonders if all patients receive radiation therapy after surgery. The nurse replies:

    A. As far as I know that is the best treatment.

    B. That is the usual treatment, although some physicians may use chemotherapy or hormonal therapy.

    C. For your kind of cancer, you must have radiation therapy in order to be cured.

    D. Radiation therapy is not usually done, but your doctor must have a reason for suggesting it.

2. Mrs. Patrick is crying and says, "I am no longer going to be a woman. I may as well die." The nurse responds:

    A. What do you mean? Of course you are still a woman.

    B. Don't be silly, you aren't going to die.

    C. You seem concerned about having this procedure.

D. Let me call your husband; you know he loves you.

3. Counseling for which of the following should be an important part of the discharge planning?

A. Teaching her to do breast self-examination

B. Teaching the side effects of chemotherapy

C. Teaching her to cough and deep breathe

D. Referring her to Reach for Recovery

Situation ■ 4

Mrs. Stetson, 55, has been diagnosed with advanced adenocarcinoma of the uterus with metastasis to the bowel and bladder. She is scheduled for a total pelvic exenteration.

1. Prior to the surgery, extensive diagnostic testing is done to:

A. Rule out any metastasis beyond the pelvis

B. Determine the usage of radiation therapy

C. Determine if her bowels will function well after surgery

D. All of the above

2. During the preoperative preparation, the nurse will be administering which of the following?

A. Laxatives and antibiotics

B. Anticholinergics and analgesics

C. Antiemetics and antibiotics

D. Antacids and antibiotics

3. The nurse explains to Mrs. Stetson that she will be kept in the ICU for several days after the surgery. The reason for this is:

A. Because of the high risk of sepsis

B. Because of the risk of shock or cardiac problems

C. Because of the risk of respiratory failure

D. Because of the risk of fluid overload

4. Following this radical surgery, the patient will be discharged with:

A. NG tube for feeding, Foley catheter

B. Hickman catheter and antibiotic therapy

C. Colostomy, ileal conduit

D. Jejunostomy

Chapter Forty-five

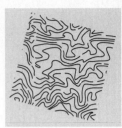

KNOWLEDGE BASIC TO THE NURSING CARE
of Men with Reproductive System Dysfunction

Learning Objectives

1.0 *Review the Anatomy and Physiology of the Male Reproductive System.*

1.1 Identify the Parts of the Male Reproductive System.
1.2 List the Functions of External and Internal Genitalia.
1.3 Identify Signs of Reproductive System Dysfunction.
1.4 Assess the Patient with an Alteration in the Male Reproductive System.

2.0 *Demonstrate an Understanding of the Assessment Data Related to Men with Reproductive System Dysfunction.*

2.1 Identify Clinical Manifestations of Men with Reproductive System Dysfunction.
2.2 Identify Diagnostic Procedures Used to Identify Problems in the Male Reproductive System.
2.3 Plan the Nursing Care for the Patient Having a Biopsy.

3.0 *Demonstrate an Understanding of the Interventions Used to Treat Men with Reproductive System Dysfunction.*

3.1 Identify Medical and Surgical Treatment Options Available for the Men with Reproductive Dysfunction.
3.2 Plan Nursing Interventions for the Patient Having Surgery.
3.3 Plan Nursing Interventions for the Patient Having a Penile Implant.

Learning Activities

Define

1. Spermatogenesis:

2. Semen:

3. Erection:

4. Ejaculation:

5. Impotence:

6. Premature ejaculation:

7. Retrograde ejaculation:

8. Infertility:

9. Cystourethroscopy:

10. Prostatic biopsy:

Identify

11. On the following diagram, identify the parts of the male reproductive system.

   A. Urethra   E. Prostate
   B. Penis   F. Testis
   C. Scrotum   G. Epididymis
   D. Prepuce

Questions

12. List two specific functions of the penis.
   1.
   2.

13. List two functions of the scrotum.
   1.
   2.

Fill In

14. The testes are the _____ glands of the male.

15. Sperm from each testis is stored in the _____ and _____ .

16. The urethra serves as a pathway for the elimination of both _____ and _____ .

17. Untreated impotence may result in _____ .

18. Impotence has been found to be of either _____ or _____ origin.

19. The treatment of choice for organic impotence would be _____ .

Questions

20. List four nonpathologic factors which have been associated with impotency.
    1.
    2.
    3.
    4.

21. List three of the physical causes of infertility.
    1.
    2.
    3.

Fill In

22. A vasectomy is performed as a method of _____ .

23. A testicular biopsy may be done on men with _____ .

24. Explain what transurethral resection syndrome is:

True or False

25. _____ Testosterone production begins during infancy.

26. _____ Testosterone production stops at about age 50.

27. _____ The vas deferens connects the epididymis with the ejaculatory duct.

28. _____ The seminal vesicles secrete an acidic fluid which helps sperm motility.

29. _____ The urethra passes through the prostate gland.

30. _____ Erection can occur by way of a spinal cord reflex mechanism.

31. _____ During the refractory period, the male cannot be aroused.

32. _____ Antihypertensive medications can cause impotence.

33. _____ A bowel prep is given prior to having surgery involving the male reproductive system.

34. _____ A patient having a vasectomy will be hospitalized for 48 hours.

35. _____ Patients should be told that a vasectomy can be reversed.

36. _____ Infertility is immediate after the vasectomy.

37. _____ Bladder spasms are normal following prostatectomy.

Questions

38. The male sex hormone is:
    A. Progesterone
    B. Testosterone
    C. Spermatozoon
    D. Estrogen

39. After ejaculation, the sperm live approximately _____ hours in the female reproductive tract.
    A. 6–8
    B. 12–15
    C. 24–28
    D. 46–48

40. What chronic medical condition is most likely to cause impotency?
    A. Diabetes
    B. Cardiac disease
    C. Chronic obstructive pulmonary disease
    D. Arthritis

41. The cause of premature ejaculation is believed to be:

    A. Organic

    B. Psychological

    C. Neurogenic

42. Treatment for premature ejaculation would be:

    A. Surgery to correct defect

    B. Medication such as testosterone

    C. Sex therapy

43. Pain in the inguinal and lower abdominal area is most generally indicative of which condition?

    A. Premature ejaculation

    B. Prostatitis

    C. Epididymitis

    D. Urinary retention

44. Urinary retention is often associated with which of the following conditions?

    A. Retrograde ejaculation

    B. Benign prostatic hypertrophy

    C. Epididymitis

    D. Impotence

45. In obtaining a history from the patient with a sexual dysfunction, which of the following questions should the nurse ask? (Check all that apply.)

    A. Ask about use of any OTC medications

    B. Ask if he is circumcised

    C. Ask him to describe his symptoms

    D. Ask if he has any urinary problems

    E. Ask if he has any GI problems

46. Prior to a male pelvic examination, which information would the nurse give to the patient?

    A. You will need to have an enema in the morning

    B. You will need to empty your bladder

    C. You will be examined in the prone position

    D. You will feel some pain during the exam

47. When an infertility problem is suspected, the nurse would expect which diagnostic procedure to be done?

    A. Rectal exam

    B. Semen analysis

    C. Radioimmunoassay

    D. Prostatic specific antigen

48. Blood analysis is often done to diagnose male reproductive disorders. Measurement of the prostate acid phosphatase is used in the diagnosis of which condition?

    A. Prostatic cancer

    B. Penile cancer

    C. Infertility

    D. Epididymitis

49. The blood test for alpha-fetoprotein (AFP) will show an elevation in which of the following conditions?

    A. Prostatic cancer

    B. Benign prostatic hypertrophy

    C. Bowel cancer

    D. Testicular cancer

50. Laboratory results indicate that a 33-year-old patient has a testosterone level of 2.5 mg/dl. How would the nurse interpret this information?

    A. This is normal for the patient

    B. This is low and may be related to infertility

    C. This is high and may be related to prostate cancer

    D. This is high and may be related to testicular cancer

51. A patient has just returned from a transperineal biopsy of the prostate. Which manifestation indicates a possible side effect of this procedure?

    A. Patient complains of discomfort in perineal area

    B. Patient voids 30 ml 8 hours after procedure

    C. Patient states that he is free from pain

    D. Patient complains of nausea

52. Which of the following nursing interventions would be appropriate following a testicular biopsy?

    A. Encourage the patient to drink fluids

    B. Schedule a physician appointment in 6 weeks

    C. Suggest the use of a scrotal support

53. A patient is to be discharged following cystourethroscopy and transurethral prostatic biopsy. Discharge instructions aimed at preventing infection would include: (Check all that apply.)

    A. Teach patient to administer antibiotics if ordered

    B. Teach patient to administer analgesics if ordered

    C. Teach patient to avoid contaminating biopsy site

    D. Instruct patient on how to clean perianal area

    E. Instruct patient to report chills, fever, or pain

54. Reasons that surgery may be done for dysfunctions of the male reproductive system include all of the following EXCEPT:

    A. Restore normal anatomy

    B. Repair structural abnormalities

    C. Treat epididymitis

    D. Restore normal sexual functioning

55. A 23-year-old male has been having problems with sexual performance. Functioning of which other system should also be studied for this patient?

    A. Gastrointestinal system

    B. Endocrine system

    C. Cardiovascular system

    D. Respiratory system

56. A patient is scheduled for prostate surgery because of an obstruction. Which of the following findings indicate a possible complication of the surgery?

    A. Patient has a urinary output of 75 ml the first hour

    B. Patient complains of pain in his leg

    C. Patient has bloody urine during the first 12 hours

    D. Patient has a respiratory rate of 24 and a pulse of 92

57. For the patient who has had a transurethral prostatic resection, which of the following complications should the nurse be alerted to observe for?

    A. Bleeding

    B. Infection

    C. Wound dehiscence

    D. Cystitis

58. One of the disadvantages of the transurethral prostatectomy over other methods is that:

    A. Hemorrhage is more common

    B. Infection is more common

    C. Urethral stricture can occur

    D. Pain is more severe

59. For the patient who has a very large prostate, and abdominal surgery is contraindicated, which approach would be preferred for removal?

    A. Perineal

    B. Transurethral

    C. Retropubic

    D. Suprapubic

60. Following removal of the prostate, a patient becomes restless, disoriented, and nauseated. Which lab values should the nurse monitor?

    A. Serum sodium, potassium, and osmolarity

    B. Hemoglobin and hematocrit

    C. White blood count, sedimentation rate

    D. BUN and creatinine

61. Management for the patient with the above symptoms might include administration of:

    A. IV of 5% dextrose and water; potassium bolus

    B. IV of 3% sodium chloride; Lasix

    C. Transfusion of packed red blood cells

    D. Antibiotics

62. A penile implant is generally used on patients with:

    A. Psychogenic impotency

    B. Organic impotency

    C. Anyone who wants one

63. To prevent a common postoperative complication following penile implant, which of the following interventions should the nurse implement?

    A. Monitor for urinary bleeding

    B. Assess for any respiratory distress

    C. Monitor temperature every 4 hours

    D. Assess for bowel sounds every 8 hours

64. Write a nursing care plan for a 25-year-old male who is an insulin-dependent diabetic and has been impotent for the past 6 months.

    Nursing Diagnosis:

    Patient Outcome:

    Nursing Interventions:

65. Plan the nursing care for the patient with a penile implant.

    Nursing Diagnosis: Anxiety related to the effect of the surgery on his sexual functioning.

    Patient Outcome:

    Nursing Interventions:

66. Write a nursing care plan for the patient who has just returned from a prostatectomy.

    Nursing Diagnosis:

    Patient Outcome:

    Nursing Interventions:

CLINICAL SITUATIONS

Situation ■ 1

Mr. Cummings is 28 years old. He and his wife have been trying for 4 years to have a family. He is in for an evaluation by the fertility expert.

1. Which of the following would be most indicative of the cause of this patient's condition?

    A. Family history of hypertension

    B. Sperm count of <20 million/ml

    C. History of intercourse less than twice a week

    D. All of the above

2. Mr. Cummings asks if there is a surgical treatment to correct his problem. What would the nurse respond?

    A. Yes, the surgeons often treat this condition.

    B. No, this is usually treated medically.

    C. No, this condition is usually treated by sex therapy.

3. Mr. Cummings is to collect a semen specimen for analysis. Which information would the nurse give him in order to have good results from this test?

    A. You need to abstain from sex for 1 week prior to this test.

    B. You need to abstain from sex for 2–5 days prior to this test.

    C. You need to have frequent intercourse prior to this test.

    D. You do not have to follow any special protocol for this test.

4. How would the nurse suggest that Mr. Cummings collect this specimen?

    A. Use a rubber condom

    B. Masturbate and collect specimen in container

    C. Use coitus interruptus

Situation ■ 2

Mr. Coleman is 66 years old and is admitted with a diagnosis of benign prostatic hypertrophy. He is scheduled for surgery.

1. The nurse obtains the health history from Mr. Coleman. Which of the following information is most likely related to his current condition?

    A. Patient has complained of constipation

    B. Patient gets up at night to urinate

C. Patient must sleep on two pillows

D. Patient complains of intermittent leg pain

2. Mr. Coleman is scheduled for a transurethral resection. The nurse should explain to him that this means:

A. Under general anesthesia, the physician will make an abdominal incision and remove the tissue.

B. In the patient's room, the physician will use a cystoscopy to excise the tumor.

C. Using local anesthesia, a resectoscope is inserted into the urethra to scrap out the enlarged gland.

D. Using general anesthesia, the physician incises the perineum to remove hypertrophied tissue.

3. Mr. Coleman wonders why he needs to have an enema. He says, "I thought they didn't do that anymore." The nurse explains that the purpose of the enema is:

A. To clean the bowel

B. To prevent straining postoperatively

C. To prevent an infection in his incision

D. To reduce pain

4. In caring for this patient, which of the following nursing diagnoses would be the most important?

A. Alteration in urinary elimination

B. Pain

C. High risk for aspiration

D. Alteration in physical mobility

5. As the primary nurse, you realize that it is important to explain to the patient that he should not try to urinate around the drainage catheter. What is the rationale for this?

A. It can cause an infection

B. It may precipitate bleeding

C. It may precipitate bladder spasms

D. It may cause TUR syndrome

6. Which information would be important to relay to this patient on discharge?

A. Normal urinary function will return immediately

B. Temporary urinary problems may occur such as dribbling and urgency

C. Bleeding during urination may occur for the next 2 weeks

D. Impotency is a common complication of this surgery

Chapter Forty-six

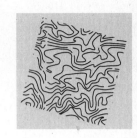

NURSING CARE
of Men with Disorders of the Reproductive System

Learning Objectives

1.0 Demonstrate an Understanding of the Inflammatory Processes of the Male Reproductive System.

1.1 Define Several Inflammations and Infections of the Male Reproductive System.
1.2 Identify the Clinical Manifestations Associated with Several Inflammatory Processes.
1.3 Write a Nursing Diagnosis for an Adult with an Infection of the Male Reproductive Organs.
1.4 Plan Nursing Interventions for the Adult with an Infection.
1.5 Identify the Teaching Needs of the Adult Male with a Reproductive System Infection.

2.0 Demonstrate an Understanding of the Structural Disorders of the Male Reproductive System.

2.1 Identify Several Structural Disorders.
2.2 Identify the Clinical Manifestations of Structural Disorders.
2.3 Plan Nursing Interventions for the Adult with a Structural Disorder.

3.0 Demonstrate an Understanding of the Types of Neoplasms that Affect the Male Reproductive System.

3.1 Identify the Clinical Manifestations of Several Neoplasms.
3.2 Identify Types of Medical Treatment Used with Neoplasms of the Male Reproductive System.
3.3 Identify Surgical Interventions Used to Treat Neoplasms of the Male Reproductive System.
3.4 Demonstrate Application of the Nursing Process when Caring for the Adult Male with a Neoplasm of the Reproductive System.

Learning Activities

Define

1. Balanitis:

2. Posthitis:

3. Epididymitis:

4. Hydrocele:

5. Orchitis:

6. Prostatitis:

7. Phimosis:

8. Meatotomy:

9. Paraphimosis:

10. Cryptorchidism:

11. Priapism:

Fill In

12. Phimosis is often the result of _____.

13. Treatment of phimosis is _____.

14. Treatment for paraphimosis is _____.

Questions

15. Two complications which can occur following a varicocelectomy are:

    1.

    2.

16. The diagnosis of penile cancer is suggested by a small lesion on the glans, and is confirmed by _____.

    A. X-ray

    B. Laboratory testing

    C. Ultrasound

    D. Biopsy

17. A contributing factor to the development of balanitis and posthitis would be:

    A. Poor nutrition

    B. Poor hygiene

    C. Sexual practices

    D. Heredity

18. Epididymitis occurs as a result of an infection which often descends from the:

    A. Urinary tract

    B. Gastrointestinal tract

    C. Integumentary system

    D. Vascular system

19. A possible complication of epididymitis is:

    A. Impotency

    B. Hemorrhage

    C. Sterility

    D. Urinary retention

20. Mr. Parsons has been diagnosed with epididymitis. All of the following are possible treatments EXCEPT:

    A. Antibiotic therapy

    B. Heat therapy

    C. Analgesics

    D. Cold therapy

21. Mr. Parsons is being discharged. The nursing diagnosis is: Knowledge deficit related to self-care after discharge and ways to prevent a recurrence. Write three nursing interventions.

    1.

    2.

    3.

22. All of the following are symptoms of prostatitis EXCEPT:

    A. Urinary frequency

    B. Pain in the rectal area

    C. Ureteral discharge

    D. Scrotal swelling

23. What is the rationale for giving anticholinergic medications to the patient with prostatitis?

    A. To relieve discomfort associated with urination.

    B. To relieve gastrointestinal discomfort.

    C. To reduce the amount of ureteral discharge.

    D. To reduce swelling.

24. A patient with epididymitis is having severe pain. An appropriate nursing intervention would be:

    A. Elevate the scrotum

    B. Apply a Bellevue bridge

C. Apply ice packs to the scrotum

D. All of the above

25. A 23-year-old male has recently recovered from mumps. He is at risk for developing:

    A. Orchitis

    B. Prostatitis

    C. Epididymitis

    D. Urinary infection

26. A patient has been admitted for incision and drainage of the scrotum. The most appropriate nursing diagnosis is:

    A. Body image disturbance

    B. High risk for infection

    C. Altered health maintenance

    D. Anxiety related to outcome of procedure

27. Medical management for acute bacterial prostatitis would include administration of:

    A. Penicillin G

    B. Corticosteroid

    C. Testosterone

    D. Co-trimoxazole DS

True or False

28. _____ Orchitis usually results in sterility.

29. _____ Orchitis occurs as a result from a primary infection.

30. _____ Drainage of a hydrocele reduces the incidence of testicular atrophy.

31. _____ Prostatitis is most often caused by a bacteria.

32. _____ Chronic bacterial prostatitis is usually treated with Bactrim.

33. _____ Priapism is considered a urologic emergency.

34. _____ Painless swelling of the scrotum is the classical sign of a hydrocele.

35. _____ Conservative treatment of a varicocele involves using a scrotal support.

Questions

36. Unsuccessful treatment of paraphimosis might result in:

    A. Urinary retention

    B. Impotency

    C. Necrosis of the penis

    D. Systemic infection

37. A complication of cryptorchidism would be:

    A. Urinary tract infection

    B. Testicular cancer

    C. Impotency

    D. Phimosis

38. In the majority of cases, the cause of priapism is unknown. Which statement best describes the pathophysiology of this condition?

    A. Penile enlargement results from an obstruction to the outflow of blood from the corpora cavernosa.

    B. Penile enlargement results from a change in neurologic enervation.

    C. Penile enlargement results from sexual overstimulation and delayed orgasm.

    D. Penile enlargement results from an endocrine dysfunction.

39. Which statement best describes the emergency treatment for priapism?

    A. The foreskin is manually retracted

    B. A venous fistula is created to shunt blood

    C. A urinary catheter is inserted and Novocain injected

    D. Anesthesia is given and the penis relaxes

40. A patient has had an orchiopexy performed. Because of the reason for and possible outcome of the surgery, the nurse should:

    A. Monitor intake and output

    B. Administer antibiotics as ordered

    C. Medicate frequently for pain

    D. Assess emotional state

41. Which statement is most accurate about the male who has Stage I cancer of the penis?

    A. It is almost 100% curable

    B. The neoplasm spreads rapidly

    C. There is no known treatment

    D. Surgery involves a radical penectomy

42. Following a total penectomy, what changes will be made in the patterns of urinary elimination?

    A. The patient will have an abdominal urethrostomy

    B. The patient will have a perineal urethrostomy

    C. The patient will have an indwelling catheter

    D. The patient will have a suprapubic catheter

43. Because of the radical nature of a penectomy, which nursing diagnosis would be most appropriate?

    A. Alteration in urination

    B. Alteration in body image

    C. Alteration in mobility

    D. Alteration in breathing

44. Which statement is true about testicular cancer?

    A. Pain is often the first symptom

    B. Most men detect the tumor

    C. Tumors can be palpated by bimanual exam of the scrotum

    D. The diagnosis is confirmed by biopsy

45. A diagnosis of Stage II testicular cancer would mean:

    A. Tumor is a hard, localized mass

    B. Tumor has spread to the retroperitoneal lymph nodes

    C. Tumor has spread beyond the retroperitoneal lymph nodes

    D. Tumor has spread to the bone and abdominal organs

46. For the patient with Stage II testicular cancer, treatment would most likely involve:

    A. Chemotherapy

    B. Radiation therapy

    C. Orchectomy

    D. Orchectomy and radiation therapy

47. To reduce the risk of postoperative paralytic ileus for a patient having a retroperitoneal lymph node dissection, the nurse would:

    A. Administer antibiotics

    B. Hold all food for 24 hours

    C. Administer mechanical bowel prep

    D. Teach the use of an incentive spirometer

48. Following a thoracoabdominal approach for retroperitoneal lymph node biopsy, nursing care would involve:

    A. Monitoring the chest tube drainage system

    B. Maintaining bedrest

    C. Administering corticosteroids

    D. Maintaining a gastric tube

True or False

49. _____ Most of the men with benign prostatic hypertrophy (BPH) are asymptomatic.

50. _____ One of the symptoms associated with BPH is urinary retention.

51. _____ Diagnosis of BPH is confirmed by biopsy.

52. _____ The most common form of prostatic cancer is adenocarcinoma.

53. _____ Prostate cancer can be palpated during a rectal exam.

Questions

54. The nurse teaching a patient about the conservative treatment for BPH would include information on:

    A. Increasing fluid intake, limiting alcohol

    B. Prostate massage, mild tranquilizers

    C. Sexual intercourse, limiting fluids

    D. Application of heat, forcing fluids

55. Surgical removal of the enlarged prostate is usually performed when symptoms of obstruction occur. An indication of this might be:

    A. Patient voids every 2 hours

    B. Patient develops a hydrocele

    C. Patient develop hydronephrosis

    D. Patient develops a bladder infection

56. Elevation of the alkaline phosphate titer in the patient who has prostatic cancer may indicate:

    A. The patient has metastasis to the bone

    B. The patient has cardiac disease

    C. The patient is responding appropriately to therapy

    D. The patient has a nutritional deficit

57. A possible side effect of radiation therapy used in the treatment of prostatic cancer would be:

    A. The patient develops alopecia

    B. The patient develops a reddish discoloration on the skin

    C. The patient develops bruises on his buttocks

    D. The patient complains of lethargy

58. Because of the high incidence of prostate cancer in the elderly male, the nurse would stress the importance of:

    A. Yearly physical exams

    B. Following a low-fat diet

    C. Quitting smoking

    D. Increasing exercise

59. Write a nursing care plan for Mr. Unger, who is in the emergency room with paraphimosis. He is complaining of pain, and his penis is bluish and swollen.

    Nursing Diagnosis:

    Patient Outcome:

    Nursing Interventions:

60. Write a nursing care plan for Mr. Masters, who has had a total penectomy for Stage III cancer.

    Nursing Diagnosis: Sexual dysfunction related to loss of penis

    Patient Outcome:

    Nursing Interventions:

CLINICAL SITUATIONS

Situation ■ 1

Mr. Herman is a 32-year-old male who is admitted with high fever and inguinal pain. The diagnosis is orchitis.

1. Which statement by Mr. Herman would suggest the cause of his infection?

    A. I had a swollen jaw last week

    B. I fell off my bike 6 weeks ago

    C. I have never been married

    D. I have severe allergies to pollen

2. Which of the following interventions should the nurse implement?

    A. Antibiotic therapy, warm moist compresses

    B. Bedrest, scrotal elevation, cold packs

    C. Analgesics, antipyretics, steroids

3. Mr. Herman wants to know why he is receiving diethylstilbestrol. The nurse would explain:

    A. To reduce swelling

    B. As a prophylactic measure

    C. To control pain

    D. To prevent spread of infection

4. Mr. Herman lives with a male roommate who has never had parotitis. Which precautions should his roommate take to avoid contracting this disease?

    A. Have a dose of gamma globulin administered

    B. Have a therapeutic dose of penicillin

    C. Refrain from sexual relations for 4 weeks

    D. Avoid contact with Mr. Herman for 2 weeks

Situation ■ 2

Mr. Smith is 33 years old and has a hard node in the left testicle. He is scheduled for an inguinal orchidectomy.

1. Before the surgery it would be important for the nurse to assess:

    A. Reproductive history

    B. Understanding about the surgery

    C. Emotional status

    D. All of the above

2. Mr. Smith is very anxious about the surgery. A patient outcome related to this problem would be:

    A. Patient states that he does not have cancer

    B. Patient asks questions about postoperative care

    C. Patient states that he will be impotent

    D. Patient can state diet restrictions

3. Mr. Smith has recently married and has no children. Which information would be important for him to know?

    A. If the remaining testis is normal, fertility is usually not affected

    B. Sterility is usually an unfortunate side effect of this surgery

    C. Many men have had the surgery without problems

    D. The doctor can answer all of his questions

4. Three days after his orchidectomy, Mr. Smith is scheduled for a retroperitoneal lymph node dissection. Nursing care in preparation for the surgery would include:

    A. Mechanical bowel prep

    B. Insertion of a nasogastric tube

    C. Insertion of a central line

    D. All of the above

5. The surgeon uses a thoracoabdominal approach to perform the surgery. The nurse's responsibility in preventing complications following surgery include:

    A. Maintaining bedrest for 3–4 days

    B. Maintaining patency of chest tubes

    C. Giving Tylenol for pain as needed

    D. Encouraging clear liquids as soon as possible

Chapter Forty-seven

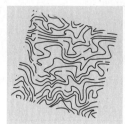

NURSING CARE
of Adults with
Sexually Transmitted Diseases

Learning Objectives

1.0 Demonstrate an Understanding of Several Types of Sexually Transmitted Diseases.

1.1 Define Several of the Sexually Transmitted Diseases.
1.2 Identify the Clinical Manifestations of the Sexually Transmitted Diseases.
1.3 Identify the Current Treatments for Sexually Transmitted Diseases.

2.0 Plan the Nursing Care for the Patient with a Sexually Transmitted Disease.

2.1 Write Several Nursing Diagnoses and Patient Outcomes.
2.2 Write Nursing Interventions for the Patient with a Sexually Transmitted Disease.
2.3 Identify the Teaching Needs of the Patient with a Sexually Transmitted Disease.

Learning Activities

Define

1. Syphilis:

2. Herpes simplex:

3. Gonorrhea:

Fill In

4. _____ is the organism which causes syphilis.

Questions

5. Describe the clinical manifestations of the four stages of syphilis.

   1. Primary syphilis:

   2. Secondary syphilis:

   3. Latent syphilis:

   4. Tertiary syphilis:

6. Why has syphilis been referred to as the "great imitator"?

7. Explain the mode of herpes simplex type I transmission.

True or False

8. _____ Use of systemic antibiotics causes increased incidence of candidiasis.

9. _____ Candidiasis is rare during pregnancy.

10. _____ The normal vaginal environment is acidotic.

11. _____ Itching is the most common symptom of genital candidiasis.

12. _____ Flagyl is the only effective drug used to treat trichomoniasis.

13. _____ Herpes simplex can be transmitted from one site on the body to another.

14. _____ Herpes viruses have the ability to remain in the body and recur later.

Matching

A. *Treponema pallidum*
B. *Chlamydia trachomatis*
C. Human papillomavirus
D. Nongonococcal urethritis
E. Condylomata acuminata
F. Pediculosis pubis

15. _____ Inflammation of the urethra in the absence of *Neisseria gonorrhoeae*.

16. _____ Major cause of nongonococcal urethritis.

17. _____ Causes 50% of the cases of acute epididymitis.

18. _____ Warts appearing in the anogenital area.

19. _____ Causes genital warts.

20. _____ Species of lice which is sexually transmitted.

Fill In

21. _____ is the recommended treatment for venereal warts.

22. _____ is the primary symptom of lice infestation.

23. _____ is the recommended treatment for pubic lice.

Questions

24. Which of the following questions is most effective in eliciting information concerning the health history of the individual suspected of having a vaginal infection. (Check all that are applicable.)

    A. Ask patient to describe the color, consistency, amount, and odor of discharge

    B. Ask patient about history of other sexually transmitted diseases

    C. Ask patient about her knowledge of normal vaginal functioning

    D. Ask patient about her personal hygiene practices

25. Choose the risk factors that often lead to the development of a fungal infection of the vagina. (Check all that apply.)

    A. Multiple sexual partners

    B. Change in the normal microbial environment

    C. Change in host resistance

    D. Poor nutrition

26. The treatment of choice for a fungal infection of the vagina would be:

    A. Mycostatin

    B. Ampicillin

    C. Cefoxitin

    D. Micronase

27. One of the most common sexually transmitted urogenital infections is:

    A. Gonorrhea

    B. Trichomoniasis

    C. Candidiasis

    D. Syphilis

28. Which of the following symptoms are generally associated with trichomoniasis?

    A. Thin, watery discharge; itching

    B. Hematuria; pruritus

    C. Greenish-gray or purulent discharge; dysuria

    D. Urinary frequency; brown drainage

29. In women that have been labeled as having non-specific vaginitis, the causative organism in 95% of them has been found to be:

    A. Candidiasis

    B. Trichomoniasis

    C. *Gardnerella vaginalis*

    D. *Neisseria gonorrhoeae*

30. During the assessment of a patient with vaginitis, the nurse reviews the personal hygienic habits because she or he realizes one of the practices which may predispose a woman to infection is:

    A. Frequent douching with solutions that alter vaginal pH

    B. Wearing of cotton underwear

    C. Taking a bath or shower immediately after intercourse

    D. Urinating every 4 hours

31. Recurrence of herpes simplex can be precipitated by:

    A. Trauma

    B. Emotional stress

    C. Menstruation

    D. Any of the above

32. The nurse suspects herpes simplex in a patient. If herpes is present, the lesions would appear:

    A. Pustular, which crust and spread along linear tracts

    B. Red, flattened lesions around genitals

    C. Raised, scaly, and crusty

    D. Erythematous maculas which change to macular to papular to vesicular to pustular to crusts

33. When caring for a patient with a herpes infection, the nurse would expect the physician to treat with:

    A. Tetracycline

    B. Hydrocortisone

    C. Acyclovir

    D. Nystatin

34. Herpes simplex has the ability to stay in the body in a latent state and cause recurrent disease. In caring for a patient with herpes, the nurse is aware that:

    A. Herpes is infectious only during the first episode

    B. Herpes is infectious during each episode of recurrence

    C. Having herpes provides immunity against another attack

    D. Having genital herpes prevents contacting herpes labialis

35. Major symptoms associated with genital herpes include:

    A. Pain, itching, dysuria, discharge, vesicles

    B. Purulent drainage, vesicular formation, ulcers

    C. Fever, nausea, lethargy

    D. Localized lesions over perineum and trunk

36. In women, the major site of infection by herpes lesions is:

    A. Vulva

    B. Vagina

    C. Cervix

    D. Uterus

37. In most individuals, there is a strong emotional reaction when they are told that they have contacted genital herpes. Which of the following reactions may occur?

    A. Shock

    B. Anger

    C. Denial

    D. All of the above

38. Medical care for the patient with genital herpes would most likely include administration of:

    A. Ampicillin

    B. Tetracycline

    C. Acyclovir

    D. Leukeran

39. Write a nursing care plan for the individual with herpes.

    Nursing Diagnosis: Ineffective individual coping related to the potential effect of having a chronic sexually transmitted disease

    Patient Outcome:

    Nursing Interventions:

40. List three factors that may precipitate a recurrence of genital herpes.

    1.

    2.

    3.

41. A patient with active genital herpes is admitted in labor. What would be an appropriate nursing action?

    A. Monitor patient carefully because of the risk of birth defects

    B. Set up for cesarean section

    C. No special precautions, normal labor routine

    D. Contact the neonatal intensive care unit

42. An important concern of the nurse is to prevent further transmission of sexually transmitted diseases. Write a nursing care plan related to this problem.

    Nursing Diagnosis: Knowledge deficit related to disease process and prevention of transmission.

    Patient Outcome:

    Nursing Interventions:

43. When counseling patients with genital herpes, the nurse is aware that much of the anxiety that individuals experience is due to:

    A. The potential for recurrent, unpredictable outbreaks of infection

    B. The problem related to dealing with an ongoing infectious process

    C. The problem related to becoming sterile

    D. The problem related to infertility

44. Which of the following medications is able to eradicate both gonorrhea and coexistent chlamydia?

    A. Procaine penicillin G

    B. Ampicillin

    C. Tetracycline

    D. Acyclovir

45. The medical treatment of choice for trichomoniasis and *Gardnerella* vaginitis is:

    A. Gentamicin

    B. Acyclovir

    C. Ampicillin

    D. Metronidazole

46. A patient complains of difficulty urinating. On further questioning, he also states he has noticed he has a yellowish urethral discharge. This information suggests:

    A. He has a urinary tract infection

    B. He has genital herpes

    C. He has contracted gonorrhea

    D. He has contracted syphilis

47. What is the most common and serious complication of gonorrhea infection in women?

    A. Pelvic inflammatory disease

    B. Acute septicemia

    C. Sterility

    D. Kidney failure

48. What diagnostic test is done to verify the presence of gonorrhea in women?

    A. Pelvic exam

    B. Cervical culture

    C. Cervical biopsy

    D. Ultrasound of reproductive organs

49. What is the rationale for using probenecid along with penicillin to treat gonorrhea?

    A. Probenecid prevents allergic reactions to penicillin

    B. Probenecid increases secretion of penicillin

    C. Probenecid decreases renal secretion of penicillin

    D. Probenecid has analgesic qualities to control discomfort

50. If the nurse suspects that disseminated gonococcal infection is present in an individual, which of the symptoms would probably be present?

    A. GI upset, nausea, vomiting, diarrhea

    B. Skin lesions on legs, arthritic symptoms, fever, anorexia

    C. Diffuse rash on trunk, flushing on face, fever

    D. Anorexia, vomiting, dehydration

True or False

51. _____ Most women with gonorrhea do not know they have it.

52. _____ Tetracycline is the best drug to treat gonorrhea.

53. _____ Individuals with gonorrhea should be recultured 7 days after treatment.

54. _____ Using condoms will not prevent transmission of gonorrhea.

55. _____ Tetracycline should be taken with meals.

56. _____ Once antibiotics are started, the individual with an STD can resume sexual relations.

Questions

57. A nurse working with a group of teenage girls is aware that certain risk factors have been identified for sexually transmitted diseases. List three risk factors which should be discussed with this group.

1.

2.

3.

58. Which statement by 18-year-old Sally would indicate that the teaching was ineffective?

   A. My boyfriend wouldn't give me any disease.

   B. Abstinence will prevent STD.

   C. Having sex can lead to a disease.

   D. I didn't know how easy it was to get an STD.

59. Which statement provides valid information about primary syphilis?

   A. It includes multiple painful genital lesions

   B. The infection heals spontaneously in 3–6 weeks

   C. If the lesions disappear, no further treatment is needed

   D. It includes lesions, discharge, fever, and lethargy

60. The classic symptom of primary syphilis is:

   A. Raised rash on the trunk

   B. Discharge from vagina or penis

   C. Painless genital ulcer at the site of entry

   D. Low-grade fever, rash on genitals

61. The nurse is aware that when a person has syphilis, there is a possibility for a false negative test to occur. What is the rationale for this?

   A. The virus hasn't fully matured

   B. It can take up to 3 weeks for the antibodies to form

   C. The antigen-antibody reaction doesn't occur with this disease

   D. The lab tests take 2 weeks to run

True or False

62. _____ Syphilis is inactive during the latent period.

63. _____ Tertiary syphilis is rare today.

64. _____ Antibodies are present in the blood 2 days after exposure to syphilis.

65. _____ Penicillin G is the drug of choice for the treatment of all stages of syphilis.

66. _____ Sexual partners of the individual who has syphilis must be contacted.

67. _____ Infections by chlamydia are more common than gonorrhea.

68. _____ In males, chlamydia causes ureteritis.

Questions

69. Noncompliance with the treatment of syphilis is a problem in society. Write a nursing care plan that relates to this.

   Nursing Diagnosis: High risk for noncompliance with the treatment regimen related to lack of knowledge, lifestyle, and distrust of health professionals

   Patient Outcome:

   Nursing Interventions:

70. Which statement is NOT true about *Chlamydia*?

   A. *Chlamydia* has a high incidence of infecting the neonate at the time of delivery.

   B. *Chlamydia* is a major cause of pelvic inflammatory disease.

   C. *Chlamydia* is a potent virus that affects both men and women.

   D. *Chlamydia* causes symptoms such as abdominal pain and vaginal bleeding and can lead to infertility.

71. List three antibiotics which have been found to be very effective in the treatment of *Chlamydia trachomatis*.

   1.

   2.

   3.

72. The patient with a suspected case of *Chlamydia* should have a thorough history taken. Which of the following information is the most significant predictor for this infection?

   A. Use of contraceptives

B. Socioeconomic status

C. Past history of STD

D. Sexual history, number of partners

73. Write a nursing care plan for the patient who has her third vaginal infection with *Candida* this year.

Nursing Diagnosis:

Patient Outcome:

Nursing Interventions:

74. Plan the nursing care for the woman with sexually transmitted vaginitis. Use the following diagnosis:

Nursing Diagnosis: Pain related to the inflammatory process

Patient Outcome:

Nursing Interventions:

CLINICAL SITUATIONS

Situation ■ 1

Ms. Spencer is 23 years old and is 3 months pregnant. She is seen in the clinic with lesions on her vulva, vagina, cervix, and perineum. She is diagnosed as having genital herpes.

1. How would the physician know if this is a primary or recurrent infection?

A. Based solely on patient history

B. Based on history and absence of antibodies to HSV

C. Based on history of exposure from sexual partner

D. Based on the presence of high WBC and ANA

2. Ms. Spencer wonders how she could have developed this problem. What information does the nurse give her?

A. Genital herpes is transmitted via sexual contact

B. Genital herpes is transmitted by contact with the virus

C. Genital herpes is transmitted because of poor hygienic practices

D. Genital herpes is always present; being pregnant caused her to have an outbreak

3. Ms. Spencer is crying when the nurse enters the room. She says, "The doctor told me there is no cure for this disease." An appropriate response is:

A. You sound upset; I'm sure that's not true.

B. Don't worry; most people never have a recurrence.

C. While it is true there is no permanent cure, there are medications to treat the symptoms.

D. Don't cry; you will only cause more stress on your pregnancy.

4. Based on Ms. Spencer's current health status, what would the nurse explain to her?

A. She will have to be monitored closely and deliver her baby by cesarean section

B. She may have a spontaneous abortion because of the severity of her symptoms

C. She will need to have weekly cultures, and if they are negative, she may be able to deliver vaginally

D. She will very likely have a child with birth defects

Situation ■ 2

Patsy is seen in the clinic with cervical discharge and abdominal pain. Testing reveals she has an infection caused by *Chlamydia*. Assessment reveals she also has a fever, vomiting, and intermittent bleeding.

1. The presence of these symptoms suggest what other problem?

A. Ascending urinary tract infection

B. Pelvic inflammatory disease

C. Septicemia

D. Gonorrhea as well as *Chlamydia*

2. The nurse would assess the patient's knowledge of the disease and its mode of transmission. Which

question would the nurse use to elicit this information?

A. What factors in your sexual lifestyle would have put you at risk for this infection?

B. Explain to me how you contracted this disease.

C. Give me a list of all your sexual partners.

D. How many children do you have?

3. Patsy is very upset and wants to know if this disease can be treated. Which information should be provided?

A. This disease has no cure, but symptoms can be treated.

B. This disease can be treated and cured, but you could be reinfected.

C. This disease will go into remission without treatment.

D. This disease will have some recurring episodes, but they lessen in severity.

4. Patsy is ready for discharge. Which statement indicates that she has a good understanding of the way this disease is spread?

A. I will tell my boyfriend I don't want to see him again.

B. I am going to find another boyfriend.

C. I am going to be more selective in my sexual partners.

D. I don't see why this happened to me.

Chapter Forty-eight

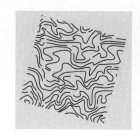

NURSING CARE
of Adults with
Breast Disorders

Learning Objectives

1.0 Review the Anatomy and Physiology of the Breast.

1.1 Identify the Structure of the Breast.
1.2 Identify Changes in Breast Structure.

2.0 Demonstrate an Understanding of Assessment Data Related to the Breast.

2.1 Review Assessment Procedures of the Breast.
2.2 Identify Clinical Manifestations of Breast Disorders.
2.3 Match Diagnostic Tests Used with Breast Disorders with the Appropriate Definition.
2.4 Choose Appropriate Interventions for the Patient having a Breast Biopsy.

3.0 Demonstrate an Understanding of the Infections and Inflammations of the Breast.

3.1 Identify Clinical Manifestations of Infectious Disorders.
3.2 Identify Treatment Modalities of the Infectious Disorders.
3.3 Identify Nursing Interventions for the patient with an Infectious Disorder of the Breast.

4.0 Demonstrate an Understanding of the Structural Disorders of the Breast.

4.1 Identify Characteristics of Several of the Structural Disorders.
4.2 Identify the Management Techniques for the Structural Disorders of the Breast.
4.3 Identify Nursing Interventions Used with Patients with Structural Disorders of the Breast.

5.0 Demonstrate an Understanding of the Neoplasms that Affect the Breast.

5.1 Identify the Etiology and Pathophysiology of Several of the Breast Neoplasms.
5.2 Identify the Clinical Manifestations of Neoplasms of the Breast.
5.3 Identify the Treatment Protocols for the Patient with a Neoplasm of the Breast.
5.4 Write a Nursing Care Plan for the Patient with Breast Cancer.

Learning Activities

Fill In

1. The breast is composed of _____, _____, and _____ tissue.

2. The _____ tissue has the ability to elongate in response to pregnancy and lactation.

3. Normal breast development requires the production of _____ and _____ hormone by the anterior pituitary.

4. Structural change in the older female breast after menopause is known as _____.

Questions

5. When the breasts are examined, the patient should be in a/an _____ position.
   A. Upright
   B. Side lying
   C. Supine
   D. Upright, then supine

Matching

Match the following diagnostic tests with their descriptions.

A. Mammography   D. Ultrasound
B. Xeroradiography   E. Breast biopsy
C. Thermography

6. _____ Takes pictures of infrared emissions.

7. _____ Provides an x-ray picture of the internal breast structure.

8. _____ May be used to differentiate a breast cyst from a tumor.

9. _____ X-ray which can reveal circulation around a tumor.

10. _____ Provides a definitive diagnosis of a breast mass.

Questions

11. A woman who must discontinue nursing her infant to return to work is at risk for:
    A. Fibrocystic breast disease
    B. Mastitis
    C. Breast cancer
    D. Gynecomastia

12. The etiology of gynecomastia is thought to be:
    A. Disturbance in the ratio of sex hormones
    B. Disturbance in growth hormone
    C. Normal process of growth
    D. Normal process of aging

13. Patient education for the woman with fibrocystic disease would include information on all the following EXCEPT:
    A. Avoid sleeping in the prone position
    B. Use heating pad for pain relief
    C. Limit use of caffeine
    D. Reduce intake of sodium

14. Clinical manifestations of fibrocystic breast disease include:
    A. Breast swelling that begins after menstruation
    B. Fever, lethargy and breast tenderness
    C. Discharge from breast; a hard, firm mass
    D. Aching pain in breast prior to menstruation

15. Medical treatment of fibrocystic breast disease (FBD) may include medication that inhibits anterior pituitary production of follicle-stimulating hormone and luteinizing hormone such as:
    A. Progesterone
    B. Danazol
    C. Estrogen
    D. Thyroxin

16. The primary symptom of intraductal papilloma is:

    A. Pain in both breasts

    B. Change in breast size

    C. Bleeding from the nipples

    D. Enlargement of lymph nodes

True or False

17. _____ Approximately 90% of all breast masses are found by women themselves.

18. _____ Approximately 50% of breast masses are malignant.

19. _____ Annual mammography should begin at age 50.

20. _____ If a breast biopsy is positive, surgery is performed immediately.

21. _____ When a woman develops mastitis, she has to stop nursing.

22. _____ Fibrocystic disease can affect 1 out of 2 premenopausal women.

23. _____ All women with FBD have an increased risk of developing breast cancer.

Questions

24. List four of the risk factors that have been associated with the development of breast cancer.

    1.

    2.

    3.

    4.

25. The most common site of breast cancer is the:

    A. Nipple area

    B. Lower quadrant

    C. Upper outer quadrant

    D. Inner quadrants

26. Staging of a primary breast tumor includes:

    1.

    2.

    3.

27. If a woman has a breast tumor less than 2 cm with tumor cells in 2 lymph nodes, she would be in which stage?

    A. Stage I

    B. Stage II

    C. Stage III

    D. Stage IV

28. The primary treatment of breast cancer is:

    A. Palliative therapy

    B. Chemotherapy

    C. Radiation therapy

    D. Surgical removal

29. When a patient has a left radical mastectomy, which procedure would be contraindicated?

    A. Doing arm exercises with both arms

    B. Taking blood pressure in left arm

    C. Drawing blood from right arm

    D. Elevating arm and hand on pillow

30. When might a lumpectomy be a suggested treatment option for the patient with breast cancer?

    A. When they are in Stage I or II

    B. When the tumor is small and has not spread

    C. When the tumor is localized in the nipple

    D. Anytime the patient wants it

31. A recommended treatment after lumpectomy is:

    A. Chemotherapy

    B. Hormonal therapy

    C. Antibiotic therapy

    D. Radiation therapy

32. The type of chemotherapeutic agents that interferes with DNA replication is known as a/an:

    A. Mitotic inhibitor

    B. Antimetabolites

    C. Alkylating agent

    D. Hormonal inhibitors

33. If a woman with Stage III breast cancer is found to be estrogen-receptor positive, she would most likely receive:

    A. Estrogen

B. Actinomycin

C. Prednisone

D. Tamoxifen

34. When a patient has a radioactive implant to treat breast cancer, the nurse would:

A. Provide frequent time for discussion

B. Explain that this will cure the cancer

C. Limit time spent in the room

D. Explain that pain medication is scheduled

35. Following breast reconstructive surgery, the nurse would monitor for:

A. Bleeding

B. Infection

C. Scar formation

D. All of the above

36. Write a nursing care plan for the patient who has had a modified radical mastectomy.

Nursing Diagnosis: Knowledge deficit: procedure; perioperative routines

Patient Outcome:

Nursing Interventions:

CLINICAL SITUATIONS

Situation ■ 1

Susan, age 32, was diagnosed with fibrocystic breast disease 6 years ago. Her condition is worsening and she is seeking more information.

1. Typical symptoms that Susan reports include:

A. Irregularity of breast with pain and tenderness

B. Greenish discharge and pain at nipple

C. Sharp pain in breast radiating to the back

D. Dimpling of breast tissue; nontender masses

2. Which one of the following behaviors by Susan would the nurse recommend she change?

A. I follow a low-cholesterol diet

B. I drink tea instead of coffee

C. I watch my salt intake

D. I exercise every day

3. In order to be sure that Susan does not have a malignant process, the physician:

A. Orders a mammogram

B. Orders an ultrasound

C. Orders a breast biopsy

D. Prepares for surgery

4. One of the more important things that the nurse will stress in talking with Susan is:

A. Need for yearly mammograms

B. Need to perform breast self-examination

C. Need to take entire course of antibiotics

D. Relationship between FBD and breast cancer

Situation ■ 2

Ms. Thomas, age 48, has just found out that she has breast cancer. She is scheduled for surgery in the morning.

1. What is the primary nursing diagnosis for the patient at this time?

A. Pain related to surgery

B. Anxiety related to uncertain outcome

C. Body image disturbance

D. High risk for infection

2. Because her tumor is 4 cm in size and the physician has found tumor cells in the lymph nodes, a decision is made to do a modified radical mastectomy. This means:

A. The tumor itself is excised along with the blood vessels

B. The breast, pectoralis minor muscle, and lymph nodes are removed

C. The breast, pectoralis minor and major muscles, and all adjacent lymph nodes are removed

D. The tumor and most of the breast and lymph nodes are removed

3. Following surgery, the nurse would explain the purpose of:

   A. IV therapy

   B. Arm exercises

   C. Drainage catheters

   D. All of the above

4. In order to inhibit swelling, the nurse would instruct the patient to:

   A. Sit with bed raised

   B. Elevate legs when out of bed

   C. Keep arm elevated on pillow

   D. Do coughing and deep breathing every 2 hours

Answers

■ CHAPTER ONE

Question

1. 1. Acute care medical centers

   2. Ambulatory care

   3. Clinics

   4. Out-patient department

   5. Urgent care setting

   6. Home care

2. 1. Nurse practitioner

   2. Clinical specialist

   3. Nurse anesthetist

3. A profession built on art and science, nursing involves caring for individuals with acute and chronic health care needs, in both illness and wellness; and the individual is viewed holistically

4. A measure used to evaluate the competency of care and the quality of service, which holds members of the health care profession accountable

5. American Nurses' Association

6. An aging society, care of the chronically ill, changes in reimbursement patterns, rising health care costs, technologic advances, expansion of nursing roles

7. Reimbursing nursing services, defining levels of nursing practice; promoting advances in nursing education through career paths; supporting health care reform; and utilizing technology such as a computer in practice

8. North American Nursing Diagnosis Association (NANDA)

9. 1. Patient assessment

   2. Establishment of nursing diagnosis

   3. Development of care plan

   4. Implementation of plan

   5. Evaluation of plan

10. A clinical judgment about actual or potential health problems that can be alleviated or prevented through nursing intervention.

11. 1. The first part is the diagnostic label or category.

    2. The second part is the etiology, which deals with the reason for the alteration.

    3. The third part includes the defining characteristics.

12. 1. Setting priorities

    2. Establishing expected patient outcomes

    3. Selecting nursing interventions

    4. Documenting the plan of care

13. By comparing the patient status with the stated outcome

14. The problem that poses the greatest threat to the patient's well-being

15. Was the assessment complete?

    Was the nursing diagnosis correct?

    Was the expected outcome realistic?

    Were the nursing interventions appropriate?

    Have the priorities or situation changed?

True or False

16. True

17. True

18. False

19. True

20. False

■ CHAPTER TWO

Questions

1. It enables the nurse to accurately differentiate between normal and abnormal findings.

2. A

3. C

4. B

5. C

6. C

7. 1. Decreased sweat production

   2. The loss of subcutaneous fat

   3. Diminished peripheral circulation

8. A

True or False

9. True

10. True

11. True

12. False

13. True

Questions

14. D

15. A

16. B

17. C

18. B

19. D

20. A

21. C

22. A

23. 1. Reduced gastric and intestinal motility increases the opportunity for drug interactions

   2. Increase in adipose tissue and impaired capillary function can affect absorption

   3. Reduction in hepatic and renal function changes excretion

24. C

25. 1. Instruction on how and when to take each medication.

   2. Information on expected effect and adverse effects.

   3. Importance of monitoring the effects of medication.

   4. Importance of reporting adverse reactions or lack of expected response.

   5. Information on any food or drugs to avoid.

   6. Avoid taking over-the-counter medication without consulting the physician.

Clinical Situations

Situation ■ 1

1. B

2. B

3. D

4. A

Situation ■ 2

1. B, C, G, H

2. Nursing Care Plan

   Nursing Diagnosis: Altered health maintenance related to lack of knowledge of medication regimen.

   Patient Outcome: Patient verbalizes understanding of the need to follow prescribed medication regimen prior to discharge.

   Nursing Interventions: Determine patient's readiness and ability to learn.
   Teach patient name, dose, frequency, and expected action and untoward side effects of medication.

Instruct patient to notify physician if side effects occur.

Situation ■ 3

1. A

2. 1. Instruct patient that visual changes occur with aging.

   2. Suggest that glasses be kept at the bedside and put on before arising.

   3. Explain circulatory changes, which may cause episodes of orthostatic hypotension. Teach patient to rise slowly to a sitting position and then sit at the bedside for several minutes before arising.

3. D

4. 1. Teach the patient that constipation is a long-term effect of laxative use due to decreased intestinal muscle tone.

   2. Teach that regular exercise, adequate fluids, and a high-fiber diet will prevent constipation.

   3. Encourage adequate fluid intake.

   4. Encourage establishment of a regular time for defecation.

5. A

6. 1. Explain that immobility increases pressure over bony prominences and impairs circulation.

   2. Instruct patient to sit in a chair with a padded seat.

   3. Use egg-crate or air mattress on bed.

   4. Instruct the patient to change her position every 2 hours.

■ CHAPTER THREE

Questions

1. A

2. B

3. C

4. D

5. B

6. C

7. A

8. B

9. B

10. C

11. A

12. C

13. C

14. A

15. B

16. B

17. C

18. C

19. A

20. D

21. C

22. A

23. A

24. C

25. D

26. A

27. B

28. B

29. C

30. A

31. B

32. A

33. B

34. B

35. C

36. A

37. B

38. 1. A

    2. D

    3. C

    4. B

39. Laboratory Values

Potassium:	3.5–5.3 mEq/L
Sodium:	135–145 mEq/L
Serum calcium:	4.5–5.5 mEq/L
Ionized calcium:	2.2–2.5 mEq/L
Magnesium:	1.5–2.5 mEq/L

True or False

40. True

41. True

42. False

43. True

44. True

45. False

46. False

47. True

48. False

49. False

50. False

51. False

52. False

Clinical Situations

Situation ■ 1

1. A

2. C

3. B

4. Nursing Care Plan

Nursing diagnosis: Fluid volume excess related to excessive fluid retention.

Patient Outcome: Vital signs are within the patient's baseline.
Breath sounds are clear.
Extremities are free of edema.

Nursing Interventions: Monitor vital signs and breath sounds.
Check for the presence of edema.
Monitor weight daily.
Restrict fluid and sodium intake.
Administer medications as ordered.

Situation ■ 2

1. A

2. A

3. A

4. C

Situation ■ 3

1. Oranges   Broccoli
   Spinach   Tomatoes
   Potatoes

2. C

3. A

4. B

Situation ■ 4

1. A

2. B

3. B

4. C

5. C

Situation ■ 5

1. A

2. C

3. A

4. C

5. C

6. B

■ CHAPTER FOUR

Define

1. Implies that the patient or legal guardian has been informed by the physician of the nature, risks, desired results, and possible complications associated with the procedure.

2. Refers to emergency treatment that is performed without written permission when it is believed that the individual would have given permission if competent.

3. An anesthetic agent that is deposited directly in the area to be anesthetized or along a nerve or nerve pathway to the CNS to block the pain stimulus.

4. Injection of anesthetic agent directly into a vein or by inhalation of the gas.

5. Rare but potentially fatal complication of surgery. It is a hypermetabolic crisis triggered by administration of certain anesthetic agents, and is characterized by a rapid rise of body temperature.

Questions

6. As a witness, the nurse is verifying that the patient has signed the form voluntarily and understands the procedure he or she is signing consent for.

7. Physician

8. Federal Patient Self Determination Act

9. 1. Extent of the surgery
   2. Urgency of the surgery
   3. Surgical approach

10. CBC

    Electrolytes

    Coagulation studies

    Chest x-ray

    Electrocardiogram

11. Narcotics: to minimize pain and supplement the action of general anesthesia

    Barbiturates: to provide sedation

    Tranquilizers: to provide sedation and reduce anxiety

    Antihistamines: to provide sedation

    Anticholinergic: to reduce oral, respiratory, and gastric secretions

12. Surgeon

    Surgical assistant

    Anesthesiologist

    Scrub assistant

    Circulating nurse

13. Topical: sprays, gargles to surface area to be anesthetized

    Local infiltrate: injection of agent into subcutaneous tissue

    Nerve block: injection of agent into and around the nerve

    Epidural block: injection of agent into epidural space for rectal or vaginal procedures

    Spinal: injection of agent into subarachnoid space

14. 1. Hypothermia

2. Hypotension

3. Hypoxia

15. 1. Stable vital signs

2. Patient must be awake and able to answer simple questions

3. Airway is patent

4. Spontaneous respirations are present

5. Gag reflex is present

6. Pain minimal

7. Postoperative complications resolved or controlled

16. 1. Patient maintains adequate tissue perfusion as evidenced by pulse 60–100

2. BP stable

3. Capillary refill < 3 seconds

4. Urine output > 30 ml/hr

5. Patient is easily aroused, oriented

17. A

18. C

19. D

20. A

21. B

22. B

23. C

24. C

25. D

26. C

27. B

28. A

29. C

30. D

31. A

32. B

33. C

34. Impaired, impaired, diminished

True or False

35. False

36. True

37. False

38. True

39. False

40. False

41. False

42. True

43. True

44. False

45. True

Clinical Situations

Situation ■ 1

1. Patient Outcome

1. Patient asks questions and verbalizes concerns.

2. Patient states feelings of apprehension have decreased.

2. Interventions

1. Provide opportunity for the patient to express thoughts and concerns.

2. Encourage questions to demonstrate interest and concern.

3. Reinforce the physician's explanation of planned surgery.

4. Provide appropriate referrals if indicated.

3. A,B,D

4. A

5. B

6. C

Situation ■ 2

1. 1. High risk for ineffective breathing patterns

   2. High risk for fluid volume deficit

   3. Pain related to surgical incision

   4. High risk for injury

   5. High risk for altered nutrition

2. C

3. C

4. B

■ CHAPTER FIVE

Questions

1. 1. Denial

   2. Anger

   3. Bargaining

   4. Depression

   5. Acceptance

2. Developing an awareness of impending death

   Balancing hope and fear

   Relinquishing the will to live

   Letting go of autonomous control

   Detaching from former relationships

   Achieving spiritual preparation

3. Patient Outcome: Patient demonstrates aware-

ness of dying through verbalization.
Patient prepares spiritually for death.

Nursing Interventions: Provide opportunities for discussion.
Use therapeutic communication.
Display respect and caring for the patient.
Provide the patient with short-term achievable goals.
Provide opportunities to discuss religious beliefs.

4. Patient Outcome: The person reaches out appropriately to others for support, comfort, and assistance.
The person openly ventilates, projects, and displaces anger and guilt.
The person gradually demonstrates an acceptance of the death.

Nursing Interventions: Provide opportunity for the family to say farewell with visual and tactile contact.
Provide strong support and protection of the bereaved.
Demonstrate empathy, patience, and tolerance during the anger phase.
Encourage contact with self-help organizations.
Provide opportunities to discuss the deceased person.
Actively listen and offer emotional support.

5. C

6. D

7. B

8. A

9. C

10. B

11. B

12. Patient Outcome: The person openly expresses unresolved feelings of guilt, anger, and despair and actively seeks ways to complete mourning.

Nursing Interventions: Listen actively.
Provide opportunities for the individual to express feelings.
Offer referrals for counseling as appropriate.
Refer the bereaved person to support groups.

True or False

13. False

14. False

15. True

16. True

17. False

18. False

19. True

20. True

21. True

22. False

Matching

23. D

24. A

25. F

26. F

27. A

28. H

29. B

30. A

31. D

32. G

33. B

34. B

35. C

Questions

36. Patient Outcome: The patient participates in religious practices with clergy. The patient openly expresses religious concerns and seeks answers from clergy, nurses, or other members of his or her faith.

Nursing Interventions: Act as an advocate in regard to religious practices.
Explore the possibility of praying with the patient.
Encourage religious practices and rituals at the patient's bedside.
Engage in open, nonjudgmental, and empathetic communication.
Encourage family visits by loved ones and other members of the religious community.

37. It should be autonomous and offer a comprehensive program of care by a health team educated in thanatology. The goal should be to control symptoms, thus enabling the patient to complete his or her lifework and die in peace and dignity.

38. A sense of peace
A freedom from pain
An awareness of leaving the physical body
A sense of floating
Movement through a tunnel into a light
A final viewing of one's life in a noncritical way.

39. 1. Unreceptivity and unresponsiveness even to pain.

2. No spontaneous breathing for 1 hour, no breathing if off ventilator for 3 minutes.

3. No reflexes.

4. A flat EEG

5. Tests are the same 24 hours later.

6. Cannot have hypothermia or a central nervous system depression from a drug overdose.

Clinical Situations

Situation ■ 1

1. A

2. B

3. C

4. D

5. D

6. C

■ CHAPTER SIX

Identify

1. Refer to text, Figure 6–1.

Matching

2. E

3. A

4. F

5. B

6. C

7. D

8. C

9. G

Questions

10. 1. Skin color

2. Turgor

3. Temperature

4. Sensation

Define

11. Macule: a flat lesion characterized by a change in skin color; flat; nonpalpable.

12. Papule: a raised lesion that is less than 1 cm; palpable; firm.

13. Cyst: an elevated, encapsulated mass in the dermis or the subcutaneous layer; fluid, semifluid, or solid content.

14. Ulcer: a deeper open lesion that is devoid of epidermis.

15. Wheal: a transient, irregularly shaped elevation of the skin.

16. Vesicle: a lesion with a cavity that contains free fluid.

Identify

17. Macule

18. Vesicle

19. Wheal

20. Papule

21. Cyst

22. Ulcer

Fill In

23. Papule

24. Staphylococcal

25. Acne

26. Hive, urticaria

27. Eczema or impetigo

28. Skin atrophy

Questions

29. B

30. A

31. C

32. D

33. A

34. B

35. A

36. D

37. C

True or False

38. True

39. True

40. True

41. True

42. True

43. False

44. True

45. True

Questions

46. A

47. B

48. C

49. B

50. C

51. C

52. C

53. Patient Outcome: Spreading erythema around the graft is absent.
    Purulent drainage is absent.
    Foul odor from the graft site is absent.

    Nursing interventions: Use aseptic technique.
    Change dressing as per order.
    Instruct patient on the proper technique.

54. C

55. C

56. D

57. A

58. A

59. A

60. D

61. C

62. C

63. B

64. B

65. A

Clinical Situations

Situation ■ 1

1. D

2. B

3. C

4. A

5. C

6. D

Situation ■ 2

1. A

2. B

3. B

4. A

5. C

Situation ■ 3

1. Wear pressure garments as directed over the recipient site.

2. Elevate the upper arm to prevent swelling.

3. Wear warm clothing; avoid exposure to sunlight or heat.

4. Massage the graft and donor sites with lanolin to soften the skin, decrease itching, and increase circulation.

■ CHAPTER SEVEN

Matching

1. I

2. G

3. A

4. D

5. J

6. C

7. F

8. H

9. B

10. E

Fill In

11. Hair follicle by *Staphylococcus aureus*

12. Staphylococci or streptococci

13. Dermatophyte (tinea) or nondermatophyte (yeast)

14. Human papillomavirus

True or False

15. True

16. False

17. False

18. True

19. False

20. False

21. False

22. True

23. True

24. True

Questions

25. B

26. D

27. C

28. B

29. C

30. E

31. B

32. C

33. B

34. C

35. A

36. A

37. C

38. C

39. B

40. C

41. A

42. C

Define

43. Flesh-colored, tan, or brown round or oval papules or plaques that appear greasy and pasted to the skin

44. Sebaceous cyst whose wall is lined with keratin-secreting epithelial cells

45. Yellowish plaques on the eyelids

46. Excessive proliferation of scar tissue in response to trauma

47. Subcutaneous fat tumor

Questions

48. Avoid sunlight between 10 am and 3 pm.
Increase exposure gradually.
Apply lip balm and a sunscreen of 15 SPF or higher.
Wear protective clothing when out in the sun.
Avoid using a tanning booth.
Perform monthly self-evaluation of skin.
Report any changes in skin lesions promptly.

49. Changes in a nevus which include: asymmetry, border irregularity, change in color, surface or sensation, diameter > 6 mm.

50. Patient Outcome: Skin lesions clear.

Nursing Interventions: Instruct the patient to apply warm moist compresses for 20 minutes three times a day.
Apply astringent compresses to promote crusting.
Instruct the patient in self-administration of antibiotics.

51. Patient outcome: Patient verbalizes positive, realistic perception of self.
Patient expresses confidence in own coping ability.

Nursing Interventions: Encourage patient to express feelings about the disease and its impact on personal appearance.
Assess for behaviors that indicate negative feelings.
Teaching ways to use clothing to conceal affected area.

52. Patient Outcome: Patient verbalizes anxiety.
Patient discusses fear of malignancy.
Patient states that anxiety is reduced.

Nursing Interventions: Support patient during diagnostic and surgical procedures.
Answer questions and correct misconceptions.
Encourage patient to verbalize fears and concerns.

53. Patient Outcome: Patient describes care of the wound.
Wound heals without excessive scarring or infection.

Nursing Interventions: Instruct patient in care of the wound.
Instruct patient in specific type of solution and dressing to be used.
Instruct patient to avoid activity that might disrupt the suture line.

Clinical Situations

Situation ■ 1

1. A

2. B

3. C

4. B

Situation ■ 2

1. A

2. C

3. C

4. B

5. C

Situation ■ 3

1. A

2. C

3. A

4. A

Situation ■ 4

1. C

2. A

3. A

■ CHAPTER EIGHT

Questions

1. 1. What time did the injury occur?

   2. Was the victim in an enclosed space?

   3. How did the accident occur?

   4. Did the patient lose consciousness?

   5. Does the patient have any chronic illnesses?

2. B

Fill In

3. Blood stream into the body tissues

4. Three, sixty

Questions

5. C

6. B

7. A

Matching

8. B

9. A

10. C

11. A

12. C

13. B

14. C

15. A

16. B

17. A

18. C

True or False

19. False

20. False

21. True

22. True

23. True

24. False

25. False

26. True

Questions

27. B

28. A

29. B

30. C

31. C

32. C

33. B

34. C

35. B

36. C

37. B

38. B

39. D

40. A

41. C

42. D

43. C

44. B

45. A

46. B

47. B

Define

48. Open wound care: Wounds are covered with a topical agent; no dressing is used. This allows for easy visualization and takes less time.

49. Closed wound care: Wounds are covered by a topical agent and then covered with gauze dressing. This provides a protective barrier against infection, but may promote growth of microor-

ganisms. In addition, it is hard to see the wound.

50. Debridement: removal of dead tissue to promote the healing process

Questions

51. Patient outcome: Patient is alert, oriented, and able to follow commands.
Patient has normal skin color.
Patient's respirations are clear, unlabored and 12–20/minute.

Nursing Interventions: Encourage deep breathing, administer high flow oxygen as ordered.
Observe for changes in level of consciousness.
Monitor arterial blood gases.
Monitor respiratory status and breath sounds to detect changes in condition.

52. Patient Outcome: Patient is alert and oriented.
Patient maintains adequate hydration.

Nursing Interventions: Establish intravenous access.
Administer and document fluid replacement.
Insert Foley catheter and monitor output.
Monitor vital signs.
Monitor daily weights.
Monitor lab results.

53. Patient Outcome: Patient expresses relief from analgesics.
Pain decreases in intensity as the wounds heal.

Nursing Interventions: Assess level of pain.
Administer narcotic analgesics as needed.
Monitor response to medication.
Explain cause of pain and feelings to patient.
Keep patient informed

of the need to do procedures.

Explore the use of other techniques to reduce anxiety and enhance pain relief.

Clinical Situations

Situation ■ 1

1. C

2. C

3. A

4. C

5. C

6. A

7. B

Situation ■ 2

1. B

2. C

3. B

4. A

5. A

6. C

Situation ■ 3

1. C

2. C

3. A

4. A

■ CHAPTER NINE

Questions

1. 1. Defense
   2. Surveillance
   3. Homeostasis

2. 1. Bone marrow
   2. Lymph nodes
   3. Spleen
   4. Liver
   5. Tonsils

3. Thymus gland

4. Bone marrow

5. Spleen

6. Cellular immunity

7. A cytolytic reaction in response to virus-infected cells

8. B cells

9. T cells

Fill In

10. IgG

11. IgM

Matching

12. C

13. D

14. A

15. B

Questions

16. N

17. N

18. N

19. S

20. N

21. 1. Blood vessels in the area dilate to become more permeable to chemical mediators. More blood and lymph go to the injured area. Monocytes also phagocytize any harmful agent.

    2. Phagocytosis and exudate formation occur.

    3. Repair and regeneration of injured tissue occurs.

Define

22. Process by which a particle is ingested and digested by a cell.

23. A substance that produces a detectable immune response when introduced into a host.

24. Specialized proteins that are formed in response to an antigen and react specifically with that antigen.

25. A complex of 20 proteins that are formed in the liver and found in the serum. These proteins interact with antigen and antibody in a complex series of reactions that result in the lysis of foreign cells.

26. A reduction or depression in any aspect of the immune system's ability to respond to an antigen.

Matching

27. B

28. A

29. D

30. C

Questions

31. A

32. B

33. A

34. B

35. B

36. B

37. C

38. Active immunity, because of the presence of memory T and B lymphocytes, which can be reactivated

39. E

True or False

40. False

41. True

42. False

43. True

44. False

45. True

46. True

Questions

47. C

48. D

49. C

50. B

51. Donor

52. B

53. D

54. A

55. Flowers harbor large numbers of bacteria

56. C

57. Nursing Care Plan

Patient Outcome: Patient states why the test is being done.
Patient states where the test is being done.
Patient understands the sensations associated with the procedure.

Nursing Interventions: Explain procedure, including reasons for test, sensations felt, equipment used, length of procedure and expected outcome.

58. A

59. C

60. Because of changes in the immune system and also age-related changes in the body's other defenses

Clinical Situations

Situation ■ 1

1. C

2. B

3. A

Situation ■ 2

1. D

2. C

3. C

■ CHAPTER TEN

Fill In

1. Produce an adequate response to an antigen

2. Frequent infections, infections with unusual organisms, minor infections that don't heal

3. Primary or congenital

4. Human immunodeficiency virus (HIV)

5. Kaposi's sarcoma

6. *Pneumocystis carinii*

Questions

7. Mononucleosis-like illness

Persistent, generalized lymphadenopathy

AIDS-related complex

AIDS

AIDS-related dementia

8. 1. An acute infection such as the flu

2. Asymptomatic period lasting 2 months to 15 years

3. Transitional or symptomatic disease period

4. Period marked by development of opportunistic infections or malignancies.

9. B

10. C

11. E

12. D

13. A

14. B

True or False

15. True

16. True

17. False

18. True

19. False

20. False

21. True

22. True

23. True

24. False

Questions

25. D

26. B

27. B

28. C

29. A

30. C

31. Patient Outcome: The patient can explain what AIDS is, how it is spread, symptoms that require attention, and medical treatment options.

    Nursing Interventions: Explain what causes the disease and its method of transmission.
    Instruct the patient in self-care.
    Explain medications.
    Instruct the patient on when to seek medical attention.

Matching

32. A

33. D

34. B

35. C

Fill In

36. I

37. IV

38. II

39. III

40. Anaphylaxis

41. Antihistamines

42. Desensitization

43. Anergy

44. Autoimmunity

Questions

45. B

46. D

True or False

47. True

48. False (intrinsic)

49. True

50. True

51. False

Questions

52. A

53. A

54. A

55. B

56. D

57. B

58. A

59. Nursing Diagnosis: Ineffective breathing pattern related to bronchoconstriction

Patient Outcome: 1. The patient maintains a patent airway.
2. The patient's respiratory rate and depth are in the normal range.
3. The patient does not exhibit respiratory distress.

60. All but B

61. Antinuclear antibodies

62. A

63. B

64. D

65. C

66. C

67. C

68. Patient Outcome: The patient will express or exhibit signs of increased comfort.

Nursing Interventions: Administer analgesic and antiinflammatory drugs.
Maintain bedrest during flareup, and support the joints.
Maintain joint mobility through active and passive range-of-motion exercises.
Keep the skin lesion clean and dry.

69. Patient Outcome: Patient expresses feelings and concerns.
Patient can set priorities for activities.
Patient schedules periods of activity and rest.

Nursing Interventions: Help patient adapt to a fatigue state.
Encourage patient to express feelings, fears, and concerns.
Guide the patient to modify activities.
Stress consistency.
Explain ways to conserve energy.

Situation ■ 1

1. A

2. C

3. B

4. D

5. A

Situation ■ 2

1. B

2. C

3. B

Situation ■ 3

1. B

2. A

3. D

4. A

Situation ■ 4

1. B

2. E

3. A

4. B

5. D

■ CHAPTER ELEVEN

Define

1. Group of cells that has an abnormal growth pattern

2. Process of transforming a normal cell into a malignant cell

3. Thought to occur when a cell has undergone a permanent change from an initiating agent and is then exposed to a chemical promoter.

4. Personality with low self-esteem who sees himself or herself as a victim, lacks resiliency, and has a narrow range of personal relationships

5. Method of identifying the extent of the disease

6. Proteins and hormones that are produced by certain tumors.

Questions

7. Individuals with specific genetic characteristics may have an increased risk of certain cancers.

8. Chemicals in the environment have been shown to contribute to certain oncologic disorders.

9. Single most preventable cause of disease and death documented is the relationship between smoking and cancer.

10. Diet is still being studied, but it may be responsible for up to one third of oncologic disorders.

11. When the immune system fails, tumors can grow and spread.

12. There is a strong relationship between stress and illness. Cancer often occurs following a major loss and depression.

Matching

13. D

14. A

15. E

16. C

17. B

Questions

18. 1. Change in bowel or bladder habits

    2. A sore that does not heal

    3. Unusual bleeding or discharge

    4. Thickening or lump in the breast or elsewhere

    5. Indigestion or difficulty swallowing

    6. Obvious change in wart or mole

    7. Nagging cough or hoarseness

19. A

20. B

21. B, C

22. A,B,C

23. C

24. B

25. D

26. B

27. C

28. A

29. D

30. Patient Outcome: Patient will state an understanding of the treatment protocol associated with cancer.

    Nursing Interventions: Review the type of cancer and associated risk factors.
    Encourage the patient to ask questions.
    Explain any diagnostic tests and treatments being planned.

31. A

32. A

33. C

34. B

Matching

35. D

36. E

37. B

38. A

39. C

Questions

40. A

41. A

42. A, D

43. Skin—erythema, dry desquamation, moist des-
    quamation
    Mouth—mucositis, stomatitis
    Head—cerebral edema, alopecia
    Chest—esophagitis, pneumonitis, pulmonary
    fibrosis

44. Nursing Interventions:
    Skin—wear loose clothing to limit effects; for dry
    desquamation, use water-soluble lubricant
    Mouth—follow liquid or high-protein diet; prac-
    tice good oral hygiene

45. D

46. Patient Outcome: The patient describes expected
    effects of radiation.

    Nursing Interventions: Reinforce the purposes
    and type of treatment.
    Instruct the patient in
    self-care and comfort
    measures.

47. D

48. C

49. D

50. A

51. C

52. It is given in time intervals that allow for drug
    effectiveness and recovery from side effects

53. A,B,C,D

54. A

55. B

56. Nausea and vomiting
    Mucositis, stomatitis, esophagitis
    Diarrhea, constipation
    Skin rashes, alopecia

57. 1. Use anti-emetics
    2. Follow a good diet, adequate fluid intake, and
       perform good oral hygiene.
    3. Use lotion; may like to use wig.

58. E

59. A

60. B

61. A

62. C

63. C

64. B

65. A,B,E,F

66. Nursing Interventions:
    1. Help the patient talk about his or her feel-
       ings; the use of therapeutic communication
       is essential.
    2. Give the patient information in clear, simple
       terms.
    3. Help the patient identify steps to reduce
       anxiety.
    4. Teach the patient guided relaxation.
    5. Teach problem-solving techniques.

67. Nursing Interventions:
    1. Differentiate between psychological conflicts
       and results of medications.
    2. Explore the mate's reaction to the treatment.
    3. Discuss alternative techniques to satisfy the
       patient's needs.
    4. Make referrals to counseling.

68. Nursing Interventions:
    1. Discuss ways to enable the patient to make
       decisions and actively participate in planning
       for the future.

2. Involve the patient in decision-making.

3. Explore support groups.

4. Explore and encourage spiritual support.

69. B

70. A

71. Pain is a subjective individualized event that represents several interrelated sensory, affective, and personal factors.

72. B

73. B

74. C

75. Patient Outcome: Patient uses appropriate methods of pain control.

Nursing Interventions: Implement measures to alleviate and control pain, such as medication and adjunct therapy.
Monitor response to intervention and any side effects.

Clinical Situations

Situation ■ 1

1. A

2. D

3. A

Situation ■ 2

1. A

2. A

3. B

4. D

Situation ■ 3

1. C

2. A

3. B

4. D

5. B

■ CHAPTER TWELVE

Questions

1. 1. Nasal cavity

2. Sinuses

3. Nasopharynx

4. Pharynx

5. Larynx

2. 1. Trachea

2. Bronchi

Identify

3. Refer to text, Figure 12–2.

Fill In

4. Active

5. Passive

6. Expands downward

7. The respiratory center in the medulla is stimulated by concentrations of carbon dioxide. It also responds slightly to a deficiency of oxygen.

8. Elastic

9. Stretched

10. Alveolar membrane

11. Cellular level

12. Hemoglobin

Questions

13. 1. Heart action
    2. Blood pressure

14. 1. Cough
    2. Excessive nasal secretions
    3. Sputum production
    4. Pain
    5. Dyspnea
    6. Fatigue

15. C

16. A

17. A

18. A

19. D

Matching

20. C

21. B

22. A

23. D

Questions

24. D

25. B

26. B

27. B

28. A

29. A

30. A

31. E

32. C

Define

33. Increase in the depth of respirations

34. Increase in both the depth and rate of respirations

35. Rapid, deep breathing

36. Cycle of apnea and hyperpnea

37. Respirations which vary in depth with irregular periods of apnea

38. Abnormal prominence of the sternum with an increased anteroposterior diameter

39. Chest appears rounded with the sternum pulled forward

40. Exaggerated curvature of the thoracic spine

41. Exaggerated curvature of the lumbar spine

42. Lateral deformity of the spine

Questions

43. B

44. C

Matching

45. C

46. A

47. B

48. B

49. A

50. C

Questions

51. C

52. A

53. A

Identify

54. D

55. A

56. A

57. B

58. C

59. A

60. A

Matching

61. B

62. A

63. C

64. D

65. E

66. F

Questions

67. B

68. A

69. C

70. B

71. C

72. B

73. Changes in vital signs; faintness; vertigo; chest tightness; uncontrolled cough; blood-tinged frothy mucus

74. 1. Pursed lip breathing
    2. Diaphragmatic breathing

75. C

76. D

Fill In

77. Vibration

78. Postural drainage

Questions

79. B

80. 1. Follow guidelines for proper inflation
    2. Avoid putting any traction on the tubing or connectors
    3. Check the cuff inflation to prevent necrosis
    4. Deflate the cuff every 2 hours if it is not a low-pressure tube

81. E

82. C

83. C

84. The patient cannot ventilate adequately to maintain proper levels of oxygen and carbon dioxide in the blood.

Define

85. Assist control—the patient's respiratory effort triggers the machine.

    Tidal volume—the volume of gas delivered

Questions

86. A

87. Call the physician immediately.

88. A

89. 10

90. B

91. Using a word board, a pad and pencil, a computer, and pictures.

92. D

93. C

94. A

95. B

96. Nursing Diagnosis: Ineffective breathing patterns

   Patient Outcome: Arterial blood gases within the patient's normal range.

   Nursing Interventions: Maintain oxygen
   Keep head of bed elevated
   Explain all procedures
   Maintain ventilator function
   Assess breathing patterns frequently

Identify

97. Refer to text, Figure 12–29.

Questions

98. B

99. C

100. B

101. Assess the patient's respiratory status every 2 hours;
   Assess the function of the drainage system;
   Assess for fluctuation; bubbling; drainage

102. Nursing Diagnosis: Ineffective breathing patterns

   Patient Outcome: Normal breath sounds, full lung re-expansion.

   Nursing Interventions: Maintain an airtight, patent, functioning chest drainage system.
   Maintain a sterile, dry, occlusive dressing.
   Encourage the patient to cough and breathe deeply.

103. A

104. D

105. C

106. The nurse should ask about the patient's smoking history.

107. A mediastinoscope is passed through an incision made between the laryngeal prominence and the sternum.

108. B

109. Nursing Diagnosis: Knowledge deficit related to breathing exercises, effective coughing, wound splinting, and arm and shoulder exercises.

   Patient Outcome: The patient describes the role of breathing, exercises, coughing, and exercises as they relate to recovery.

   Nursing Interventions: Explain the rationale for coughing and breathing to remove secretions and facilitate ventilation.
   Demonstrate effective diaphragmatic and pursed-lip breathing.
   Demonstrate splinting of the chest.
   Demonstrate arm exercises and their rationale.

Clinical Situations

Situation ■ 1

1. B

2. A

3. C

4. B

Situation ■ 2

1. B

2. C

3. D

4. D

5. C

6. D

■ CHAPTER THIRTEEN

Matching

1. D

2. B

3. E

4. F

5. C

6. A

7. G

True or False

8. False

9. True

10. False (penicillin)

11. True

12. True

13. False

Questions

14. A

15. C

16. A

17. C

18. B

19. D (may indicate rheumatic fever)

20. B (due to difficulty swallowing)

21. C

22. D

23. A

24. C (must complete the entire course of therapy)

25. B

26. A

27. A

28. Nursing Diagnoses: High risk for aspiration
    Pain related to the surgical trauma.
    Impaired tissue integrity related to the trauma suture line.

29. D

30. B

31. B

32. C

Fill In

33. Nasal polyps

34. Submucous resection

35. Rhinoplasty

Questions

36. A

37. B

38. Heavy smoking and ingestion of alcohol

39. D

True or False

40. True

41. False

42. False

43. False

Questions

44. Patient Outcome: Patient can cough up sections. Patient has a normal respiratory rate and respiratory patterns.
    Nursing Interventions: Have patient cough and deep breathe every 2 hours.
    Use lintfree wipes to remove secretions.
    Suction as needed to keep the airway clear.
    Administer humidified air or oxygen.
    Provide tracheostomy care as needed.

Clinical Situations

Situation ■ 1

1. D

2. B

3. A

4. D

5. A

Situation ■ 2

1. C

2. B

3. C

Situation ■ 3

1. A

2. B

3. C

4. B

5. C

■ CHAPTER FOURTEEN

Define

1. Inflammation of the larger bronchi

2. An acute inflammation of the gas-exchanging units of the lungs

3. Collection of pus in the pleural cavity

4. An acute inflammation of the pleural surfaces

5. Chronic disorder with which there is an enlargement of the air spaces and destruction of the alveolar walls

Questions

6. All but C

7. B

8. D

9. A

10. D

11. C

12. C

13. 1. Hydration
    2. Proper nutrition
    3. Oxygenation
    4. Analgesic
    5. Antibiotics

14. C

15. C

16. B

17. C

18. A

19. B

20. Patient Outcome: Patient will have normal blood gases.
Patient will have normal breathing patterns, as evidenced by normal respiratory rate and rhythm and clear breath sounds.

Nursing Interventions: Turn the patient every 2 hours
Encourage coughing and deep breathing every 2 hours
Suction the lungs if needed
Promote adequate fluid intake
Administer supplemental oxygen as ordered

21. 1. Elevate the bed at least 30 degrees

2. Check for proper tube placement

3. Check the amount of residual every 4 hours

22. A

23. C

24. B

25. A and D

26. B and C

27. B

28. A

Fill In

29. Mycobacterium

True or False

30. True

31. True

32. False

33. False (only in about 10%)

34. True

Questions

35. C

36. D

37. B (medical chemotherapy often lasts more than a year)

38. Patient Outcome: Patient can state when the disease is infectious.
Patient can explain the method of transmission.
Patient can describe precautions to take to prevent transmission.

Nursing Interventions: Teach the patient how tuberculosis is spread and how to protect others from it. Explain the principles of handwashing, avoiding face-to-face contact, and ways to prevent droplet transmission.

39. D

40. A

41. B

42. A

43. C

44. E

45. B

46. D

47. D

48. A

49. B

50. B

51. A

52. A

53. D

54. A, C, D

55. C

True or False

56. True

57. False

58. True

59. False

60. True

61. False

Questions

62. 1. Patient Outcome: The patient uses the nebulizer and medication as ordered.
The patient uses effective breathing techniques.

   Nursing Interventions: Administer bronchodilator drugs as needed.
Administer aerosol as needed.
Instruct the patient on the proper use of medication.
Explain the need to monitor therapeutic effect of medication. Force fluids, up to 2 to 3 liters per day, to replace fluid loss.

   2. Patient Outcome: The patient practices consciously controlling the inspiration: expiration ratio when short of breath.
Patient uses diaphragmatic breathing to control dyspnea.

   Nursing Interventions: Teach breathing techniques, which promote good ventilation, ease the work of breath-

ing, and control dyspnea.

Define

63. The permanent abnormal dilation and distortion of the bronchi

64. Partial or complete collapse of the lung tissue

65. Occlusion of the pulmonary artery or branches

66. The presence of air in the pleural cavity

67. The presence of blood in the pleural cavity

68. Air that has escaped from the lung enters the subcutaneous space.

69. A specific disease that is produced by exposure to silica.

70. A disease that is the result of prolonged exposure to coal dust.

Questions

71. C

72. B

73. C

74. C

75. D

76. A

77. D

78. A, B, D

79. A, B, D

80. Chest tube; intrapleural

81. Patient Outcome: The patient will exhibit arterial blood gases within the normal range.

   Nursing Interventions: Position the patient in a semi-Fowler's position

Encourage the patient to cough and breathe deeply

Administer oxygen therapy

Maintain a proper setup of an intrapleural drainage system

82. A

83. B

84. D

85. C

True or False

86. True

87. True

88. False

89. False

Questions

90. Patient Outcome: Patient discusses concerns and feelings with a support person.

Nursing Interventions: Provide opportunities for the patient to express anxieties.
Instruct the patient in relaxation techniques.
Provide diversional therapy.
Assist the patient in identifying available support systems.

Clinical Situations

Situation ■ 1

1. C

2. A

3. B

4. A

5. B

6. A

7. D

Situation ■ 2

1. A

2. B

3. C

4. B

5. A

Situation ■ 3

1. B, C, D

2. D

3. C

4. B

■ CHAPTER FIFTEEN

Questions

1. 1. It transports oxygen to the cells and carries carbon dioxide to the lungs for removal.

2. It carries nutrients to the tissues and removes waste products.

3. It transports hormones from the endocrine glands.

4. It protects against infection by carrying leukocytes and antibodies to the site of infection.

5. It regulates the body temperature.

2. 1. Blood

2. Lymph nodes

3. Bone marrow

4. Spleen

5. Liver

Matching

3. D

4. B

5. E

6. A

7. F

8. C

9. B

Questions

10. A

11. C

Fill In

12. WBC	5–10000 cu mm
13. RBC	4.2–5.4 million/cu mm (male)
	3.6–5.0 million/cu mm (female)
14. Hematocrit	40–54% (male)
	37–47% (female)
15. Hemoglobin	14–16.5 g/100 ml (male)
	12–15 g/100 ml (female)
16. Platelet count	150,000–350,000/cu mm
17. PT	8–12 seconds
18. PTT	30–45 seconds
19. Serum iron	80–160 μ/dl (males)
	50–150 μ/dl (females)

Matching

20. D

21. C

22. E

23. A

24. C

25. B, D, E

26. B

27. B, C, D

Questions

28. B

29. A

30. D

31. C

32. A

33. D

34. B

35. B

36. D

37. B

38. A

39. A

40. D

41. B

42. B

Define

43. Caused by an infusion of ABO-incompatible blood

44. Caused by sensitivity to the donor's platelets, proteins, or white blood cells

45. Caused by sensitivity to plasma protein

46. Caused by the infusion of a specific protein to a patient who is deficient in the protein but who has antibodies to it

47. Occurs when a patient receives contaminated blood

True or False

48. True

49. False

50. False

51. True

52. True

53. True

Questions

54. Patient Outcome: Patient follows regimen of planned activities and rest periods.
Patient can complete daily activities without signs of fatigue.

    Nursing Interventions: Instruct the patient to develop a regimen of activity with frequent rest periods.
Teach patient energy saving techniques and ways to conserve energy. Encourage good nutrition.

55. Patient Outcome: Patient's extremities are warm with good color and palpable pulses.
Patient's laboratory studies are within normal limits.

    Nursing Interventions: Encourage rest periods to conserve oxygen. Administer oxygen if needed. Elevate the bed. Utilize range of motion to stimulate circulation. Discourage smoking. Avoid constrictive clothing.

Clinical Situations

Situation ■ 1

1. B

2. A

3. C

4. D

Situation ■ 2

1. A

2. B

3. A

4. C

Situation ■ 3

1. B

2. A

3. B

4. A

■ CHAPTER SIXTEEN

Matching

1. F

2. C

3. A

4. D

5. G

6. B

7. E

8. H

Questions

9. D

10. C

11. B

12. A

13. A

14. D

15. B

16. B

17. C

18. C

19. B

20. D

21. B

22. B

23. C

24. A

25. A

26. D

27. D

28. C

29. C

30. B

31. C

32. B

33. A

34. B

35. A

36. D

Matching

37. C

38. A

39. A

40. B

41. C

42. C

Questions

43. Patient Outcome: Patient's vital signs and laboratory studies are within normal limits for the patient. Patient exhibits no signs of infection.

    Nursing Interventions: Restrict visitors. Use protective isolation. Monitor the vital signs frequently. Promote good nutrition. Provide good oral care. Teach patient the signs of infection.

44. Patient Outcome: Patient's vital signs are within normal ranges for patient with no signs of cyanosis dyspnea, tachypnea, or tachycardia. The patient can perform activities of daily living without respiratory distress.

    Nursing Interventions: Instruct the patient to turn and cough and deep breathe every hour to prevent respiratory infection and increase oxygen intake. Teach the patient to use full chest expansion. Keep head of bed elevated. Promote good nutrition. Administer oxygen as needed.

Clinical Situations

Situation ■ 1

1. C

2. B

3. A

4. B

5. D

Situation ■ 2

1. B

2. A

3. C

4. B

Situation ■ 3

1. C

2. A

3. D

4. B

■ CHAPTER SEVENTEEN

Identify

1–14. Refer to text, Figure 17–3.

Questions

15. The heart's function is to pump blood through the vessels to all body tissues.

16. Venous (unoxygenated) blood returns to the right atrium, passes through the tricuspid valve to the right ventricle, through the pulmonary valve and the pulmonary artery and into lungs, where carbon dioxide is exchanged for oxygen. Oxygenated blood returns by the pulmonary veins to the left atrium, through the mitral valve, to the left ventricle. It is then pumped through the aortic valve through the aorta to the body.

Fill In

17. Coronary arteries

Questions

18. 1. Intrinsic method of control: the more blood in the ventricles, the more blood that will be pumped during systole

    2. Neutral control: results from a combination of sympathetic, parasympathetic, and baroceptor reflex nerve function

    3. Humoral control: accomplished by the release of epinephrine and norepinephrine

Identify

19. Refer to text, Figure 17–7.

Questions

20. 1. P wave: atrial depolarization

    2. PR interval: time it takes impulse to pass from SA node to AV node to ventricular myocardium

    3. QRS complex: ventricular depolarization as well as the period of atrial repolarization

    4. T wave: repolarization (recovery) of ventricular muscle

Matching

21. C

22. A

23. D

24. B

25. D

26. C

Define

27. CVP: right atrial pressure

28. PAP: gives information about the pressure in the left side of the heart

29. PWP: indication of the left ventricular end diastolic pressure

30. CO: amount of blood propelled forward by the heart

Questions

31. 1. Nonmodifiable: positive family history; increasing age; male sex

    2. Modifiable: hyperlipidemia; high blood pressure; diabetes mellitus; obesity; smoking; use of oral contraceptives; sedentary lifestyle; stress

32. B

33. D

34. A

35. B

36. D

37. A

38. B

39. B

40. B

41. C

42. A

43. D

44. C

45. B

46. A

47. Patient Outcome: The patient maintains adequate cardiac output as evidenced by hemodynamic monitoring normal for patient.

    Nursing Interventions: Monitor vital signs and hemodynamic indicators every 2 to 4 hours. Encourage frequent rest periods. Instruct the patient to stop activity if pain occurs. Monitor cardiac rhythm. Monitor intake and output. Monitor peripheral pulses.

48. Patient Outcome: Patient verbalizes decreased feelings of fatigue and demonstrates an increased activity level.

    Nursing Interventions: Instruct the patient on energy-saving techniques. Allow for planned periods of rest. Encourage good nutrition. Administer medication that improves the oxygen supply.

49. Patient Outcome: Patient relates accurate information about signs and symptoms of complications and when to seek medical attention.

    Nursing Interventions: Describe the potential complications of surgery such as bleeding, cardiac arrhythmias, respiratory distress, or infection. Explain home-care restrictions. Explain the need to avoid lifting heavy objects. Explain the need for good nutrition.

Clinical Situations

Situation ■ 1

1. A
2. D
3. D
4. A

Situation ■ 2

1. C
2. B
3. D
4. A
5. D

■ CHAPTER EIGHTEEN

Define

1. Inflammation of the endocardium and the heart valves

2. Inflammation of the heart muscle

3. Inflammation of the sac surrounding the heart, the pericardium

4. Occurs when the cardiac output is not sufficient to meet the body's demands

5. Results from complete obstruction of a coronary artery

6. Disease of the heart muscle

7. Organized method of providing cardiac or respiratory support to a victim of cardiac arrest

Questions

8. B
9. A
10. D
11. B
12. D
13. D
14. C
15. A
16. B
17. A
18. A
19. C
20. B
21. C
22. A
23. B
24. D
25. C
26. B
27. D
28. D
29. A
30. B
31. A
32. C
33. B
34. D
35. A
36. B
37. A

True or False

38. True

39. False

40. True

41. False

42. True

43. True

44. True

Questions

45. Patient Outcome: Patient's vital signs are within acceptable range for this patient.
Patient is free of dysrhythmias.

Nursing Interventions: Monitor vital signs at rest and upon activity.
Encourage rest periods.
Keep the environment quiet.
Monitor cardiac status.
Monitor intake and output.
Monitor urine output.

46. Patient Outcome: Patient verbalizes an understanding of heart disease and his or her current condition.
Patient verbalizes an understanding of the need to make lifestyle changes.

Nursing Interventions: Explain the cause and effects of myocardial infarction.
Instruct patient on medication, diet, and any lifestyle changes.
Alert patient to signs and symptoms of complications.

Clinical Situations

Situation ■ 1

1. D

2. B

3. A

4. A

5. C

6. D

Situation ■ 2

1. A

2. B

3. D

4. B

■ CHAPTER NINETEEN

Matching

1. E

2. B

3. A

4. F

5. D

6. C

Questions

7. 1. Diameter of the vessel
   2. Elastic recoil
   3. Viscosity of the blood

8. C

9. C

10. A

11. C

12. A

13. C

14. B

15. B

16. B

17. C

18. B

19. A

20. C

21. D

22. C

Fill In

23. Sympathectomy

24. Embolectomy

25. Endarterectomy

26. Amputation

Questions

27. Patient Outcome: Patient verbalizes a decrease in the level of pain.

    Nursing Interventions: Assess things which precipitate pain.
    Position the patient for pain relief:
    Keep extremities dependent for arterial insufficiency;
    Keep extremities elevated for venous disorders.
    Administer and evaluate the effectiveness of analgesics.
    Teach relaxation exercises.
    Teach a gradual exercise program to the patient.

28. Patient Outcome: Patient exhibits a palpable pulse, adequate temperature sensation, and color in extremities.

    Nursing Interventions: Monitor neurocirculatory status for signs of reocclusion.
    Assess pulses.
    Assess extremities for color, sensation, and temperature.
    Keep extremity straight for 24 hours and position patient off the graft site.
    Notify physician of any abnormalities.

Clinical Situations

Situation ■ 1

1. C

2. B

3. B

4. D

Situation ■ 2

1. D

2. A

3. D

4. C

5. D

■ CHAPTER TWENTY

Questions

1. 1. A diet high in sodium, fats

   2. Smoking

   3. A sedentary lifestyle

   4. Obesity

   5. Heredity

Matching

2. H
3. E
4. I
5. D
6. A
7. B
8. F
9. G
10. C

Questions

11. B
12. C
13. C
14. C
15. B
16. D
17. D
18.
  1. Avoid exposure to cold temperatures or dampness
  2. Wear protective clothing when out in the cold
  3. Use relaxation exercises to reduce stress
  4. Cease smoking
  5. Stop activity during an episode of vasospasm
19. A
20. B
21. A
22. C
23. B
24. C
25. A
26. A
27. C
28. A
29. C
30. B
31. D
32. B
33. A
34. A
35. A
36. C
37. A
38. C

True or False

39. True
40. True
41. True
42. False
43. False
44. True
45. True

Questions

46. Patient Outcome: Patient has increased perfusion as evidenced by warm, dry skin, strong pulses, absence of edema, and cyanosis in the extremities.

Nursing Interventions: Encourage balanced periods of rest and activity.
Discourage smoking.
Remove constrictive clothing.
Administer vasodilators as ordered.
Teach lifestyle changes that will promote good circulation.

47. Patient Outcome: Patient describes the cause, effects, and risk factors associated with thrombophlebitis.
Patient describes the self-care and the need to treat the disorder and prevent complications.

Nursing Interventions: Explain the cause, effects, and course of disease.
Teach the patient the signs and symptoms of the disease and its possible complications.
Teach the type, dosage, and side effects of medications.
Teach comfort and therapeutic measures.

Clinical Situations

Situation ■ 1

1. C

2. B

3. C

4. A

5. B

6. C

7. B

Situation ■ 2

1. B

2. B

3. D

4. C

■ CHAPTER TWENTY-ONE

Fill In

1. Saliva

2. Peritoneum

3. Peristalsis

4. Pyloric sphincter

5. Vitamin B_{12}

6. Negative; pH

7. Chyme

8. Duodenum, jejunum, and ileum

9. Small intestine

10. Bile

11. Large intestine

12. 1. Storage and metabolism of nutrients
    2. Detoxication of noxious substances
    3. Production of bile

13. Store and concentrate

14. Pancreas

Matching

15. B

16. A

17. D

18. C

Questions

19. C

20. E

21. B

22. A

23. C

24. C

25. A

26. B

Matching

27. D

28. F

29. B

30. E

31. B

32. C

33. G

34. D

35. A

36. C

Questions

37. D

38. C

39. C

40. B

41. C

42. A

43. B

44. C

Matching

45. C

46. A

47. B

48. C

49. B

Questions

50. 1. To remove contents by suction or drainage
    2. To instill irrigating solution or medications
    3. To administer enteral feedings

51. B

52. A

53. C

54. C

55. A

56. D

57. B

58. D

59. C

60. B

61. B

62. 1. Infection
    2. Hypoglycemia
    3. Hyperglycemia

63. A

64. B

65. C

66. C

67. 1. Infection

    2. Wound dehiscence

    3. Paralytic ileus

    4. Atelectasis

    5. Urinary infection

68. A

69. A, B, D, E

70. A

71. D

72. C

73. D

74. B

75. A

76. D

77. B

78. C

79. E

80. C

81. B

82. B

83. A

84. Nursing Diagnosis: Knowledge deficit related to appearance and function of the colostomy, and the need for learning self-care measures

    Patient Outcome: The patient will be able to demonstrate how to care for the colostomy.

Nursing Interventions: Provide the patient with basic information about the function of the colostomy; include a drawing. Define terms such as stoma, appliance, and pouch. Explain the daily routine for self-care. Demonstrate the procedure. Allow the patient time to ask questions. Have the patient practice the procedure.

85. Patient Outcome: Patient practices relaxation as instructed. Patient expresses an optimistic view about the surgical outcome.

    Nursing Diagnosis: Anxiety

    Nursing Interventions: Reassure patient that anxiety is normal. Reassure patient about the surgical outcome, if appropriate. Discuss surgery in general terms, including the frequency that the physician performs the operation, and positive outcomes. Review relaxation techniques. Maintain a quiet, calm environment.

    Patient Outcome: Patient describes pre- and postoperative procedures. The patient describes the importance of coughing and deep breathing.

    Nursing Diagnosis: Knowledge deficit

    Nursing Interventions: Review the preoperative preparation. Explain all tests and procedures as appropriate. Explain the specifics of the postoperative course, including the equipment (IV, NG, dressing, etc.). Explain the usual diet and activity orders.

86. Nursing Diagnosis: Pain

Patient Outcome: Patient moves without signs of severe pain.
Patient rests quietly without signs of discomfort.
Patient states that pain is relieved.

Nursing Interventions: Administer pain medications as ordered. Keep the bed elevated to decrease the pull on the incision. Splint the incision when the patient is turning or coughing. Encourage relaxation.

Nursing Diagnosis: Ineffective breathing

Patient Outcome: The patient can cough and breathe deeply as instructed. The patient has no cyanosis. The patient has a normal respiratory rate and normal arterial blood gases.

Nursing Interventions: Have the patient turn, cough, and deep breathe every 2 hours. Splint the incision. Medicate as needed. Encourage ambulation.

87. Patient Outcome: Patient consumes a 1200-calorie diet per day.

Nursing Interventions: Offer foods that are well liked and that meet the patient's nutritional needs. Encourage the patient's family to provide favorite foods. Serve food in small portions in an attractive setting. Keep the environment calm, neat, and free of odors or offensive sights.

88. Patient Outcome: Oral mucous membrane is pink and moist. Lips are supple, moist, and free of cracks.

Nursing Interventions: Provide good mouth care. Use a soft toothbrush to avoid trauma. Avoid lemon and glycerine swabs and mouthwash that contains alcohol. Apply a water-soluble lubricant to lips. Use saline gargle and anesthetic throat lozenges as ordered.

Clinical Situations

Situation ■ 1

1. A
2. B
3. C
4. B
5. C

Situation ■ 2

1. A
2. B
3. A
4. B
5. A

Situation ■ 3

1. A
2. C
3. A
4. B

■ CHAPTER TWENTY-TWO

Define

1. Inflammation of the esophagus

2. Inflammation of the stomach mucosa

3. Break in the mucosa in any part of the GI tract

4. Unique form of a peptic ulcer, caused by stress

5. Protrusion of part of the stomach into the thoracic cavity

6. A motor disorder of the lower two-thirds of the esophagus, where the lower esophageal sphincter cannot relax and allow food to pass into the stomach

7. Abnormal increase in nonperistaltic contractions and overall weak muscular contraction in the esophagus

8. Absence of hydrochloric acid

Questions

9. 1. Smoking
   2. Intake of alcohol
   3. Ingestion of spicy food
   4. Ingestion of caustic agents

10. 1. Burning
    2. Retrosternal discomfort
    3. Pain on swallowing
    4. Eructation

Matching

11. B

12. B

13. C

14. A

15. C

16. A

Questions

17. All

18. A, C, D

19. B

20. D

21. B

22. C

23. A

24. C

25. B

True or False

26. False (they cause constipation)

27. True

28. True

29. False (there is no specific treatment)

30. True

31. False

32. True

33. False

34. False

35. False

36. True

37. False

38. False

Questions

39. C

40. A

41. D

42. A

43. C

44. C

45. A

46. D

47. A

48. B

49. A, B, C

50. C

51. D

52. C

53. B, C

54. D

55. B

56. A

57. B

58. C

59. A

60. D

61. A

62. B

63. C

64. A

65. All are factors

66. C

67. B

68. C

69. D

70. B

71. B (avoid sticky foods)

72. Patient Outcome: Patient can state proper self-administration of medi- cations. Patient states that discomfort has been de- creased.

Nursing Interventions: Administer antacids or other prescribed medi- cations. Encourage the use of relaxation tech- niques. Teach the pa- tient not to smoke or drink alcohol. Have the patient follow a diet that includes nonirri- tating foods.

73. Nursing Diagnosis: Pain related to the irritating effects of gastric juices on in- jured tissue

Patient Outcome: Patient states that pain is re- lieved (in acute phase of illness).

Nursing Interventions: Administer medications as ordered (antacids, histamine antagonists, analgesics). Encourage patient to avoid smok- ing. Teach patient to avoid those foods which cause an exacerbation of pain. Teach patient to drink 6–8 glasses of wa- ter daily.

74. Nursing Diagnosis: Alteration in nutrition: less than body requirements

Patient Outcome: The patient will take in enough calories to meet basic body requirements.
The patient will maintain normal body weight.
The patient will maintain normal nitrogen balance.

Nursing Interventions: Provide a high protein, high caloric diet.
Provide supplemental tube feeding or TPN if needed.
Teach the patient to eat slowly and eat a small amount.
Provide privacy and an environment conducive to eating.

Clinical Situations

Situation ■ 1

1. A

2. C

3. B

4. A

Situation ■ 2

1. B

2. C

3. D

4. A, B, C

Situation ■ 3

1. B

2. A

3. B

Situation ■ 4

1. A

2. A

3. B

4. C

■ CHAPTER TWENTY-THREE

Define

1. Inflammation of the peritoneum (a thin membrane which lines the abdominal cavity)

2. Acute inflammation of vermiform appendix

3. Movement of intestinal contents is impaired

4. Inflammation of the mucosal outpouches on the muscular walls of the intestine

5. Protrusion of peritoneum, omentum, and intestine out of the abdominal cavity through an abnormal opening

6. Bands of fibrous tissue that develop as a result of trauma or infection within the peritoneal cavity.

7. Dilated swollen rectal veins

Fill In

8. Intraluminal; bacterial

9. 1. Straining at stool
   2. Prolonged sitting on the toilet
   3. Heavy lifting
   4. Pregnancy

10. Peristalsis; obstruction

11. A hydrogen breath test

Questions

12. 1. Avoid chronic strenuous coughing
    2. Avoid heavy lifting or straining
    3. Avoid becoming overweight

13. A

14. D

15. B

16. B

17. D

18. B

19. A

20. D

21. A

22. C

23. C

True or False

24. True

25. False

26. True

27. True

28. False

Questions

29. A

30. B

31. D

32. D

33. C

34. B

35. C

36. C

37. E

38. D

39. B

40. C

41. A

42. C

43. A

44. B

Matching

45. A

46. C

47. B

48. A

Questions

49. C

50. C

51. A

52. C

53. B

54. B

55. B and C

56. B

57. D

58. B

59. A

60. B

61. C

62. C

63. B

64. D

65. B

True or False

66. False

67. True

68. True

69. False

70. True

71. True

72. False

73. True

74. True

75. True

Questions

76. D

77. C

78. A

79. Clean skin with soap; remove all fecal material; apply a skin barrier to protect the exposed skin; avoid oily soaps or emollients; monitor for leakage; institute immediate treatment should irritation occur.

80. Patient Outcome: Patient can tolerate a sitting position 24 hours postoperatively.

    Nursing Interventions: Administer prescribed analgesics.
    Keep patient in a side-lying position for 24 hours.
    Give sitz baths or warm compresses.
    Administer a high-fiber diet and stool softeners.

81. Patient Outcomes: Vital signs are within normal range for patient.
    Urine output is >50 ml/hour.
    Serum electrolyte levels are normal.

    Nursing Interventions: Administer replacement fluids and electrolytes.
    Monitor CVP and vital signs.
    Monitor input and output, and urine output.
    Monitor hydration status.

82. Nursing Diagnosis: Constipation related to scant stool with prolonged transit time in colon

    Patient Outcome: The patient passes soft, formed stool of normal size.

    Nursing Interventions: Explain the importance of a high-fiber diet.
    Teach the importance of food and fluid intake.
    Teach the need for a scheduled time for food intake and defecation to promote good bowel function. Instruct the patient to use bulk-forming laxatives and stool softeners.

83. Nursing Diagnosis: Knowledge deficit related to surgery, postoperative course and routines

    Patient Outcome: Patient can describe the surgery and its expected effects.

    Nursing Interventions: Review the surgical procedure and the expected effect on the cancer. Include information on preoperative preparations and postoperative routines. Provide information about pain control. Provide information about colostomy care.

84. Nursing Diagnosis: Pain related to surgical trauma to anal area

    Patient Outcome: Patient states pain is relieved by analgesics.

    Nursing Interventions: Administer analgesics as ordered. Provide a floatation pad. Give sitz baths. Apply ice packs, warm compresses, or analgesic ointments as ordered.

Clinical Situations

Situation ■ 1

1. D

2. A

3. C

4. A

5. A

6. C

Situation ■ 2

1. C

2. A

3. A

4. D

Situation ■ 3

1. D

2. B

3. A

4. B

5. A

6. C

7. C

8. C

■ CHAPTER TWENTY-FOUR

Define

1. Inflammation of the gallbladder

2. Inflammation of the pancreas

Fill In

3. Intolerance to fatty foods

4. Bile, cholesterol, infection

5. Trypsin

Questions

6. D

7. C

8. A, C, D

9. C

10. B

11. C

12. D

13. C

14. C

15. A

16. A

17. B

18. B

19. D

20. B

21. A

22. C

23. D

24. B

25. B

26. B

27. D

28. B

29. D

30. C

31. D

True or False

32. True

33. True

34. False

35. True

36. True

37. False

38. False

39. True

Questions

40. A

41. B

42. C

43. D

44. D

45. Patient Outcome: Vital signs and hemodynamic measures within normal limits for the patient.

    Nursing Interventions: Monitor vital signs every hour or as ordered. Monitor serum electrolytes. Monitor fluid status, intake and output. Measure nasogastric tube drainage and urine output. Maintain IV and administer as ordered.

46. Nursing Diagnosis: Noncompliance related to medication regimen and diet

    Patient Outcome: The patient accurately explains the correct administration of medication and its rationale. The patient correctly describes the dietary regimen.

    Nursing Interventions: Review the prescribed medications. Review the diet. Explain the rationale for taking pancreatic enzymes and antacids. Explain that pain will subside and stools will return to normal when the regimen is followed. Involve the patient's family in teaching sessions.

47. Nursing Diagnosis: Alteration in nutrition: less than body requirements

    Patient Outcome: Patient will take in calories needed to maintain weight

    Nursing Interventions: Administer parenteral fluid, electrolytes, and nutrients as ordered. Administer TPN or diet as ordered. Offer a small feeding in a clean environment. Assess factors that affect the metabolic rate.

Clinical Situations

Situation ■ 1

1. B

2. B

3. A

4. B

5. A

6. A

Situation ■ 2

1. B

2. B

3. A

4. B

5. C

Situation ■ 3

1. D

2. C

3. D

4. A

■ CHAPTER TWENTY-FIVE

Identify

1. Refer to text, Figure 25–2.

Questions

2. 1. Excretion of metabolic waste products.
   2. Regulation of fluid and electrolyte balance.
   3. Maintenance of acid-base balance.
   4. Assist with calcium metabolism.
   5. Assist with blood pressure maintenance.
   6. Regulate red blood cell production.

Fill In

3. Glomerulus

Questions

4. 1. Permeability of the glomerular capillary walls
   2. Blood pressure
   3. Effective filtration process

5. 1. Appropriate bladder sensations during filling
   2. Closed bladder outlet during rest
   3. Absence of involuntary bladder contractions
   4. Strong and well-maintained bladder contractions
   5. Absence of any obstruction

Define

6. Frequency of urination

7. Sudden desire to urinate

8. Painful urination

9. Involuntary release of urine at night

10. Involuntary loss of urine

Fill In

11. Creatinine

12. Renin-angiotensin-aldosterone

Matching

13. E

14. C

15. A

16. F

17. D

18. B

Questions

19. B

20. B

21. D

22. A

23. B

24. C

25. A

26. A

27. B

28. C

29. D

30. B

31. B

32. C

33. C

34. C

35. C

36. B

37. D

38. A

39. B

40. C

41. C

42. D

43. B

44. A

45. D

46. C

47. D

48. B

49. B

50. A

51. C

52. B

True or False

53. True

54. False

55. True

56. True

57. False

58. True

59. False

Questions

60. 1. Maintain aseptic technique.
    2. Maintain a closed drainage system.
    3. Keep the drainage bag below the level of the bladder.
    4. Change the catheter only if it is contaminated.
    5. Empty the catheter every 8 hours.
    6. Assess the patient on a routine basis.

61. Patient Outcome: Patient voids adequate amounts within reasonable intervals.
    Patient has no visible bladder distention.

    Nursing Interventions: Determine normal elimination patterns. Assess for signs of retention. Monitor intake and output. Instruct the patient to void when the urge is felt. Provide privacy. Encourage adequate intake.

62. Patient Outcome: Patient will reestablish a normal pattern of urination within 24 hours.

    Nursing Interventions: Increase fluid consumption. Encourage ambulation. Encourage the patient to empty the bladder every 2 to 3 hours.

Clinical Situations

Situation ■ 1

1. B

2. C

3. A

4. A

5. A

Situation ■ 2

1. B

2. C

3. A

■ CHAPTER TWENTY-SIX

Define

1. Infection of the upper urinary tract

2. Infection of the bladder

3. Inflammation of the urethra

4. Inflammation of the kidney, affecting the capillary loops in the glomeruli

5. Sudden loss of kidney function that is usually reversible

6. Chronic progressive loss of renal function that is irreversible

7. Acute renal failure, renal in nature owing to ischemia or toxins

8. Build-up of nitrogenous waste products in the blood

Questions

9. D

10. C

11. D

12. D

13. B

14. B

15. A

16. A

17. B

18. C

19. C

20. D

21. D

22. D

23. B

24. B

25. C

26. A

27. C

28. C

29. B

30. B

31. 1. It maintains a steady state of blood chemistry.
   2. It provides an opportunity for patient independence in therapy.
   3. The procedure is simple to learn.
   4. There are fewer dietary restrictions.
   5. Patients have more control over daily life.

32. 1. Removal of metabolic wastes
   2. Maintain safe levels of electrolytes
   3. Correct the acid-base balance
   4. Remove excess fluids

33. B

34. D

35. D

36. B

True or False

37. True

38. True

39. False

40. False

41. False

42. False

43. True

Questions

44. B

45. A

46. A

47. C

48. B

49. A

50. C

51. B

52. B

53. C

54. C

55. B

56. A

57. B

58. C

59. C

Fill In

60. Blunt or penetrating

Questions

61. D

62. C

63. B

64. B

65. A

True or False

66. False

67. True

68. False

69. True

70. True

Questions

71. A

72. A

73. B

74. C

75. Patient Outcome: Patient reports relief of symptoms.
Patient resumes a normal voiding pattern.

Nursing Interventions: Administer antimicrobial medications as ordered. Increase oral intake up to 3000 ml per day. Encourage voiding at regular intervals.

76. Patient Outcome: The patient will have decreased manifestations of chronic renal failure.

Nursing Interventions: Monitor fluid and electrolyte status
Provide extensive education.

Provide   psychological support.

Clinical Situations

Situation ■ 1

1. A

2. B

3. A

Situation ■ 2

1. B

2. C

3. D

4. B

Situation ■ 3

1. D

2. A

3. A

Situation ■ 4

1. C

2. A

3. B

■ CHAPTER TWENTY-SEVEN

Identify

1. Refer to text, Figure 27–1.

Questions

2. 1. Metabolizes carbohydrates, lipids, and fats

   2. Produces and secretes bile

   3. Filters foreign substances from the blood

   4. Detoxifies drugs, toxins, and hormones

   5. Stores glycogen, certain vitamins, and minerals

3. 1. Jaundice

   2. Ascites

   3. Portal hypertension

   4. Hepatic encephalopathy

   5. Clotting disorders

   6. Nutritional deficiencies

Matching

4. D

5. A

6. C

7. B

Fill In

	Value	Increase	Decrease
8. Urine urobilinogen	1 to 4 mg/24 hrs	x	
9. Total serum protein	6.6 to 7.9 g/dl		x
10. Serum albumin	3.3 to 4.5 g/dl		x
11. Blood ammonia	40 to 100 μ/dl	x	
12. Total cholesterol	less than 200 mg/dl		x
13. Prothrombin time	9.5 to 11.8 sec	x	
14. Alpha-fetoprotein	less than 30 ng/ml	x	
15. AST or SGOT	8 to 46 U/L men 7 to 34 U/L women	x	

Questions

16. C

17. B

18. B

19. C

20. D

21. A

22. A

23. B

24. A

25. C

26. B

27. D

28. C

29. A

30. C

31. C

32. A

33. D

34. B

35. D

36. B

37. D

38. C

39. B

40. B

41. Patient Outcome: Patient's abdominal girth decreases daily.

   Nursing Interventions: Restrict intake and output daily.
   Monitor fluid restrictions.
   Administer diuretics.
   Weigh daily.
   Measure abdominal girth daily.

42. A

43. C

44. C

45. A

46. Patient Outcome: Patient experiences no injury.

   Nursing Interventions: Monitor the level of orientation every 4 hours.
   Restrict the intake of protein.
   Monitor daily laboratory results.
   Keep the bed siderail up at all times.

47. Nursing Diagnosis: Alteration in nutrition: more than body requirements

    Patient Outcome: Patient has a steady weight gain with no evidence of fluid retention.

    Nursing Interventions: Provide small feedings with consideration to food preferences.
    Administer antiemetic prior to meals if indicated.
    Teach the patient basic dietary information.

Clinical Situations

Situation ■ 1

1. A

2. C

3. B

4. A

Situation ■ 2

1. B

2. B

3. C

4. D

5. D

■ CHAPTER TWENTY-EIGHT

Questions

1. A

2. B

3. A

4. D

5. B

6. C

7. B

8. D

9. A

10. A

11. B

12. C

13. C

True or False

14. True

15. True

16. False

17. True

18. False

19. True

Questions

20. C

21. C

22. C

23. B

24. D

25. Patient Outcome: Patient verbalizes an understanding of the cause of viral hepatitis and the ways to prevent transmission.

    Nursing Interventions: Explain the mode of transmission to the patient and family (via fecal/oral route).

Explain the importance of handwashing.
Institute enteric precautions.
Teach the patient to refrain from drugs and alcohol.

26. B

27. B

28. C

29. A

30. D

31. C

32. A

33. D

34. D

35. A

36. C

37. B

38. B

39. Patient Outcome: The patient experiences no injury.

Nursing Interventions: Monitor orientation, speech, asterixis.
Restrict protein intake.
Monitor potassium intake.
Administer neomycin and lactulose as ordered.
Protect the patient from injury.

40. A

41. B

42. C

43. D

44. B

45. A

46. D

Clinical Situations

Situation ■ 1

1. D

2. A

3. C

4. A

5. C

Situation ■ 2

1. C

2. C

3. B

4. A

5. B

■ CHAPTER TWENTY-NINE

Identify

1. Refer to text, Figure 29–4.

Fill In

2. Target organ

3. Negative feedback control

4. Hypophysis

5. Islets of Langerhans

6. Thymus gland: Thymine, thymosin

7. Pineal gland: Melatonin

8. Hypothalamus: ADH, oxytocin

9. Pituitary gland: STH, GH, ACTH, LH, TSH, FSH

10. Thyroid: T_4, T_3

11. Adrenal glands: Glucocorticoids, mineralocorticoids, sex hormones

12. Pancreatic islets: Insulin, glucagon

Matching

13. I

14. F

15. D

16. H

17. J

18. A

19. G

20. C, D

21. E

22. B

True or False

23. True

24. False

25. True

26. True

27. False

Questions

28. A

29. C

30. D

31. B

32. B

33. A

34. A

Clinical Situation

Situation ■ 1

1. B

2. D

3. A

4. E

5. C

■ CHAPTER THIRTY

Questions

1. C

2. B

3. A

4. D

5. A

6. C

7. B

8. D

9. B

10. B

11. C

12. A

13. C

14. A

15. B

16. B

17. C

18. C

19. B

20. A

21. C

22. B

23. B

24. B

25. A

26. C

27. C

28. B

29. A

30. C

31. D

True or False

32. True

33. True

34. False

35. False

36. True

37. True

38. False

39. False

40. False

Questions

41. Patient Outcome: Patient verbalizes a basic understanding of the pathophysiology of diabetes mellitus.

Patient Outcome: Patient demonstrates a willingness to learn about the disease and to participate in self-care activities.

Nursing Interventions: Explain the pathophysiology of diabetes at patient's level of understanding.
Reinforce diet teaching. Demonstrate how to adjust the diet for changes in the activity level.
Explain the reason for insulin and how to administer it.
Teach patient how to test blood glucose.
Teach the patient the signs of hypoglycemia and hyperglycemia.

Clinical Situations

Situation ■ 1

1. A

2. A,B,C

3. B

4. A

Situation ■ 2

1. A,B

2. B

3. C

4. B

Situation ■ 3

1. C

2. A

3. B

4. A

■ CHAPTER THIRTY-ONE

Questions

1. C

2. A

3. A

4. B

5. C

6. D

7. E

8. B

9. D

10. C

11. A

12. A

13. B

14. B

15. A

16. D

True or False

17. True

18. True

19. True

20. False

21. False

22. True

23. False

Questions

24. Patient Outcome: Patient remains alert and oriented.

    Nursing Interventions: Elevate the head of the bed 30–45 degrees. Provide rest periods (decrease external stimuli). Administer oxygen as ordered. Assess the patient's neurologic status every 2 hours. Instruct the patient not to cough, sneeze, or hyperflex the head. Administer antiemetic to avoid vomiting. Monitor for early signs of increased ICP.

Clinical Situation

Situation ■ 1

1. D

2. B

3. B

4. C

■ CHAPTER THIRTY-TWO

Matching

1. A

2. C

3. B

4. A

5. B

6. B

True or False

7. True

8. False

9. True

10. False

11. True

12. True

Questions

13. B

14. B

15. C

16. D

17. B

18. D

19. A

20. B

21. C

22. B

23. D

24. A

25. B

26. C

27. D

28. B

29. C

30. A

31. A

32. B

33. C

34. C

35. Patient Outcome: Patient demonstrates adequate extracellular fluid volume.

Nursing Interventions: Administer intravenous hydrocortisone and isotonic dextrose and saline as prescribed.
Monitor vital signs, neurologic status, and urine output frequently.
Administer antiemetics as needed.

36. Patient Outcome: Patient identifies activities that will reduce the risk of infection.

Nursing Interventions: Protect patient from contracting infection.
Discuss the effect of excess cortisol on the immune system.
Stress proper handwashing.
Monitor temperature every 4 hours.
Monitor the white blood count.
Administer antibiotics as prescribed.

37. Patient Outcome: Patient identifies the disease process as the cause of feeling of anxiety.

Nursing Interventions: Provide information on the effects of catecholamines.
Encourage patient to identify and describe feeling.
Assist patient in utilizing relaxation techniques.
Stay with patient if hypertensive crisis occurs.

Clinical Situation

Situation ■ 1

1. C

2. A

3. B

4. B, C, D

5. D

■ CHAPTER THIRTY-THREE

Fill In

1. Iodine; protein

2. Thyroid stimulating hormone

3. 1. Regulate cell metabolism
   2. Energy production

4. Calcitonin

5. Hashimoto's thyroiditis

Questions

6. B

7. C

True or False

8. False

9. True

10. False

11. False

12. True

13. True

14. False

Matching

15. B

16. A

Questions

17. D

18. D

19. B

20. D

21. B

22. C

23. A

24. E

25. A

26. D

27. A

28. All

29. C

30. D

31. D

32. C

33. F

34. Patient Outcome: Patient verbalizes an understanding of the effects of the disease and the need to follow prescribed treatment.

Nursing Interventions: Offer an explanation of disease and its treatment in easily understood terms. Encourage the patient to ask questions and verbalize concerns. Teach patient the name, dose, and side effects of the medication. Teach patient to take medication in the morning. Teach patient to take pulse and notify physician if > 100. Instruct patient to wear MedicAlert identification.

35. Patient Outcome: Patient maintains adequate tissue perfusion as evidenced by normal temperature, vital signs within normal limits, adequate urine output, and normal neurologic state.

    Nursing Interventions: Monitor the vital signs, pulse pressure, capillary refill, and neurologic and urine outputs as indicated by condition. Monitor for signs of thyroid crises and institute any needed interventions.

Clinical Situations

Situation ■ 1

1. A, B, C, F

2. B

3. C

4. A

Situation ■ 2

1. D

2. C

3. B

4. D

5. B, C, D

■ CHAPTER THIRTY-FOUR

Fill In

1. Regulate serum calcium and phosphate levels

2. Rise

Questions

3. Bones: stimulates osteoclasts' activity, which causes a breakdown of bone and calcium resorption

   Kidney: acts on the renal tubules to increase reabsorption of calcium and promote phosphate excretion

   Intestine: activates vitamin D, which acts directly on the intestinal mucosa to increase calcium absorption.

4. D

5. C

6. A

7. B

8. B

9. C

10. A

11. D

12. B

13. C

True or False

14. True

15. True

16. False

17. True

Questions

18. Patient Outcome: Patient maintains normal neuromuscular activity and respiratory function.

    Nursing Interventions: Monitor calcium levels and vital signs. Monitor for signs of neuromuscular irritability. Provide a quiet environment.

Clinical Situation

Situation ■ 1

1. A

2. A

3. C

4. B

■ CHAPTER THIRTY-FIVE

Questions

1. 1. Bones
    2. Joints
    3. Ligaments
    4. Muscles
    5. Tendons

2. 1. Produces locomotion
    2. Supports and protects body structures

3. 1. Formation of clot or hematoma forms. Fibroblasts and capillaries invade the clot to form granulation tissue.
    2. Proliferation of cell formation where the periosteum is torn. Fibroblasts develop and osteogenic cells proliferate at the site to form a callus across damaged bone.
    3. Cells differentiate into bone or cartilage.
    4. Ossification stage. Inorganic salts are deposited in the new bone matrix to calcify the bone.
    5. Consolidation and remodeling of the new bone occurs.

4. 1. Age
    2. Physical condition of the individual
    3. Type of injury
    4. Degree of displacement of bone fragments
    5. Presence of infection
    6. Adequate immobilization after injury vascular sufficiency
    7. Functional periosteum

Fill In

5. Ossification

6. Puberty

7. Osteoblasts; osteoclasts

8. Periosteum

9. Compact; cancellous

10. Central nervous system

11. Movement

12. Adenosine triphosphate

Matching

13. B

14. C

15. A

16. C

17. D

18. A

19. E

20. C

21. F

22. B

True or False

23. True

24. True

25. False

26. True

27. False

28. True

29. False

30. False

Questions

31. B

32. A

33. B

34. C

35. C

36. A

37. D

38. C

39. B

40. D

41. B

42. B

43. C

44. A

45. D

46. C

47. D

48. B

49. B

50. E

51. Patient Outcome: Patient can state accurate information about the potential problems related to immobility.
Patient can state the signs of complications of immobility. Patient can relate the measures necessary to lessen the risk of complications.

Nursing Interventions: Instruct patient about the effects of immobility such as elimination difficulty, discoloration of the skin; diminished pulses, and symptoms of infection. Teach patient when to seek medical assistance. Explain safety measures. Teach patient to drink adequate fluids. Teach patient to follow a high-fiber diet.

52. Patient Outcome: Patient states appropriate information about the care and management of the device. Patient can demonstrate correct pin site care. Patient moves safely with the fixation device intact.

Nursing Interventions: Teach patient how to care for the device. Demonstrate pin care. Reinforce information about activity. Teach proper use of assistive devices. Provide information on ways to modify clothing.

Clinical Situations

Situation ■ 1

1. B

2. D

3. C

4. A

Situation ■ 2

1. C

2. A

3. A

4. D

■ CHAPTER THIRTY-SIX

Define

1. Infection of the bone with necrosis of bone and marrow tissue

2. Inflammation of a joint

3. Degenerative, nonsystemic joint disease

4. Chronic, progressive inflammatory disease of the spine and sacroiliac joint

5. Inflammatory joint reaction caused by the accumulation of uric acid crystals in the joints

6. Chronic inflammatory disease that is transmitted by the bite of a tick

7. Metabolic bone disorder characterized by a decrease in calcium and phosphorus deposits in bone matrix

8. Metabolic bone disorder characterized by thinning, less dense, or porous bone mass

True or False

9. True

10. False

11. True

12. True

13. False

14. False

15. True

16. True

Questions

17. B

18. D

19. A

20. C

21. B

22. A

23. C

24. D

25. A

26. D

27. C

28. A

29. B

30. B

31. A

32. A

33. B

34. D

35. A

36. B

37. C

38. C

39. D

40. B

Matching

41. A

42. D

43. B

44. A

45. B

46. C

47. A

Questions

48. D

49. B

50. D

51. C

52. B

53. A

54. C

55. D

56. A

57. A

58. C

Define

59. A common tumor that develops near an epiphyseal growth plate during adolescence. Symptoms include a palpable nodule and mild pain.

60. Highly vascular cavernous tumor filled with red blood cells. Frequently found on the face, skull, or neck.

61. Most common malignant bone tumor, characterized by extreme pain, rapid growth, and metastasis.

62. Tumor that arises from fibrous connective tissue.

63. Primary tumor that arises in the plasma cells in the bone marrow. Pain is the most common symptom.

Questions

64. D

65. B

66. A

67. Patient Outcome: Patient can perform passive range-of-motion exercises to maintain strength.
Patient maintains mobility with the assistance of an ambulatory aid.

Nursing Interventions: Teach the patient passive and active range-of-motion exercises. Instruct patient to change position frequently. Use ambulatory aids to assist with mobility. Involve the patient in a physical therapy program. Give analgesics to decrease pain levels.

68. Patient Outcome: Patient's extremity has good color, sensation, and pulses with no signs of compromised circulation.

Nursing Interventions: Help conserve oxygen by encouraging rest. Monitor for signs of compromised circulation. Prevent edema by elevating the extremity. Utilize range-of-motion exercise.

Clinical Situations

Situation ■ 1

1. B

2. A

3. C

4. A

Situation ■ 2

1. B

2. B

3. A

4. C

Situation ■ 3

1. B

2. All

3. C

4. B

5. D

■ CHAPTER THIRTY-SEVEN

Identify

1. Refer to text, Figure 37–8.

Fill In

2. Brain; spinal cord

3. 1. Cranial nerves
   2. Spinal nerves
   3. Autonomic nervous system

4. Dendrites; axons

5. Meninges

6. Choroid plexus

7. To provide a cushion for the CNS, prevent injury.

8. Venous system

9. Ascending; descending

10. Dermatones

Questions

11. Pressure exerted within the cranial cavity by its contents

12. 80–180 mm of water or 0–15 mm of mercury

13. Damage to brain tissue due to lack of nutrition or oxygen

Matching

14. A

15. F

16. B

17. C

18. G

19. H

20. I

21. D

22. E

23. J

Questions

24. C

25. A

26. C

27. C

28. A

29. B

30. C

31. B

Matching

32. B

33. A

34. C

35. C

36. B

Questions

37. D

38. B

39. B

40. B

41. A

42. A

43. C

44. A

45. B

46. D

47. D

48. A

49. C

50. B

51. A

52. D

53. Patient Outcome: Patient demonstrates adequate cerebral perfusion.

    Nursing Interventions: Assess patient every 1–2 hours.
    Elevate the head of the bed 30–45 degrees as ordered.
    Instruct patient to refrain from any activity which can increase ICP.
    Minimize the number of invasive procedures.

54. Patient Outcome: Patient maintains joint mobility.

    Nursing Interventions: Perform range-of-motion exercises for all joints every 4 hours.
    Position properly in side-lying position.
    Turn and reposition every 2 hours.
    Teach family to participate in care.

Matching

55. B

56. A

57. C

Questions

58. Nursing Diagnosis: Impaired verbal communication related to expressive aphasia

    Patient Outcome: Patient demonstrates alternative methods of communication.

    Nursing Interventions: Use alternative communication devices such as pantomime, communication boards, flash cards, computers.
    Provide patient with choices that can be answered with yes or no.
    Allow patient time to answer.
    Allow patient to ventilate frustrations and provide an accepting atmosphere to learn and test communication skills.

59. Patient Outcome: Patient uses assistive devices and compensatory techniques

to compensate for sensory dysfunction.

Nursing Interventions: Maintain a consistent environment.
Keep personal belongings within reach.
Explore the use of assistive devices that will increase awareness of the environment.
Teach patient that his or her awareness and visualization of activities is essential.

Matching

60. A

61. C

62. A

63. D

64. B

65. C

Questions

66. A

67. D

68. B

69. C

70. B

71. A

72. Patient Outcome: Patient verbalizes a satisfactory level of comfort.

Nursing Interventions: Medicate as needed and at least one half-hour prior to position changes.
Log roll from side to side to avoid tension on the operative area.
Monitor for side effects of analgesics.

Clinical Situations

Situation ■ 1

1. C

2. B

3. B

4. C

Situation ■ 2

1. C

2. A

3. D

4. B

■ CHAPTER THIRTY-EIGHT

Define

1. An inflammation of the brain.

2. An acute, rapidly progressive inflammation and demyelination of the nerve endings of the peripheral nervous system.

3. Progressive degeneration and loss of both upper and lower motor neurons.

4. Progressive neurologic condition characterized by the demyelination and scarring of sites along the central nervous system.

5. Autonomic disturbance of the bladder characterized by incontinence and recurrent urinary infections.

6. Hereditary neurologic condition characterized by progressive degeneration and weakness of the voluntary muscles.

7. Chronic, progressive, neurodegenerative condition characterized by marked cognitive dysfunction.

8. State of recurrent seizure activity without interictal recovery between seizures.

Questions

9. A

10. C

11. D

12. C

13. B

14. B

15. Nursing Diagnosis: Alteration in nutrition: less than body requirements, related to anorexia, nausea, vomiting

   Patient Outcome: Nausea and vomiting are minimized and adequate nutritional status is maintained.

   Nursing Interventions: Administer IV fluids as necessary to prevent dehydration.
   Provide supplemental feedings by NG or TPN.
   Monitor intake and output and weight.
   Monitor laboratory values.
   Administer antiemetics.

16. A

17. C

18. B

19. A

20. C

21. B

22. B

23. A

24. C

25. D

26. E

27. C

28. A

29. Nursing Diagnosis: Alteration in urinary elimination related to neurogenic bladder

   Patient Outcome: Patient can empty bladder completely and remains free of urinary infections.

   Nursing Interventions: Maintain a schedule for bladder training.
   Monitor intake and output.
   Establish appropriate bladder regimen such as intermittent catheterization, Crede's maneuver.
   Instruct patient on signs and symptoms of urinary tract infections.
   Instruct patient to eat a high-acid diet.

30. C

31. A

32. B

33. A, D

34. C

35. C

36. D

37. A

38. C

39. C

40. Nursing Diagnosis: Impaired physical mobility

   Patient Outcome: Patient maintains the current level of mobility with assistance as needed.

   Nursing Interventions: Encourage the patient to be as physically independent as possible.
   Provide active and passive range-of-motion exercises every 6 hours.
   Allow for sufficient time

to perform activities of daily living.
Administer medication to control symptoms.
Provide assistive devices as needed.

41. A

42. D

43. C

44. C

45. B

46. D

47. A

48. B

49. B

50. A

51. D

52. B

53. A

54. A

55. C

56. C

57. Patient Outcome: Patient participates in activities of daily living.

Nursing Interventions: Perform range-of-motion every 6 hours.
Assist the patient in being as independent as possible.
Obtain supportive and assistive devices.
Provide good skin care.

Patient Outcome: Patient can successfully communicate needs.

Nursing Interventions: Identify alternative strategies to facili-

tate communication.
Decrease environmental distractions when communicating.
Allow patient time to interpret messages and express needs.

True or False

58. True

59. True

60. True

61. False

62. False

Questions

63. C

64. B

65. C

66. B

67. A

68. A

69. C

70. B

71. A

72. B

73. Patient Outcome: Deviations in baseline neurologic functioning will be identified.

Nursing Interventions: Establish a baseline neurologic status and reevaluate every 2 hours.
Monitor the patient according to the Glasgow coma scale.

Monitor for signs of increased intracranial pressure.
Administer medication to decrease cerebral edema.

74. Patient Outcome: Baseline neurologic function is maintained.

Nursing Interventions: Maintain cervical traction as ordered.
Logroll the patient when positioning.
Monitor neurologic status frequently and report any changes immediately.

Clinical Situations

Situation ■ 1

1. B

2. D

3. B

4. A

Situation ■ 2

1. C

2. A

3. A

4. B

5. D

6. B

Situation ■ 3

1. B

2. C

3. A

Situation ■ 4

1. D

2. C

3. D

4. C

■ CHAPTER THIRTY-NINE

Identify

1. Refer to text, Figure 39–3.

Fill In

2. Lacrimal

3. Iris

4. Choroid

5. Retina

6. Aqueous humor

7. Lens

Questions

8. Light rays stimulate the retina and initiate the nerve impulses, which travel to the optic nerve. The impulses pass through the right or left optic tract to the geniculate nucleus of the thalamus, where the neurons conduct the impulse to the right and left occipital lobes.

9. It means "Pupils equal, round, reactive to light and accommodation."

10. 1. III
    2. IV
    3. VI

Matching

11. B

12. D

13. A

14. C

15. F

16. E

17. F

18. E

19. D

20. B

21. C

22. A

Questions

23. A

24. B

25. C

26. A

27. A

28. C

29. B

30. B

31. B

32. D

33. A

34. B

Matching

35. A

36. C

37. B

38. D

Fill In

39. Mydriatics; dilation

40. Miotics; constriction

41. Lower; aqueous humor

42. Osmosis

Questions

43. C

44. B

45. A

True or False

46. True

47. False (mydriatic)

48. True

49. False

50. True

51. True

52. True

Define

53. Removal of the vitreous by suction

54. Removal of a small portion of the iris

55. Indentation of the sclera by means of an implant to reposition the retina.

56. Corneal transplant or grafting

57. Complete removal of the globe

Questions

58. 1. Magnifying glasses

    2. Prisms which can be attached to eyeglasses

    3. Electronic vision enhancement aids

59. Patient Outcome: Patient will be able to describe the procedure and expected outcome.

    Nursing Interventions: Review the surgical procedure.
    Describe the preoperative preparations (NPO, hair shampoo, draping during procedure, etc.).
    Review the postoperative care.
    Explain that improvement in vision may not be immediate.

Clinical Situations

Situation ■ 1

1. B

2. A

3. C

Situation ■ 2

1. A

2. C

3. A, D, E

■ CHAPTER FORTY

Define

1. Chronic inflammation of the eyelid

2. Chronic inflammation of the meibomian gland

3. Inflammation or infection of the conjunctiva

4. Infection of the nasolacrimal sac or duct

5. Inflammation or infection of the cornea

6. Infection or inflammation of the internal eye

Questions

7. B

8. C

9. C

10. D

11. C

12. C

13. A

14. E

15. B

16. A

Matching

17. A

18. C

19. D

20. B

21. E

Questions

22. B

23. D

24. Patient Outcome: Patient reports improved visual acuity.

    Nursing Interventions: Use strict aseptic technique.
    Administer ophthalmic drops or ointments.

Remove any drainage from the eye; irrigate if needed. Follow universal precautions.
Assess patient's current visual acuity.
Adjust the environment to facilitate independence.

25. B

26. D

27. A

28. A

29. A

30. Patient Outcome: Patient's eye heals without evidence of trauma.
Patient avoids injury.

Nursing Interventions: Explain to patient how patching one eye changes depth perception. Use adaptive devices when necessary. Orient patient to surroundings. Keep call light within reach. Remove all hazards in the environment.

31. C

32. B

33. D

34. B

35. B

36. A

37. C

38. C

39. D

40. A

41. C

42. A

43. C, D

Clinical Situations

Situation ■ 1

1. B, D

2. B, C

3. D

Situation ■ 2

1. C

2. D

3. B

4. B

5. C

■ CHAPTER FORTY-ONE

Identify

1. Refer to text, Figure 41–3.

Define

2. Pain in ear

3. Drainage from ear

4. Sensation of buzzing or ringing in one or both ears

5. Sensation of imbalance, unsteadiness, or faintness

6. Progressive sensorineural hearing loss associated with age.

Fill In

7. Cochlea

8. Hertz (Hz)

9. Decibels (dB)

10. Otoscope

Questions

11. Air waves from the environment enter the external auditory canal and set the tympanic membrane in motion. The vibrations pass to the bony ossicle and through the oval window to the perilymph. Receptor cells in the cochlea are stimulated, which then send electric impulses to the brain.

12. 1. Hearing loss
    2. Ear pain
    3. Discharge
    4. Tinnitus
    5. Vertigo

Matching

13. B

14. C

15. A

Questions

16. D

17. All

18. A

19. B

20. A

21. B

22. D

Matching

23. D

24. A

25. E

26. C

27. B

28. F

Questions

29. C

30. C

31. B

32. C

33. C

34. A

35. B

36. B

37. A

38. D

39. B

40. A

41. D

42. B

True or False

43. True

44. True

45. False (infection)

46. True

47. True

48. False

Questions

49. Patient Outcome: Patient reports vertigo, dizziness, or unsteadiness and takes medications as ordered.

    Nursing Interventions: Administer medications as ordered. Explain the purpose of medications. Explain that symptoms are not uncommon after surgery. Keep environment dim and quiet. Instruct patient to avoid sudden movements.

Clinical Situations

Situation ■ 1

1. E

2. B

3. A

4. C

Situation ■ 2

1. B

2. C

3. B

4. A, D, E, F

■ CHAPTER FORTY-TWO

Define

1. Inflammation of the skin of the auricle and/or the outer ear canal

2. Fungus infection of the outer ear

3. A boil; a localized suppurative inflammation of the skin and underlying tissue

4. Infection of the inner ear

5. Inflammation of the spongy cells of the mastoid bone

6. Inflammation of the labyrinth of the inner ear

7. Recurrent and usually progressive disorder of the labyrinth of the inner ear

Questions

8. 1. Recurrent attacks of severe vertigo
   2. Sensorineural hearing loss
   3. Tinnitus

Matching

9. C

10. D

11. B

12. A

Questions

13. A

14. C

15. B

16. D

17. C

18. A

19. B

20. D

21. C

22. D

23. B

24. C

True or False

25. True

26. True

27. False

28. True

29. True

30. False (formation of a white mass of dead skin)

31. True

32. True

33. True

Questions

34. D

35. C

36. C

37. Patient Outcome: Patient demonstrates ways to help open the eustachian tube and permit air to enter the middle ear.

    Nursing Interventions: Teach patient how to perform Valsalva's maneuver.
    Teach patient how to blow the nose to open the tubes.
    Teach patient to take decongestants as ordered.

38. Nursing Diagnosis: Pain related to tissue disruption in the ear.

    Patient Outcome: The patient takes analgesic as prescribed, states relief of pain.

Nursing Interventions: Explain the disease process and expected outcomes. Explain the administration of analgesics. Explain other comfort measures.

39. Patient Outcome: Patient expresses confidence in his ability to cope.

    Nursing Interventions: Allow patient opportunities to express concerns. Encourage independent problem-solving. Assist patient in identifying support systems.

40. Patient Outcome: Patient instructs others on ways to increase effective communication.

    Nursing Interventions: Provide a quiet, calm environment.
    Face the patient when speaking; speak slowly and clearly.
    Use normal conversational tone. Use gestures or written communication as needed.

Clinical Situations

Situation ■ 1

1. C

2. A

3. B

4. C

Situation ■ 2

1. A

2. C

3. A

4. B

5. D

■ CHAPTER FORTY-THREE

Identify

1. Refer to text, Figure 43–1.

2. Refer to text, Figure 43–2.

Fill In

3. Vagina

4. Uterus

5. Ligaments

6. Fallopian tubes

7. Ovaries

8. To prepare the body for pregnancy

Questions

9. 1. Illness
   2. Fatigue
   3. Stress
   4. Anxiety
   5. Environmental change

10. 1. Hot flashes
    2. Insomnia
    3. Weakness
    4. Dizzy spells
    5. Palpitations
    6. Nervousness
    7. Headaches
    8. Weight gain

Matching

11. C

12. A

13. B

14. D

True or False

15. False

16. True

17. True

18. True

19. True

20. False

21. True

22. True

23. False

24. False

Questions

25. C

26. D

27. B

28. F

Matching

29. C

30. E

31. G

32. F

33. A

34. D

35. B

Questions

36. B

37. A

38. E

39. B

40. D

41. A

Matching

42. B

43. C

44. A

Questions

45. D

46. B

47. C

48. D

True or False

49. True

50. True

51. False

52. True

53. True

54. False

55. False

Questions

56. B

57. C

58. C

59. A

60. D

61. A

62. 1. Early movement

    2. Adequate hydration

    3. Routine examination of the calves to provide for early recognition

63. Patient Outcome: Patient defines menopause. The patient can describe the effects of menopause on lifestyle. Patient can describe the health practices relevant to the menopausal woman.

    Nursing Interventions: Explain what menopause is. Discuss the symptoms and treatment options. Instruct patient in related health care practices. Provide information to prevent misconceptions.

64. Patient Outcome: Patient expresses feelings of anxiety.

    Nursing Interventions: Provide patient with needed information. Encourage patient to express feelings. Provide privacy for communication. Explore coping strategies.

Clinical Situations

Situation ■ 1

1. A

2. C

3. B

4. C

Situation ■ 2

1. A, D

2. B

3. C (burns can lead to necrosis, bowel perforation, and peritonitis)

4. F

Situation ■ 3

1. A

2. C

3. C

4. C

5. B

6. C

■ CHAPTER FORTY-FOUR

Define

1. Inflammation of the vagina

2. Inflammation of the vulva (external genitalia)

3. Inflammation of the endometrium (membrane that lines the inner surface of the uterus)

4. Vaginal mucosa protrudes outside the vagina

5. Urethra protrudes into the vagina

6. Rectum protrudes into the vagina

7. Bladder protrudes into the vagina

Questions

8. 1. Mechanical irritation
   2. Infection

9. 1. Tampons
   2. Douching
   3. Contraceptive creams

10. 1. Rinse thoroughly to clean vulva
    2. Avoid soap that leaves residue
    3. Keep area dry
    4. Avoid tight clothing
    5. May use a sitz bath or hot compresses

11. 1. Fever
    2. Vomiting
    3. Diarrhea
    4. Muscle aching
    5. Shock
    6. Impaired cardiopulmonary function
    7. Hepatic and renal function

12. 1. Gastrointestinal symptoms
    2. Breast swelling and tenderness
    3. Pain
    4. Neurologic sensitivities
    5. Tachycardia
    6. Back pain
    7. Joint pain
    8. Emotional symptoms (See text, Table 44–2)

13. 1. Progesterone
    2. Androgen
    3. Antigonadotropic

Fill In

14. Childbirth

15. Bladder; rectum

Questions

16. Physical: Assist in cleansing the perineal area. Change pads. Use deodorizer. Remove soiled material promptly. Clean with mild soap and water. Use ointments and heat therapy. Use a good diet. Monitor intake and output.

Psychological: Promote a positive self-concept; encourage an attractive appearance. Keep the environment clean. Avoid social isolation. Spend time with the patient. Encourage ambulation.

17. A

18. B

19. E

20. D

21. A

22. A

23. C

24. B

25. A

26. D

27. C

28. D

29. C

30. B

True or False

31. False

32. True

33. True

34. False

35. True

36. True

37. False (after family is complete)

38. False

Questions

39. Patient Outcome: The patient identifies the disease as real and identifies ways to cope with it.

    Nursing Interventions: Affirm that the disease

is real and other women suffer from it.
Explain the role of stress and PMS.
Explore family support and coping strategies.

40. Rest and activity: adequate rest, naps, with periods of exercise

    Diet: high in protein, complex carbohydrate, green vegetables

    Fluids: limit

    Anxiety: avoid tobacco, coffee, caffeine

41. B

42. C

43. C

44. C

45. A

46. A, B, C, E

47. A, C, E, F

48. B

49. C

50. C

51. A

52. D

53. B

54. A

55. B

56. C

57. B

58. C

Matching

59. B

60. D

61. A

62. C

Questions

63. A

64. C

65. B

66. B

67. Patient Outcome: Suture line remains intact.

   Nursing Interventions: Use a low Fowler's or a side-lying position.
   Place a pillow to support the back and between the knees.
   Have patient use a trapeze bar to move in bed.
   Use a bed cradle.
   Prevent constipation to prevent pressure on the suture line.

68. B

69. A

70. E

71. C

72. E

73. A

74. Patient Outcome: Patient describes radiation procedures which will be observed by staff and visitors.

   Nursing Interventions: Patient will be on bedrest with a catheter and a low-residue diet.
   Explain limited contact by staff and visitors.
   Explain that nausea, vaginal cramps, and discharge are normal.

75. B

76. A

77. Patient Outcome: Patient demonstrates interest in her appearance.

   Nursing Interventions: Allow patient to express her feelings.
   Discuss the meaning of the surgery with the patient.
   Discuss coping strategies.
   Elicit family support.

Clinical Situations

Situation ■ 1

1. C

2. B

3. C

Situation ■ 2

1. C

2. A

3. A

Situation ■ 3

1. B

2. C

3. A

Situation ■ 4

1. A

2. A

3. B

4. C

■ CHAPTER FORTY-FIVE

Define

1. The process by which the germ cells become transformed into mature spermatozoa

2. Milky viscid fluid which contains sperm

3. The enlargement and hardening of the penis in response to stimuli

4. Expulsion of the semen from the urethra

5. A persistent inability to obtain or maintain an erection

6. Premature expulsion of sperm

7. Propulsion of seminal fluid from the posterior urethra into the bladder

8. Failure to conceive within a period of time (usually 1 year)

9. Direct visualization of the bladder and urethra

10. Insertion of a needle into the prostate gland to obtain aspirate

Identify

11. Refer to text, Figure 45–1.

12. 1. Organ for copulation (sexual intercourse)
    2. Urination

13. 1. Covers the testes
    2. Protects the testes
    3. Regulates the temperature of the testes

Fill In

14. Reproductive

15. Epididymis; vas deferens

16. Urine; semen

17. Infertility

18. Organic; psychogenic

19. A penile implant

Questions

20. 1. Aging
    2. Anxiety
    3. Boredom
    4. Depression
    5. Fear

21. 1. Endocrine dysfunction
    2. Sexual dysfunction
    3. Structural anomalies
    4. Medications

Fill In

22. Sterilization

23. Aspermia (to determine if sperm are being produced)

24. A dilutional hyponatremia, due to the irrigation fluid used during surgery, which enters the vascular compartment

True or False

25. False

26. True

27. True

28. False

29. True

30. True

31. True

32. True

33. True

34. False

35. False

36. True

37. True

Questions

38. B

39. D

40. A

41. B

42. C

43. C

44. B

45. All are relevant

46. C

47. B

48. C

49. D

50. B

51. B (may indicate urinary retention)

52. C

53. A, C, D, E

54. C

55. B

56. B (may indicate deep venous thrombosis)

57. A

58. C

59. A

60. A

61. B

62. B

63. C (infection is very common)

64. Nursing Diagnosis: Sexual dysfunction related to impotence

    Patient Outcome: Patient describes alternative methods of sexual expression.

    Nursing Interventions: Suggest noncoital activities as a means of obtaining sexual gratification.
    Suggest physical exercise as an alternative release of sexual energy.
    Encourage the expression of concerns and feelings related to his sexual dysfunction.
    Suggest a referral to a sexual support group.

65. Patient Outcome: Patient expresses thoughts and concerns.
    Patient states that anxiety is decreased.

    Nursing Interventions: Acknowledge that his anxiety is normal.
    Encourage expression of his feelings.
    Assure the patient that his privacy will be maintained.
    Explain the normal outcome of this surgery.

66. Nursing Diagnosis: Urinary retention related to obstruction of the drainage catheter

    Patient Outcome: Urinary drainage tubes remain patent and output is adequate.

    Nursing Interventions: Maintain the flow of the normal saline irrigant.
    Empty the urinary drainage bag frequently.
    Keep the tube in a

straight   line;   avoid kinks.

Irrigate the catheter as ordered.

Clinical Situations

Situation ■ 1

1. C

2. B

3. B

4. B or C

Situation ■ 2

1. B

2. C

3. B

4. A

5. C

6. B

■ CHAPTER FORTY-SIX

Define

1. Inflammation of the glans penis

2. Inflammation of the foreskin

3. Inflammation or infection of the epididymis

4. Collection of clear fluid in the tunica vaginalis

5. Inflammation of one or both of the testes

6. Inflammation of the prostate gland

7. A disorder with which the foreskin is unable to be retracted over the penis

8. Making a dorsal slit in the foreskin

9. A condition with which the uncircumcised foreskin is retracted over the penis and cannot be easily returned to its normal position

10. The failure of one or both testicles to descend into the scrotum before birth

11. A prolonged, uncontrolled erection that is not associated with stimulation or desire

Fill In

12. Recurrent infection of the glans and foreskin or congenital condition

13. Circumcision

14. Manual reduction

Questions

15. 1. Infection
    2. Hydrocele

16. D

17. B

18. A

19. C

20. B

21. 1. Explain the cause of epididymitis.
    2. Stress the need to continue antibiotics after discharge.
    3. Instruct patient to maintain daily fluid intake of 2000 ml.
    4. Instruct patient to empty bladder frequently.

22. D

23. A

24. D

25. A

26. B

27. D

True or False

28. True

29. False

30. True

31. False

32. True

33. True

34. True

35. True

Questions

36. C

37. B

38. A

39. B

40. D

41. A

42. B

43. B

44. C

45. C

46. D

47. D

48. A

True or False

49. True

50. True

51. False

52. True

53. True

Questions

54. C

55. C

56. A

57. C

58. A

59. Nursing Diagnosis: Pain related to constricted, retracted foreskin

Patient Outcome: Patient states that relief of pain has been obtained.

Nursing Interventions: Administer a narcotic analgesic prior to reduction. Instruct the patient to elevate the penis after treatment. Apply cool compresses for edema and discomfort.

60. Patient Outcome: Patient identifies alternative ways of dealing with sexual expression.

Nursing Interventions: 1. Encourage patient to express his concerns. 2. Provide privacy for visits between patient and his partner. 3. Encourage alternative methods of sexual expression. 4. Refer patient to a sex therapist or counselor if needed.

Clinical Situations

Situation ■ 1

1. A

2. B

3. C

4. A

5. D

Situation ■ 2

1. D

2. B

3. A

4. A

5. B

■ CHAPTER FORTY-SEVEN

Define

1. Infectious, chronic venereal disease characterized by lesions that can affect an organ

2. Infectious disease caused by the herpes simplex virus I

3. Contagious, catarrhal inflammation of the genital mucous membrane of either sex

Fill In

4. *Treponema pallidum*

Questions

5. 1. Chancre develops 3 to 4 weeks after exposure

   2. Skin lesion; flu-type symptoms develop 6 to 8 weeks after stage 1

   3. No symptoms; only positive serology

   4. Affects almost any system; leads to disability and death

6. Because of the variety of skin lesions seen in secondary syphilis, which can mimic other conditions.

7. It is transmitted by direct skin-to-skin contact with an infected lesion or infected secretions.

True or False

8. True

9. False

10. True

11. True

12. True

13. True

14. True

Matching

15. D

16. B

17. B

18. E

19. C

20. F

Fill In

21. Topical application of podophyllin, or cryosurgery

22. Itching

23. Application of Kwell

Questions

24. All

25. B and C

26. A

27. B

28. C

29. C

30. A

31. D

32. D

33. C

34. B

35. A

36. C

37. D

38. C

39. Patient Outcome: The patient describes changes in lifestyle that may prevent a recurrence.

    Nursing Interventions: Identify strategies for self-management to help patient feel in control of this disease.
    Review the factors which may precipitate outbreaks.
    Discuss with the patient the need to inform prospective partners about the disease.

40. 1. Exposure to heat

    2. Stress

    3. Sexual intercourse

41. B

42. Patient Outcome: Patient states the disease's cause and mode of transmission.
    Patient states methods to prevent transmission to others.

    Nursing Interventions: Assess patient's learning needs and current level of understanding.
    Correct any misconceptions about the disease.
    Provide materials, both written and verbal, to provide information and as a way of reinforcement later.

43. A

44. C

45. D

46. C

47. A

48. B

49. C

50. B

True or False

51. True

52. False

53. True

54. False

55. False

56. False

Questions

57. 1. Early onset of sexual activity can lead to STDs.

    2. Frequent sexual partners can lead to STDs.

    3. Use of contraceptives will decrease risk of STD.

58. A

59. B

60. C

61. B

True or False

62. False

63. True

64. False

65. True

66. True

67. True

68. True

Questions

69. Patient Outcome: Patient lists potential long-term effects of untreated syphilis.
Patient can state the recommended treatment regimen.

    Nursing Interventions: Explain treatment plan and rationale in detail.
Review all medications, dosage, and side effects.
Provide a resource to call if patient has questions.
Educate patient on long-term effects if the disease is not treated effectively.
Caution the patient to avoid sex until he or she is free of transmitting the disease.

70. C

71. 1. Tetracycline

    2. Erythromycin

    3. Sulfisoxazole

72. D

73. Nursing Diagnosis: Knowledge deficit related to ways to prevent the reoccurrence of infection

    Patient Outcome: Patient identifies factors which may predispose her to infection.
Patient describes methods for preventing recurrence of infection.

    Nursing Interventions: Review the cause, symptoms, and treatment of infection. Review factors that promote the growth of *Candida*. Review the use of medications that may predispose to the development of candidiasis.

74. Patient Outcome: Patient reports that using recommended measures do reduce discomfort.

    Nursing Interventions: Review medications and the treatment plan.
Make sure patient uses all medication as ordered and does not stop when the symptoms abate.
Recommend cool compresses and sitz baths.
Recommend the use of cotton undergarments.

Clinical Situations

Situation ■ 1

1. B

2. A

3. C

4. C

Situation ■ 2

1. B

2. A

3. B

4. C

■ CHAPTER FORTY-EIGHT

Fill In

1. Glandular; fibrous; fat

2. Fibrous

3. Prolactin; growth

4. Involution

Questions

5. D

Matching

6. C

7. A

8. D

9. B

10. E

Questions

11. B

12. A

13. B

14. D

15. B

16. C

True or False

17. True

18. False

19. True

20. False

21. False

22. True

23. False

Questions

24. 1. Family history of breast cancer
    2. Early menarche
    3. Delayed pregnancy
    4. Environmental factors
    5. Estrogen therapy

25. C

26. 1. The size of the primary tumor
    2. The presence or absence of a tumor in the lymph nodes
    3. The presence or absence of organ metastases

27. B

28. D

29. B

30. B

31. A

32. C

33. D

34. C

35. D

36. Patient Outcome: Patient states the reason for surgery, pre- and postoperative activities.

    Nursing Interventions: Review all information on the procedure with patient. Clarify the postoperative appearance. Demonstrate breathing exercises. Demonstrate arm exercises. Explain all postoperative equipment.

Clinical Situations

Situation ■ 1

1. A

2. B

3. C

4. B

Situation ■ 2

1. B

2. B

3. D

4. C